Principles of
ASSESSMENT IN MEDICAL EDUCATION

Principles of
ASSESSMENT IN MEDICAL EDUCATION

Second Edition

Tejinder Singh MD DNB MAMS FIMSA FIAP
MSc (Health Professions Education) (Maastricht; Hons)
MA (Distance Education); PG Dip Higher Education (Gold Medal)
Diploma Training and Development (Gold Medal)
PG Diploma in Human Resource Management (Gold Medal)
Certificate Course Evaluation Methodology and Examinations (AIU)
FAIMER Fellow, IFME Fellow, IMSA Fellow

Professor
Department of Pediatrics and Medical Education
SGRD Institute of Medical Sciences and Research
Amritsar, Punjab, India

Anshu MD DNB, MNAMS
MSc (Health Professions Education) (Maastricht; Hons.)
FAIMER Fellow, IFME Fellow, Commonwealth Fellow

Professor
Department of Pathology
Mahatma Gandhi Institute of Medical Sciences
Sevagram, Wardha, Maharashtra, India

Forewords
John Dent
Lambert Schuwirth

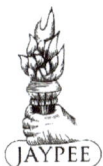

JAYPEE BROTHERS MEDICAL PUBLISHERS
The Health Sciences Publisher
New Delhi | London

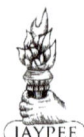 **Jaypee Brothers Medical Publishers (P) Ltd**

Headquarters

Jaypee Brothers Medical Publishers (P) Ltd
EMCA House, 23/23-B
Ansari Road, Daryaganj
New Delhi 110 002, India
Landline: +91-11-23272143, +91-11-23272703
+91-11-23282021, +91-11-23245672
Email: jaypee@jaypeebrothers.com

Corporate Office

Jaypee Brothers Medical Publishers (P) Ltd
4838/24, Ansari Road, Daryaganj
New Delhi 110 002, India
Phone: +91-11-43574357
Fax: +91-11-43574314
Email: jaypee@jaypeebrothers.com

Overseas Office

J.P. Medical Ltd
83 Victoria Street, London
SW1H 0HW (UK)
Phone: +44 20 3170 8910
Fax: +44 (0)20 3008 6180
Email: info@jpmedpub.com

Website: www.jaypeebrothers.com
Website: www.jaypeedigital.com

© 2022, Jaypee Brothers Medical Publishers

The views and opinions expressed in this book are solely those of the original contributor(s)/author(s) and do not necessarily represent those of editor(s) of the book.

All rights reserved. No part of this publication may be reproduced, stored or transmitted in any form or by any means, electronic, mechanical, photocopying, recording or otherwise, without the prior permission in writing of the publishers.

All brand names and product names used in this book are trade names, service marks, trademarks or registered trademarks of their respective owners. The publisher is not associated with any product or vendor mentioned in this book.

Medical knowledge and practice change constantly. This book is designed to provide accurate, authoritative information about the subject matter in question. However, readers are advised to check the most current information available on procedures included and check information from the manufacturer of each product to be administered, to verify the recommended dose, formula, method and duration of administration, adverse effects and contraindications. It is the responsibility of the practitioner to take all appropriate safety precautions. Neither the publisher nor the author(s)/editor(s) assume any liability for any injury and/or damage to persons or property arising from or related to use of material in this book.

This book is sold on the understanding that the publisher is not engaged in providing professional medical services. If such advice or services are required, the services of a competent medical professional should be sought.

Every effort has been made where necessary to contact holders of copyright to obtain permission to reproduce copyright material. If any have been inadvertently overlooked, the publisher will be pleased to make the necessary arrangements at the first opportunity.

Inquiries for bulk sales may be solicited at: jaypee@jaypeebrothers.com

Principles of Assessment in Medical Education

First Edition: 2012
Second Edition: 2022

ISBN 978-93-5465-247-9

Cover design: **Dinesh N Gudadhe**

Contributors

Abhishek V Raut
MD DNB (SPM)
Professor
Department of Community Medicine
Mahatma Gandhi Institute of Medical Sciences
Sevagram, Maharashtra, India
abhishekraut@mgims.ac.in

Anshu
MD DNB MNAMS MSc (HPE) IFME Fellow
FAIMER Fellow
Professor
Department of Pathology
Mahatma Gandhi Institute of Medical Sciences
Sevagram, Wardha, Maharashtra, India
dr.anshu@gmail.com

Ara Tekian
PhD MHPE
Professor
Department of Medical Education
Associate Dean, Office of International Education
College of Medicine, University of Illinois at Chicago
Chicago, USA
tekian@uic.edu

Balachandra V Adkoli
MSc MEd PhD MMEd (Dundee)
Director
Centre for Health Professions Education
Professor
Department of Medical Education
Sri Balaji Vidyapeeth (Deemed University)
Puducherry, India
bvadkoli@gmail.com

Chinmay Shah
MD PhD (Physiology) PGDHPE PGDHMM
Fellow (GSMC-FAIMER)
Professor and Head
Coordinator MEU
Government Medical College
Bhavnagar, Gujarat, India
chinmay.ffri@gmail.com

Ciraj Ali Mohammed
PhD MHPE FAIMER Fellow
Professor
Department of Microbiology
Melaka Manipal Medical College (MMMC)
Director
MAHE-FAIMER Institute
Manipal Academy of Higher Education
Manipal, Karnataka, India
cirajam@gmail.com

Jyoti Nath Modi
MD FICOG Fellow (CMCL-FAIMER)
Associate Professor
Department of Obstetrics and Gynecology
Member Secretary
Centre for Medical Education Technology
All India Institute of Medical Sciences (AIIMS)
Bhopal, Madhya Pradesh, India
modijn@gmail.com

KA Narayan
MD DPH
Professor
Department of Community Medicine
Mahatma Gandhi Medical College and Research Institute
Professor
Health Professions Education
Sri Balaji Vidyapeeth
Puducherry, India
narayan.ka@gmail.com

KK Deepak
MD PhD FAMS DSc
Dean (Examinations)
Professor and Head
Department of Physiology
All India Institute of Medical Sciences (AIIMS)
New Delhi, India
kkdeepak@gmail.com

Medha Anant Joshi
MD MHPE IFME Fellow
Director
Medical Education Unit
International Medical School, MSU
Bengaluru, Karnataka, India
medhajoshi11@gmail.com

Piyush Gupta
MD FIAP FNNF FAMS
Professor
Department of Pediatrics
University College of Medical Sciences
New Delhi, India
prof.piyush.gupta@gmail.com

Pooja Dewan
MD MNAMS FIAP
Professor
Department of Pediatrics
University College of Medical Sciences
New Delhi, India
poojadewan@hotmail.com

Rajiv Mahajan
MD Dip Clin Res FIMSA Fellow (CMCL-FAIMER)
Professor (Department of Pharmacology) and Principal
Adesh Institute of Medical Sciences and Research
Dean, Academic Affairs
Chairperson, HPEU
Adesh University
Bathinda, Punjab, India
drrajivmahajan01@gmail.com

Rita Sood (Late)
MD MMEd FAMS
Professor
Department of Medicine
All India Institute of Medical Sciences
New Delhi, India
ritasood@gmail.com

Subodh S Gupta
MD (Paed) DNB (SPM) DNB (MCH)
Professor and Head
Department of Community Medicine
Mahatma Gandhi Institute of Medical Sciences
Sevagram, Maharashtra, India
subodh@mgims.ac.in

Tejinder Singh
MD DNB FIAP MSc HPE PGDHE
MA (Distance Education) PGDHRM FAIMER Fellow
Founder Director, CMCL-FAIMER;
National Convener, and Consultant ACME (MCI);
Expert Group Member (MCI)
Professor
Department of Pediatrics and Medical Education
SGRD Institute of Medical Sciences and Research
Amritsar, Punjab, India
drtejinder22@gmail.com

Upreet Dhaliwal
MS Fellow (CMCL-FAIMER)
Former Director-Professor
Department of Ophthalmology
University College of Medical Sciences
University of Delhi
New Delhi, India
upreetdhaliwal@gmail.com

Vinay Kumar
MD FRCPath
Lowell T Coggeshall Distinguished Service Professor of Pathology
Pritzker School of Medicine and the Biologic Sciences Division
University of Chicago
Chicago, IL, USA
vkumar@bsd.uchicago.edu

Foreword

"Students can, with difficulty, escape the effects of poor teaching, but they cannot (by definition, if they want to graduate) escape the effects of poor assessment."
—***Boud, 1995***

Unfortunately, authentic assessment can be the weak link in our curriculum. We tend to use approaches with which we are familiar and to assess too much, but at the same time fail to assess what is important for future clinical practice. In seeking to change our approach to assessment our questions may include:

What should we assess? Do we just aim to measure retention of factual knowledge or to measure clinical reasoning? At what level on Miller pyramid are we assessing? Do we focus assessment on agreed learning outcomes, including attitudes?

When should we assess? At the end of the course, during the course, throughout the course, or with an annual progress test?

How should we assess? What instruments should we choose to put in our assessment "toolkit"?

Who should assess? Should assessment be by faculty or should it be a wider, 360-degree, workplace based assessment?

And, what about assessment becoming part of learning?

Finding answers to these questions may lead us in different directions, but here, the second edition of *Principles of Assessment in Medical Education* provides an accessibly, comprehensive and convenient source of answers. In this book, the editors present a readable digest of key topics covering both the underlying theories of assessment as well as practical illustrations of how to apply a range of assessment instruments and the crucial role of feedback.

The topics are clearly presented in 28 chapters introduced by Key Points. There are six new chapters and others which have been extensively updated and rewritten. The format is clear, the pages are not too crowded, and the book is not over-long or too large or heavy to handle.

There is a great deal that we should know about the extensive and sometimes perplexing topic of assessment. But if we want to help our students by providing good assessment, I am confident that you will find this book a valuable "go-to" resource to learn more about assessment in medical education. But remember, our aim in assessment should be less about trying to trip students up, and more about giving them the chance to shine!

John Dent MMEd MD FAMEE FHEA FRCS (Ed)
International Relations Officer
Association for Medical Education in Europe
Hon Reader in Postgraduate Medicine, University of Dundee, UK

Foreword

What a rich history research and development of assessment in medical education have! Since the 1960s, an increasingly productive stream of ideas, developments, methods and research projects have found their way into the medical education literature.

This is not surprising. Assessment is important. It is not only what guides, steers and drives student learning but it also helps to certify the quality of our graduates and reassure the public.

Developing assessment in medical education is certainly not an easy task; medical competence has many facets, and all are important at various times. It is, therefore, only logical that our views on what constitutes good assessment have evolved. Originally, assessment was seen purely as a measurement process. Competence was treated the same way that test psychology approached personality characteristics, with structured and standardized testing. So, in that perspective, the measurement characteristics of assessment were the hallmark of quality: reproducibility or reliability, and construct validity.

Around the mid-1990s, the views changed. Instead of purely looking at assessment as a measurement process, it was acknowledged that every assessment involves human judgment. Even the most structured multiple-choice test is preceded by phases in which human judgments are used; blueprinting, standard setting, selection of items, options and specific wordings are all based on human judgments.

The distinguishing feature though, was that in authentic and workplace-based assessment human judgment must take place simultaneously with the observation of the candidate, in real-time, so to speak. Consequently, the focus of much research and development shifted to the examiner, because it was recognized that even the best designed rubrics or scales could not replace examiner expertise. So, a significant amount of research was now focused on human decision-making, assessment literacy and how to combine multiple perspectives of different assessors. Where, for example, in the measurement perspective, different views of assessors on the same candidate were seen as error and had to be eliminated, they are now seen as complementary and a logical phenomenon given the multifaceted nature of competence, as long as they can be relied upon as being well-informed, expert judgments. This assessor expertise has been and still is the focus of a considerable amount of research.

This evolved further in the mid-2000s, and our current views are best described as seeing assessment as a system or total program. Now, much of our research and development are focused at understanding how quantitative and qualitative information, formative and summative and assessment *FOR*, and assessment *OF* learning can be combined in an integral system. And how this can be used to optimally 'diagnose' competence and the development of each student in the more bespoke manner. In this system thinking the assessment as measurement views and the assessment as judgment views come together in a true synthesis.

This book provides a comprehensive overview of all the issues around assessment and will greatly support any reader who wants to develop a system of assessment in ensuring that they will be able to base this on the best available evidence.

Lambert Schuwirth MD PhD FANZHPE
Professor of Medical Education
Director, Prideaux Centre for Research in Health Professions Education
College of Medicine and Public Health
Flinders University, South Australia

Professor for Innovative Assessment
Department of Educational Development and Research
Maastricht University, Maastricht, The Netherlands

Distinguished Professor of Medical Education
Chang Gung University, Taiwan

Professor of Medicine (Adjunct)
Uniformed Services University for the Health Sciences
Bethesda, Maryland, USA

Preface to the Second Edition

It is with a sense of pride and satisfaction that we present this second edition of *Principles of Assessment in Medical Education*. The first edition of this book has been received extremely well by teachers of health professions in India. The present edition has been revised to address assessment issues related to competency-based medical education, especially in the Indian settings. Many chapters have been re-written, and many new ones have been added. A number of graphics have also been added to make concepts clear. We do hope that this book will continue to serve its intended purpose.

We are grateful to Professor John Dent and Professor Lambert Schuwirth for contributing Forewords to this edition. We are also grateful to the Editors of *Indian Pediatrics* and *National Medical Journal of India* for allowing us to reproduce some of our earlier works, which have been acknowledged at appropriate places in the book.

We would be happy to receive suggestions to make this book better.

Tejinder Singh
Anshu

Preface to the First Edition

The earlier book *Principles of Medical Education* has been very well received going by the fact that it has entered into its third edition. The book was targeted towards orienting medical teachers to the art and science of educational methods. To a great extent, it also served as a 'how to' manual for various educational tasks required of a teacher. However, it was increasingly being felt that it may not satisfy the academic appetite of many readers, more so, with the spotlight shifting to the science of medical education in the recent times.

The present book is a sequel to the earlier book. It focuses on the specific area of student assessment, especially on using assessment as a tool for learning. The emphasis has shifted from 'how' to 'why' for most of the tools with the presumption that the readers of the book have already received a basic orientation to assessment methods. Plenty of literature support has been provided to help the readers take a broader view of the practice of assessment and a number of further readings have also been added. A chapter on evaluation of teaching by students titled "Student feedback" has also been included with the belief that it will help to improve the standard of assessment and teaching.

A number of international and national experts have shared their expertise in this area and we are extremely grateful to them for letting us use their work. We are also grateful to the editors of *Indian Pediatrics* and the *National Medical Journal of India* for allowing us to reproduce some of the chapters published earlier in their journals. We hope that the readers will benefit from seeing more than one perspective on assessment. Let us hasten to add that it is not a treatise on assessment. It has a very focused audience, *i.e.* those from India, and a very focused objective, *i.e.* to make the teachers competent in the use of assessment for learning.

The book shares some of the problems of multiauthor books. Readers may find occasional repetitions in some chapters. Although as editors, we could have cut down many of them, a deliberate omission was made for some important topics like validity and reliability or Miller's pyramid to let the readers get a multifaceted view of these important concepts.

We do hope that the book will be accepted like its predecessor and help to raise the level of knowledge and skills of medical teachers regarding student assessment. We also hope that better assessment will ultimately translate to better learning for students and better health care for the masses.

Comments and suggestions to make this book more useful are welcome.

Tejinder Singh
Anshu

Contents

Chapter 1: Assessment: The Basics   1
Tejinder Singh
- Terminology Used in Assessment   1
- Types of Assessment   3
- Attributes of Good Assessment   6
- Utility of Assessment   15
- Easing Assessment Stress   16

Chapter 2: Assessment of Clinical Competence: A Curtain Raiser   18
Tejinder Singh, Jyoti N Modi, Rita Sood
- Assessment of Learning   20
- Assessment for Learning   25
- Assessment as Learning   26

Chapter 3: Assessment of Knowledge: Free Response Type Questions   30
Anshu
- Written Assessment Methods   31
- Essay Questions   34
- Modified Essay Questions   35
- Short Answer Questions   36
- Key Points in Framing Questions for Written Assessment   38

Chapter 4: Assessment of Knowledge: Selection Type Questions   39
Ciraj AM
- Selection Type Questions   40
- True-false Questions   40
- Multiple Response Questions   40
- Ranking Questions   41
- Assertion-reason Questions   41
- Matching Questions   42
- Extending Matching Questions   43
- Key Feature Test   44
- Computer-based Objective Forms   45
- What's New in the Arena?   45

Chapter 5: Assessment of Knowledge: Multiple Choice Questions   47
Ciraj AM
- Strengths of MCQs   48
- Why is there Opposition to Use of MCQs in Written Assessment?   48
- Structure of an Item   49

- Guidelines for Writing Flawless Items 50
- Construction of Items Based on Bloom Taxonomy 56
- Introducing MCQ Formats in Written Assessment 58
- Approaches to Scoring 59
- Why is Negative Marking Such an Contentious Issue 60
- Standard Setting 62

Chapter 6: Question Paper Setting 65
BV Adkoli, KK Deepak, KA Narayan
- Existing Practices in India 65
- Steps for Effective Question Paper Setting 67
- Determining Weightage 68
- Blueprinting 71

Chapter 7: The Long Case 83
Tejinder Singh
- Process 83
- Assessment Issues 84
- Building on the Positives 85
- Objective Structured Long Examination Record 87
- What Lessons can we draw? 88

Chapter 8: Objective Structured Clinical Examination 91
Piyush Gupta, Pooja Dewan, Tejinder Singh
- What is an OSCE 93
- Types of OSCE Stations 93
- OSCE Setup: Traditional Design 97
- Preparing for OSCE 98
- Conducting the OSCE 102
- Setting Standards 103
- Checklists versus Global Rating 105
- Modifications and Innovations 109

Chapter 9: Direct Observation-based Assessment of Clinical Skills 114
Jyoti N Modi, Tejinder Singh
- Objective Structured Clinical Examination 116
- Mini-Clinical Evaluation Exercise 117
- Direct Observation of Procedural Skills 125
- Acute Care Assessment Tool 126
- Professionalism Mini-evaluation Exercise 127
- Multisource Feedback 127
- Objective Structured Long Examination Record 129
- Utility and Implementation of Observation-based Methods 130

Chapter 10: Oral Examinations 138
Anshu
- Abilities that can be Tested by Oral Examination 139

- ❖ Flaws of the Traditional Oral Examination   *139*
- ❖ Strategies to Improve the Oral Examination   *142*
- ❖ Oral Examinations for High-stakes Selection Process: Multiple Mini-interviews   *143*
- ❖ Faculty Development   *147*

Chapter 11: Portfolios for Assessment 151
Medha A Joshi
- ❖ What is a Portfolio?   *151*
- ❖ Portfolios for Learning   *152*
- ❖ Portfolios for Assessment   *157*
- ❖ Advantages and Limitations of Portfolios   *159*
- ❖ Steps in Implementing the Portfolios   *161*
- ❖ Challenges and Issues   *162*
- ❖ Place of Portfolio in Medical Education   *163*

Chapter 12: Assessment of Professionalism and Ethics 165
BV Adkoli
- ❖ What is Professionalism?   *165*
- ❖ Some Interesting Facts about Professionalism   *167*
- ❖ General Principles and Specific Challenges in the Assessment of Professionalism   *167*
- ❖ Methods, Tools and Techniques   *169*
- ❖ Assessment of Professionalism in the Workplace: Workplace-based Assessment   *171*
- ❖ Narrative-based Approaches to the Assessment of Professionalism   *173*
- ❖ Future of Assessment of Professionalism: Professional Identity Formation   *174*

Chapter 13: Workplace-based Assessment 178
Upreet Dhaliwal
- ❖ Need for WPBA   *178*
- ❖ Prerequisites for an Ideal WPBA   *179*
- ❖ Terminology in Relation to WPBA   *179*
- ❖ Setting-up WPBA in your Discipline   *181*
- ❖ Tools for WPBA   *184*
- ❖ Newer Additions to WPBA   *194*
- ❖ Roles and Responsibilities in WPBA   *196*
- ❖ Quality Parameters of WPBA   *197*
- ❖ Faculty Development for WPBA   *199*
- ❖ Potential Problem Areas in WPBA   *199*

Chapter 14: Competency-based Assessment 206
Upreet Dhaliwal, Jyoti N Modi, Piyush Gupta, Tejinder Singh
- ❖ What is a Competency?   *206*
- ❖ Competency Frameworks to Facilitate Competency-based Medical Education   *207*
- ❖ Designing Entrustable Professional Activities   *208*
- ❖ Prerequisites for Assessment in Competency-based Medical Education   *210*
- ❖ Designing a System of Competency-based Assessment   *212*

Chapter 15: Community-based Assessment — 221
Subodh S Gupta, Abhishek V Raut
- What is Community-based Medical Education? *221*
- Special Features of Assessment in Community Settings *222*
- Worley's Framework for Community-based Medical Education *223*
- Building Student Assessment for Community-based Medical Education *224*
- Portfolio Assessment *226*
- Assessment of Reflections *228*
- Assessment of Projects *229*
- Direct Observation of Learners for Professional Skills *230*
- Multisource Feedback or 360-Degree Assessment *231*

Chapter 16: Assessment for Learning — 233
Rajiv Mahajan, Tejinder Singh
- Assessment for Learning versus Assessment of Learning *234*
- Detrimental Effects of Summative Assessment *234*
- Strength of Assessment for Learning *235*
- Cycle of Assessment for Learning *236*
- Attributes of the Assessment for Learning System *237*
- Opportunities for Assessment for Learning *240*
- SWOT Analysis of Assessment for Learning *242*
- Incorporating Assessment for Learning in Undergraduate Medical Training *242*

Chapter 17: Assessment for Selection — 247
Tejinder Singh, Jyoti N Modi, Vinay Kumar, Upreet Dhaliwal, Piyush Gupta, Rita Sood
- What Works and to What Extent? *248*
- Need for Change in the Selection Procedures for Medical Courses in India *251*
- Single Entrance Examination for Selection Decisions—A Critique *253*
- Can Strengthening Internal Assessment Offset Negative Consequences of PG Entrance Examination? *255*
- Some Suggestions for Alleviating Limitations of a Single Entrance Examination *256*

Chapter 18: Programmatic Assessment — 261
Tejinder Singh, Jyoti N Modi, Rajiv Mahajan
- Rationale for Programmatic Assessment *262*
- Programmatic Assessment: Principles and Components *264*
- Implementing Programmatic Assessment *271*
- Challenges to Implementation of Programmatic Assessment *273*
- Adaptation of Programmatic Assessment to the Indian Context *274*

Chapter 19: Internal Assessment: Basic Principles — 278
Tejinder Singh, Anshu
- Is Internal Assessment Formative or Summative? *280*
- Is Internal Assessment a Pre-university Examination? *280*
- Should Internal Assessment be based on Theory and Practical Tests Only? *281*
- Is Internal Assessment Reliable? *281*
- Is Internal Assessment Valid? *282*
- Should Internal Assessment be an Aggregate of All Tests? *282*

Chapter 20: The Quarter Model — 285
Tejinder Singh, Anshu, Jyoti N Modi
- Problems with Internal Assessment in India *286*
- Proposed Quarter Model *289*
- Utility of the Model *293*

Chapter 21: Assessment in Online Settings — 296
Anshu
- Designing Online Assessment *297*
- Alternative Question Formats in Online Assessment *298*
- Assessment in Clinical Settings *302*
- Implementing Online Assessment *304*
- Plagiarism and Cheating *305*
- Concept of Triage in Medical Education During a Crisis *306*

Chapter 22: Item Analysis and Question Banking — 308
Ciraj AM
- What is Item Analysis? *308*
- Process *309*
- Facility Value *309*
- Discrimination Index *310*
- Distractor Efficiency *311*
- Point-biserial Correlation *311*
- Test Analysis *313*
- Standard Error of Measurement *317*
- Question Banking *318*

Chapter 23: Standard Setting — 322
Tejinder Singh, Ara Tekian
- The Need *322*
- Absolute or Relative? *323*
- Compensatory or Non-compensatory? *324*
- Effect on Learning *324*
- Methods of Standard Setting *325*
- Standard Setting for Knowledge Tests *325*
- Standard Setting for Practical/Clinical Skills *327*

Chapter 24: Educational Feedback to Students — 329
Rajiv Mahajan
- What is Feedback? *329*
- Feedback Loop: Corollary with the Human Body *330*
- Hierarchy of Role-categorization of Educational Feedback *332*
- Attributes of Effective Educational Feedback *332*
- Types of Educational Feedback *334*
- Models for Giving Educational Feedback to Students *335*
- Feedback Opportunities During Undergraduate Training *336*

- Issues with Giving Educational Feedback to Students *338*
- Strategies for Enhancing Value of Educational Feedback *339*

Chapter 25: Student Ratings of Teaching Effectiveness   342
Anshu, Tejinder Singh
- Student Ratings of Teaching: Misconceptions and Misuses *342*
- Process of Collecting and Interpreting Student Ratings *343*
- Purposes of Student Ratings of Teaching *348*
- Prospects of Using Student Ratings in India *348*

Chapter 26: Is Objectivity Synonymous with Reliability?   352
Tejinder Singh, Anshu
- Validity and Reliability: A Quick Recap *353*
- Countering Variability *356*
- The Impact of 'Objectification' and the Value of 'Subjective' Expert Judgment *357*
- Checklists versus Global Rating Scales *358*
- Is Subjective Expert Judgment Reliable? *359*
- Implications for Educational Practice *360*

Chapter 27: Faculty Development for Better Assessment   364
Tejinder Singh
- Formal Approaches to Faculty Development *367*
- Informal Approaches to Faculty Development *367*
- Promoting Application: Transfer-oriented Training *368*
- Model Program for Training *368*

Chapter 28: Online Resources for Assessment   371
Chinmay Shah, Anshu
- Learning Management Systems which offer Resources for Integrated Learning and Assessment *372*
- Resources for Creating, Distributing and Grading Assessments *373*
- Interactive Tools for Formative Assessment and Enhanced Student Engagement in Online Sessions *373*
- Resources to Create Customized Quizzes and Gamification Apps *376*
- Resources to Create Interactive Videos *377*
- Resources to Create Online Polls and Surveys *378*
- Resources for Online Collaboration *379*
- E-Portfolios *379*
- Resources to Conduct OSCEs and Simulation *380*
- Resources to Create Rubrics *381*
- Resources for High-stakes Examinations, Online Security and Proctor Devices *381*

Index   385

Chapter 1

Assessment: The Basics

Tejinder Singh

KEY POINTS

- Assessment is an important component of the educational system.
- Good assessment should be valid, reliable, and acceptable to all stakeholders, and have a positive educational impact. These attributes of assessment can compensate for each other.
- It requires more than one assessment tool to derive meaningful assessment results.
- Validity and reliability depend on adequacy and representativeness of the sample.

It is said that "assessment is the tail that wags the curriculum dog" (Hargreaves, 1989). This statement amply underscores the importance of assessment in any system of education. However, it also cautions us about the pitfalls that can occur when assessment is improperly used. When poorly conducted, students may view assessment as pointless and just another hurdle to jump over (McDowell & Mowl, 1995; Ramsden, 1997). Students focus on learning what is asked in the examination. As teachers, we can exploit this potential of assessment to give a direction to student learning. Simply stated, it means that if we ask them questions based on factual recall, they will try to memorize facts; but if we frame questions requiring application of knowledge, they will learn to apply their knowledge.

In this chapter, we will introduce the basic concepts related to assessment of students and how we can maximize the effect of assessment in giving a desired shape to learning.

Terminology Used in Assessment

Let us first clarify the terminology. You may have read terms such as measurement, assessment, evaluation, etc. and seen them being used interchangeably. There are subtle differences between these terms. They need to be used in the right context with the right purpose, so that they convey the same meaning to everyone. Interestingly these terms also tell the story about how educational testing has evolved over the years.

Measurement was the earliest technique used in educational testing. It meant assigning numbers to the competence exhibited by the students. For example, marking a multiple-choice question paper is a form of measurement. Since measurement is a physical term, it was presumed that it should be as precise and as accurate as possible. As a corollary, it also implied that anything which could not be measured (objectively!) should not form part of the assessment package. The entire emphasis was placed on objectivity and providing standard conditions so that the results represented only student learning (also called true score) and nothing else.

While such an approach may have been appropriate to measure physical properties (such as weight, length, temperature, etc.), it certainly did not capture the essence of educational attainment. There are several qualities which we want our students to develop, but which are not amenable to precise measurement. Can you think of some of these? You may have rightly thought of communication, ethics, professionalism, etc., which are as important as other skills and competencies, but which cannot be precisely measured.

Assessment has come to represent a much broader concept. It includes some attributes which can be measured precisely and others which cannot be measured so precisely (Linn & Miller, 2005). Some aspects such as scores of theoretical tests are objectively measured, while other aspects such as clinical-decision making are subjectively interpreted, and then combining these, a judgment is formed about the level of student achievement. Thus, viewing assessment as a combination of measurement and non-measurement gives a better perspective from teachers' point of view. Several experts favor this approach, defining assessment as "any formal or purported action to obtain information about the competence and performance of a student" (Vleuten & Schuwirth, 2019).

Evaluation is another term which is used almost synonymously with assessment. However, there are subtle differences. Though both these terms involve passing a value judgment on learning, traditionally the term 'assessment' is used in the context of student learning. Evaluation, on the other hand, is used in the context of the educational programs. So, you will *assess* the performance of students in a particular test, while you will *evaluate* the quantum to which a particular course is equipping the students with desired knowledge and skills. Assessment of students is a very important input (though not the only one) to judge the value of an educational program.

Let us also clarify some more terms that are often loosely used in the context of student assessment. "Test" and "tool" are two such terms. Conventionally, a **"test"** generally refers to a written instrument which is used to assess learning. Test can be paper/pencil-based or computer-based. On the other hand, a **"tool"** refers to an instrument used to observe skills or behavior to assess the extent of learning. Objective Structured Clinical Examination (OSCE) and mini-Clinical Evaluation Exercise (m-CEX) are examples of assessment tools.

Why do we need to assess students?

The conventional answer given to this question is: so that we can categorize them as "pass" or "fail". But more than making this decision, several other advantages accrue from assessment. Rank ordering the students (e.g., for selection), measuring improvement over a period of time, providing feedback to students and teachers about areas which have been learnt well and others which require more attention, and maintaining the quality of educational programs are some of the other important reasons for assessment **(Table 1.1)**.

Assessment in medical education is especially important because we are certifying students as fit to deal with human lives. The actions of doctors have the potential to make a difference between life and death. This makes it even more important to use the most appropriate tools to assess their learning. You will also appreciate that medical students are required to learn a number of practical skills, many of which can be lifesaving. Assessment is also a means to ensure that all students learn these skills.

Table 1.1: Purposes of assessment

Summative (to prove)	Formative (to improve)
To ensure that minimum required standard or competence has been attained	To give feedback about performance to students
For certification: as pass/fail, to award a degree	To give feedback about performance to teachers
Rank ordering for competitive selection	To evaluate the quality of an educational program

Types of Assessment

Assessment can be classified in many ways depending on the primary purpose for which it is being conducted. Some of the ways of classifying assessment are as follows:
1. Formative and summative assessment
2. Criterion- and norm-referenced testing.

1. Formative assessment and summative assessment

As discussed in the preceding paragraphs, assessment can be used not only for certification, but also to provide feedback to teachers and students. Based on this perspective, assessment can be classified as formative or summative.

Formative assessment is the assessment which is conducted with the primary purpose of providing feedback to students and teachers. Since the purpose is diagnostic (and remedial), it should be able to reveal strengths and weaknesses in student learning. If students disguise their weaknesses and try to bluff the teacher, the purpose of formative assessment is lost. This feature has important implications in designing assessment for formative purposes. To be useful, formative assessment should happen as often as possible—in fact, experts suggest that it should be almost *continuous*. Remember, when we give formative feedback, we do not give students a single score, but we give students a complete profile of their strengths and weaknesses in different areas. Since the purpose is to help the student learn better, formative assessment is also called assessment *for* learning.

Formative assessment should not be used for final certification. This implies that certain assessment opportunities must be designated as formative only, so that teachers have an opportunity to identify the deficiencies of the students and undertake remedial action. A corollary of this statement is that all assignments need not be graded, or that, all grades need not be considered during the calculation of final scores. From this perspective, all assessments are *de facto* summative; they become formative only when they are used to provide feedback to the students to make learning better. Formative assessment has been discussed in more detail in Chapter 16.

Summative assessment, on the other hand, implies testing at the end of the unit, semester or course. Please note that summative does not refer only to the end-of-the-year University examinations. Assessment becomes summative when the results are going to be used to make educational decisions. Summative assessment is also called assessment *of* learning.

Summative assessment intends to test if the students have attained the objectives laid down for a specified unit of activity. It is also used for certification and registration purposes (e.g., giving a license to practice medicine). Did you notice that we said "attainment of listed objectives"? This implies that students must be informed well in advance, right at the beginning of the course, about what is expected from them when they complete the course, so that they can plan the path of their learning accordingly. Most institutions ignore this part, leaving it for students to make their own interpretations based on inputs from various sources (mainly from senior students). No wonder then, that we often end up frustrated with the way the students learn.

The contemporary trend is towards blurring the boundary between formative and summative assessment. Purely formative assessment without any consequences will not be taken seriously by anybody. On the other hand, purely summative assessment has no learning value or opportunity for improvement. There is no reason why the same assessment cannot be used to provide feedback, as well as to calculate final scores. We will discuss this aspect in more detail in Chapter 18.

We strongly believe that every teacher can play a significant role in improving student learning by the judicious use of assessment for learning. Every teacher may not be involved with setting high-stake question papers, but every teacher is involved with developing assessment locally to provide feedback to the students. Throughout this book, you will find a tilt toward the formative function of assessment.

Sometimes, assessment itself can be used as a learning task, in which case, it is called assessment *as* learning.

2. Criterion-referenced and norm-referenced testing

Yet another purpose of assessment that we listed above was to rank order the students (e.g., for selection purposes). From this perspective, it is possible to classify assessment as criterion-referenced testing (CRT) and norm-referenced testing (NRT).

Criterion-referenced testing involves comparing the performance of the students against pre-determined criteria. This is particularly useful for term-end examinations or before awarding degrees to doctors, where we want to ensure that students have attained the minimum desired competencies for that course or unit of the course. Competency-based curricula largely require criterion-referenced testing.

Results of CRT can only be a pass or a fail. Let us have an example. If the objective is that the student should be able to perform a cardio-pulmonary resuscitation, then he must perform all the essential steps to be declared as pass. The student cannot pass if he performs only 60% of the steps! CRT requires establishment of an absolute standard *before* starting the examination.

Norm-referenced testing, on the other hand, implies rank ordering the student. Here each student's results set the standard for those of others. NRT only tells us how the students did in relation to each other—it does not tell us "what" they did. There is no fixed absolute standard, and ranking can happen only *after* the examination has been conducted.

Again, there can be variations to this, and one of the commonly employed means is a two-stage approach, i.e. first use CRT to decide who should pass and then use NRT to rank order them. Traditionally in India we have been following this mixed approach. However, we do not seem to have established defensible standards of performance so far and often arbitrarily take 50% as the cut-off for pass/fail. This affects the validity of assessment. It is important to have defensible standards. Standard setting has been discussed in Chapter 23.

Attributes of Good Assessment

We have argued for the importance of assessment as an aid to learning. This is related to many factors. The provision of feedback (e.g., during formative assessment) improves learning (Burch et al, 2006; Rushton, 2005). Similarly, the test-driven nature of learning again speaks for the importance of assessment (Dochy & McDowell, 1997). What we would like to emphasize here, is that the reverse is also true, i.e. when improperly used, assessment can distort learning. We are all aware of the adverse consequences on the learning of interns that occurs when selection into postgraduate courses is based only on the results of one MCQ-based test.

There are several attributes that good assessment should possess. Rather than going into the plethora of attributes available in literature, we will restrict ourselves to the five most important attributes of good assessment as listed by Vleuten & Schuwirth (2005). These include:
1. Validity
2. Reliability
3. Feasibility
4. Acceptability, and
5. Educational impact.

Validity

Validity is the most important attribute of good assessment. Traditionally, it has been defined as "measuring what is intended to be measured" (Streiner & Norman, 1995). While this definition is correct but, it requires a lot of elaboration (Downing, 2003). Let us try to understand validity better.

The traditional view was that validity is of various types: content validity, criterion validity (this was further divided into predictive validity & concurrent validity), and construct validity (Crossley, Humphris & Jolly, 2002) **(Fig. 1.1)**. This concept had the drawback of seeing assessment as being valid in one situation but not in another. With this approach, a test could cover all areas and have good content validity; but may not be valid when it comes to predicting future performance. Let us draw a parallel between validity and honesty as an attribute. Just as it is not possible for a person to be honest in one

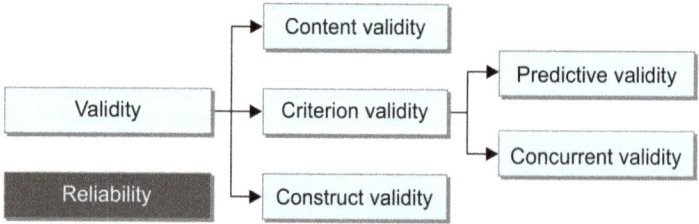

Fig. 1.1: Earlier concept of validity.

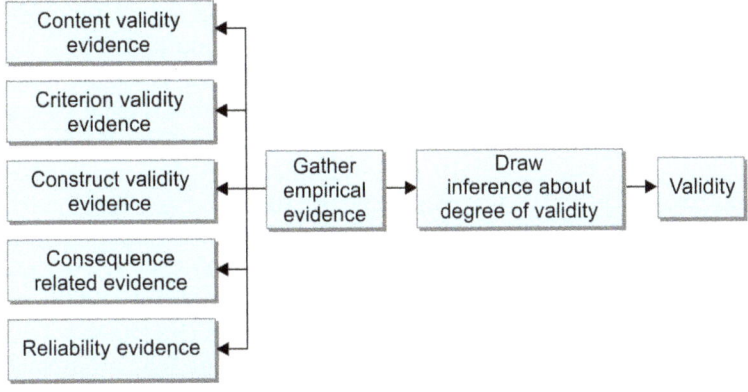

Fig. 1.2: Contemporary concept of validity.

situation and dishonest in another (then he would not be called honest!), so is true for validity.

Validity is now seen as a *unitary concept*, which must be inferred from various evidences **(Fig. 1.2)**. Let us come back to the "honesty" example. When would you say that someone is honest? One would have to look at a person's behavior at work, at home, in a situation when he finds something expensive lying by the roadside, or how he pays his taxes, and only then make an inference about his honesty. Validity is a matter of *inference*, based on available evidence.

Validity refers to the interpretations that we make out of assessment data. Implied within this is the fact that validity does not refer to the tool or results—rather, it refers to the interpretations we make from the results obtained by use of that tool. From this viewpoint, it is pertinent to remember that no test or tool is inherently valid or invalid.

Let us explain this further. Suppose we use a 200-question MCQs test to select the best students to get into postgraduate medical courses. We could interpret that the highest scorers of the test have the best content knowledge. To do this, we would have to gather evidence to check if all relevant portions of the syllabus had received adequate representation in the paper. We could also state that the students with the best aptitude have been selected for the course. For this we will need to present evidence that the test was designed to assess aptitude also. As you can see, *validity is contextual*. So here, it is not the tool (MCQ), which is valid or invalid, but the interpretations that we infer from the results of our assessment which matter.

Inferring validity requires empirical evidence. What are the different kinds of evidence that we can gather to determine if the interpretations we are making are appropriate and meaningful?

As **Figure 1.2** shows, we need to gather evidence from different sources to support or refute the interpretations that we make from our assessment results. Depending on the situation, we might look for one or two types of evidence to interpret validity of an assessment.

But ideally, we would need to look for evidence in the following four categories (Waugh & Gronlund, 2012):
a. *Content-related evidence:* Does the test adequately represent the entire domain of tasks that is to be assessed?
b. *Criterion-related evidence:* Does the test predict future performance? Do the test results compare to results of some other simultaneously conducted test (this has been explained below in more detail)?
c. *Construct-related evidence:* Does this test measure the psychological or educational characteristics that we intended to measure?
d. *Consequence-related evidence:* Did the test have a good impact on learning and avoid negative effects?

To do this, one has to be fully aware of: why we are performing a particular assessment; the exact nature of construct being assessed; what we are expecting to obtain by conducting this exercise; what the assessment results are going to be used for; the exact criterion which are going to be used to make decisions on assessment results; and the consequences of using this assessment. Let's understand this in more detail.

Evidence Related to Content Validity

Generally, we look for content-related evidence to see if the test represents the entire domain of the content, competencies, and objectives set for a course. If an undergraduate student is expected to perform certain basic skills (e.g., giving an intramuscular injection or draining an abscess) and if these skills are not assessed in the examination, then content-related validity evidence is lacking. Similarly, if the number of questions is not proportional to the content [e.g., if 50% weightage is given to questions from the central nervous system (CNS) at the cost of anemia, which is a much more common problem], the assessment results might not be meaningful.

Thus, *sampling* is a key issue in assessment. Always ask yourself if the test is representative of the whole domain that you are assessing. For this, look at the learning outcomes, prepare a plan (blueprint) and prepare items which correspond to these specifications. More on this will be dealt with in Chapter 6.

Evidence Related to Criterion Validity

The reasons why we look for evidence related to criterion validity are to see whether the test scores correspond to the criterion which we seek to predict or estimate. Let us take an example. Suppose we conduct an entrance examination to select the best undergraduate students into a postgraduate surgical course. Here, the purpose of the test is to predict future performance. To infer that this test was appropriate, we would perhaps need to gather data about the students' performance after they qualify as surgeons and see if these test results correspond to their performance. Here we are using future performance as the criterion. This is an example of how evidence about predictive validity can be gathered.

Now suppose we are introducing a new assessment method A and we want to see how it works in comparison to an existing assessment method B for the same purpose and in the same setting. To do this we can compare the results obtained from both tools in the same setting to see how effective method A is in comparison to the previous method B. Here we are concurrently judging the results of two methods to see if they are comparable. This is the concept of concurrent validity.

Evidence Related to Construct Validity

Validity also requires construct-related evidence. What do we understand by 'construct'? The dictionary meaning of construct is "a complex idea resulting from a synthesis of simpler ideas". A construct has also been defined in educational or psychological terms as "an intangible collection of abstract concepts and principles which are inferred from behavior and explained by educational or psychological theory" (Downing, 2003). Thus, a construct is a collection of inter-related components, which when grouped together as a whole gives a new meaning.

If we were to consider the construct 'beauty', we might use attributes such as physique, complexion, poise, confidence, and many such attributes to decide if one is beautiful. Similarly, in educational settings, subject knowledge, its application, data gathering, interpretation of data and many other things go into deciding the construct 'clinical competence'. In medicine, educational attainment, intelligence, aptitude, problem-solving, professionalism, and ethics are some other examples of constructs.

All assessment in education aims at assessing a construct. It is the theoretical framework which specifies the hypothetical qualities that we seek to measure. For instance, we are not interested in knowing if students can enumerate five causes of hepatomegaly. But we are interested in knowing, if they can take a relevant history based on those causes. In this context, construct-related evidence becomes most important way to infer validity. Simply stated, results of assessment will be more valid, if they told us about the problem-solving ability of a student, rather than about his ability to list five causes of each of the symptoms shown by the patient. As a corollary, it can also be said that if the construct is not fully represented (e.g., testing only presentation skills, but not physical examination skills during a case presentation), validity is threatened. Messick (1989) calls this *construct under-representation* (CU).

While content and construct seem to be directly related to the course, the way a test is conducted can also influence its validity. A question may be included in an examination to test understanding of certain concepts, but if the papers are marked based on a student's handwriting, validity is threatened. If a test is conducted in a hot, humid, and noisy room, its validity becomes low, because then, one is also implicitly testing candidates' ability to concentrate in the presence of distractions rather than their educational attainment. Notice here, that the construct that we were assessing has changed. Suppose an MCQ is framed in complicated language and if the students must spend more time in understanding the complex language of an MCQ, rather than on its content, then validity is threatened. Here besides content, one is testing vocabulary and reading comprehension. Similarly, leaked question papers, incorrect key, equipment failure, etc. can have a bearing on the validity. Messick (1989) calls this *construct irrelevance variance* (CIV).

Let us try to explain this concept in a different way. Let us say you conduct an essay type test and try to assess knowledge, skills, and professionalism from the same. We would expect that there would be low correlation between the scores on the three domains. On the other hand, if we conduct three different tests, say for example, essays, MCQs, and oral examination to assess knowledge, we would expect a high correlation between scores. If we were to get just the opposite results—i.e., high correlation in the first setting and low in the second, construct irrelevance variance would be said to exist. You can think of many common examples from your own settings, which induce CIV in our assessment. Too difficult or too complicated questions, use of complex language which is not understood by students, words which confuse the students and "teaching to the test" are some of the factors which will induce CIV. Designing OSCE stations which test only analytical skills will result in invalid interpretation about practical skills of a student by inducing CIV.

The contemporary concept of validity is that *all validity is construct validity* (Downing, 2003). It is the most important of all the evidences that we gather to determine validity.

Evidence Related to Consequential Validity

When we design an assessment, it is always pertinent to ask about the consequences of using that format. Did it motivate students to learn differently? Did it lower their motivation to study, or did it encourage poor study habits? Did it lead them to choose surface learning over deep learning? Did it make them think about application of the knowledge or did they resort to mere memorization of facts? Evidence about these effects needs to be collected.

These main concepts on validity have been summarized in **Box 1.1**.

BOX 1.1: Key concepts of validity

- Validity is a unitary concept.
- Validity refers to the interpretations that we make from assessment data.
- The degree of validity must be inferred from different sources.
- Multiple evidences must be gathered to support or refute the appropriateness of our interpretations.
- All validity is construct validity.

How can we *build in* validity?

Validity should be built in right from the stage of planning and preparation. Assessment should match the contents of the course and provide proportional weightage to each of the contents. Blueprinting and good sampling of content is a very helpful tool to ensure content representation (see Chapter 6). Also, implied is the need to let students know right in the beginning about what is expected from them at the end of the course. Use questions, which are neither too difficult nor too easy, which are worded in a way appropriate to the level of the students. Validity also involves proper administration and scoring. Maintaining transparency, fairness, and confidentiality of the examinations are some methods of building validity. Similarly, the directions, scoring system, test format all have a bearing on the validity **(Table 1.2)**.

Table 1.2: Factors which lower validity and their remedies

Factors	Remedies
Too few items or cases	Increase the number of items/cases; Increase the frequency of testing
Unrepresentative or irrelevant content	Blueprinting; Subject experts' feedback; Moderation
Too easy or too difficult questions	Better framing of questions; Test and item analysis
Items violating standard writing guidelines	Screening of items, faculty training
Problems with test administration (leakages, wrong papers, wrong keys, administrative issues)	Appropriate administrative measures, monitoring mechanisms
Problems with test construction, scoring, improper instructions	Faculty training, screening and monitoring mechanisms

We have for long, followed the dictum of "assessment drives learning," which often results in extraneous factors distorting learning. A better way would be to let "learning drive assessment" so that validity is built into assessments. This concept of *Programmatic Assessment* has been discussed in detail in Chapter 18.

Similarly, the assessment tools should aim to test broad constructs rather than individual competencies like knowledge or skills. It is often better to use multiple tools to get different pieces of information on which a judgment of student attainment can be made. It is also important to select tools, which can test more than one competency at a time. There is no use of having one OSCE station to test history taking, another for skills, and yet another for professionalism. Each station should be able to test more than one competency. This not only provides an opportunity for wider sampling by having more competencies tested at each station but also builds validity.

Reliability

Let us now move to the second important attribute of assessment—reliability. Commonly, reliability refers to *reproducibility of the scores*. Again, like in the case of validity, this definition needs a lot of elaboration (Downing, 2004).

A commonly used definition of reliability is *obtaining same results under similar conditions*. The concept of obtaining same results under similar conditions might be true of a biochemical test. However, it is not completely true of an educational test. Let us say, during the final professional MBBS examination, we allot a long case to a student in a very conducive setting, where there is no noise or urgency, and the patient is very cooperative. But we know that in actual practice, this seldom happens. Similarly, no two patients with same diagnosis will have similar presentation. In the past, educationists have tried to make the examinations more and more controlled and standardized (e.g., OSCE and standardized patients), so that the results represent only student attainment and nothing else. We argue that it might be better to work in reverse— i.e., conduct examinations in settings as close to actual ones as possible so that reproducibility can be ensured. This is the concept of *workplace based* and *authentic assessment*.

We often tend to confuse between the terms 'objectivity' and 'reliability'. *Objectivity* refers to reproducibility of the scores so that anyone marking the test would mark it the same way. There are certain problems in equating reliability with objectivity in this way. For example, if the key to an item is wrongly marked in a test, everyone would mark the test similarly and generate identical scores. But are we happy with this situation? No, because it leads to faulty interpretation of the scores. Let us add some more examples. Suppose at the end of final professional MBBS, we were to give the students a test paper containing only 10 MCQs. The results will be very objective, but they will not be a reliable measure of students' knowledge. There is no doubt that objectivity is a useful attribute of any tool, but it is more important to have items (or questions) which are fairly representative of the universe of items which are possible in a subject area, and at the same time sufficient number of items so that the results are generalizable. In other words, in addition to objectivity we also need an *appropriate* and *adequate* sample to get reliable results. This example also shows how reliability evidence contributes to validity.

We will also like to argue that objectivity is not *sine-qua-non* of reliability. A subjective assessment can be very reliable if based on adequate content expertise. We all make predictions— subjective— about potential of our students and we rarely go wrong! The point that we are trying to make is that in educational testing there is always a degree of prediction involved. Will the student whom we have certified as being able to handle a case of mitral stenosis in the medical college be able to do so in practice? To us, reliability is therefore the *degree of confidence that we can place in our results* (try reading reliability as *rely-ability*).

A common reason for low reliability is the content specificity of the case. Many examiners will prefer to have a neurological case in the final examination in medicine. It is presumed that a student who can satisfactorily present this case can also present a patient with anemia or malnutrition. This could not be farther from the truth. Herein lies the importance of including a variety of cases in the examination to make them representative of what the student is going to see in real life. You will recall what we said earlier that a representative and adequate sampling is also important to build validity.

Viewing reliability of educational assessment differently from that of other tests has important implications. Let us suppose that we give a test of clinical skills to a final year student. If we look at reliability merely as reproducibility— or in other words, getting same results if the same case is given again to the student under same conditions— then we will try to focus on precision of scores. However, if we conceptualize reliability as confidence in our interpretation, then we will like to examine the student under different conditions (outpatients, inpatients, emergency, community settings, etc., and by different examiners) and on different patients so that we can generalize our results. We might even like to add feedback from peers, patients, and other teachers to infer about the competence of the student.

We often go by the idea that examiner variability can induce a lot of unreliability in the results. To some extent this may be true. While examiner training is one solution, it is equally useful to have multiple examiners. We have already discussed about need to include a variety of content in assessment. It may not be possible to use many assessment formats at one occasion, but this can happen when we carry out assessment on multiple occasions. The general agreement in educational assessment is that a single assessment, howsoever perfect, is flawed for making educational decisions. Therefore, it is important to collect information on several occasions using a variety of tools. The key dictum to build reliability (and thereby validity) for any assessment is to have multiple *tests* on multiple *content* areas by multiple *examiners* using multiple *tools* in multiple *settings*. The concept of *Programmatic Assessment* discussed in Chapter 18 largely follows this approach.

Validity and reliability of a test are very intricately related. To be valid, a test should be reliable. Reliability evidence contributes to validity. A judge cannot form a valid inference if the witness who is being examined is unreliable. Thus, reliability is a precondition for validity. But let us caution you that it is not the only condition. Please also be aware that generally there is a trade-off between validity and reliability: the stronger the bases for validity, the weaker the bases for reliability (and *vice-versa*) (Fendler, 2016).

An *application-oriented* perspective on validity and reliability of assessments has been discussed in Chapter 26.

Feasibility

The third important attribute of assessment is feasibility. We may like to assess every student by asking them to perform a cardiopulmonary resuscitation on an actual patient, but it may not be logistically possible. Same is true of many other skills and competencies. In such situations, one needs to think of other alternatives like simulations or tie up with other professional organizations for such assessments.

Acceptability

The next attribute of assessment is acceptability. Several assessment tools are available to us and sometimes we can have a variety of methods to fulfill the same objective.

Portfolios, for example, can provide as much information as can be provided by rating scales. MCQs can provide as much information about knowledge as can be obtained by oral examinations. However, acceptability by students, raters, institutions and society, at large, can play a significant role in accepting or rejecting a tool. MCQs, despite all their problems, are accepted as a tool for selecting students for postgraduate courses, while methods like portfolios, which provide more valid and reliable results may not be. This is not to suggest that we should sacrifice good tools based on likes or dislikes, but to suggest that all stakeholders need to be involved in the decision-making process about use of assessment tools.

Linked to the concept of acceptability is also the issue of feasibility. While we may have developed very good tools for assessing communication skills of our students, resource crunch may not allow us to use this tool on a large scale.

Educational Impact

The educational impact of assessment is a very significant issue. The impact of assessment can be seen in terms of student learning, consequences for the students and consequences for the society. We have already referred to the impact of MCQ-based selection tests on student learning. For students, a wrong assessment decision can act as a double-edged sword. A student who has wrongly been failed has to face consequences in terms of time and money. On the other hand, if a student is wrongly passed when he does not deserve to, society must deal with the consequences of having an incompetent physician.

Assessments do not happen in vacuum. They happen within the context of certain objectives. For each assessment, there is an expected use—it could be making pass/fail judgments, selecting students for an award or simply to provide feedback to teachers. Asking these three questions visually brings a lot of clarity in the process and helps in selecting appropriate tools.
1. Who is going to use this data?
2. At what time? and,
3. For what purpose?

Utility of Assessment

Before we end this chapter, let us introduce you to the concept of utility of assessment. Vleuten (1996) has suggested a conceptual model for the utility of any assessment.

> Utility = Validity × Reliability × Acceptability × Educational impact × Feasibility

This is not a mathematical formula but a *notional* one. This concept is especially important because it shows us how to compensate for deficiencies in assessment tools by their strengths. Results of some tools may be low on reliability but can still be useful if they are high on their educational impact. For example, results of MCQs have a high reliability, but little educational value. Results of mini-clinical evaluation exercise (mini-CEX), on the other hand, may be low on reliability, but have a higher educational value due to the feedback component. Still, both are equally useful to assess students. Similarly, if certain assessment has a negative value for any of the parameter, (e.g., if an assessment promotes unsound learning habits), then its utility may be zero or even negative.

The above five criteria contributing to utility of assessment were accepted by consensus in 2010 as the criteria for good assessment along with two additional criteria (Norcini et al., 2011). While we have retained the earlier nomenclature of "criteria," there have been some modifications to it. Later at the 2018 Ottawa consensus meeting, the nomenclature was changed from "criteria" to "framework" for good assessment emphasizing the essential structure that these elements provide (Norcini et al., 2018). The alternative nomenclature of these seven elements was provided as: (1) Validity or coherence; (2) Reproducibility, Reliability, or Consistency; (3) Equivalence (the same assessment yields equivalent scores or decisions when administered across different institutions or cycles of testing); (4) Feasibility; (5) Educational Effect; (6) Catalytic effect (the assessment provides results and feedback in a fashion that motivates all stakeholders to create, enhance, and support education; it drives future learning forward and improves overall program quality); (7) Acceptability (Norcini et al., 2018). The same paper well summarizes the relationship between these elements of framework and purpose of assessment (formative or summative) rather well. Validity is essential for both the formative and summative purposes. While reliability and equivalence are more important for the summative assessments, the educational and catalytic effects are key to formative use. Feasibility and acceptability considerations are a must for both. Whatever nomenclature we may adopt, assessment can never be viewed in terms of a single criterion, framework or attribute.

Easing Assessment Stress

Assessments induce a lot of stress and anxiety amongst students (and teachers). Assessment should be like a moving ramp rather than like a staircase with a block at each stage. Many approaches can be used to reduce examination stress. A COLE framework has been proposed (Siddiqui, 2017) to smoothen out assessment problems. This stands for *Communication* to the stakeholders about the need and purpose of a tool; *Orientation* to ensure that the tool is used as intended, by teachers and students alike; *Learning orientation* in the tool so that all assessments contribute to better learning and *Evaluation* of the tool itself to see if it is serving the intended purpose.

The other approach is to reduce stakes on individual assessments and take a collective decision based on multiple low stake assessments, spread throughout the course. This is the basis of *programmatic assessment* and will be discussed in Chapter 18.

As we go through the subsequent chapters, we will be discussing about assessment methods and assessment design in greater detail.

REFERENCES

Burch, V.C., Saggie, J.C, & Gary, N. (2006). Formative assessment promotes learning in undergraduate clinical clerkships. *South African Medical Journal, 96*, 430–33.

Crossley, J., Humphris, G., & Jolly, B. (2002). Assessing health professionals. *Medical Education, 36(9)*, 800–4.

Dochy, F.J.R.C., & McDowell, L. (1997). Assessment as a tool for learning. *Studies in Educational Evaluation, 23*, 279–98.

Downing, S.M. (2003). Validity: on the meaningful interpretation of assessment data. *Medical Education, 37*, 830–7.

Downing, S.M. (2004). Reliability: on the reproducibility of assessment data. *Medical Education, 38 (9)*, 1006–12.

Downing, S.M., Park, Y.S., & Yudkowsky, R. (2019). *Assessment in health professions education. (2nd ed.)* New York: Routledge.

Fendler, A. (2016). Ethical implications of validity-vs.-reliability trade-offs in educational research, *Ethics & Education, 11:2*, 214–29.

Hargreaves, A. (1989) *Curriculum & Assessment Reform*. Milton Keynes, UK: Open University Press.

Linn, R.L., & Miller, M.D. (2005). *Measurement & assessment in teaching*. New Jersey: Prentice Hall.

McDowell, L. & Mowl, G. (1995). Innovative assessment: Its impact on students. In G. Gibbs (Ed.) *Improving student Learning. Through assessment & evaluation*. Oxford: The Oxford Centre for Staff Development.

Messick, S. (1989). Validity. In R.L. Linn (Ed.). *Educational measurement*. New York: American Council on Education. pp. 13–104.

Norcini, J., Anderson, M.B., Bollela, V., Burch, V., Costa, M.J., Duvivier, R., et al. (2011). Criteria for good assessment: consensus statement & recommendations from the Ottawa 2010 Conference. *Medical Teacher, 33*, 206–11.

Norcini, J., Anderson, M.B., Bollela, V., Burch, V., Costa, M.J., Duvivier, R., et al. (2018) 2018 consensus framework for good assessment. *Medical Teacher 40*, 1102–9.

Ramsden, P. (1997). The context of learning in academic departments. In F. Marton, D. Hounsell, N. Entwistle (Eds.) *The Experience of Learning: Implications for Teaching & Studying in Higher Education*, (2nd ed.) Edinburgh: Scottish Academic Press.

Rushton, A. (2005). Formative assessment: a key to deep learning? *Medical Teacher, 27,* 509–13.

Schuwirth, L.W.T., & van der Vleuten, C.P.M. (2019). How to design a useful test: The principles of assessment. In: Swanwick, T., Forrest, K., O'Brien, B.C. (Ed.) *Understanding medical education: evidence, theory & practice.* West Sussex: Wiley-Blackwell.

Siddiqui, Z.S. (2017). An effective assessment: From Rocky Roads to Silk Route. *Pakistan Journal of Medical Sciences Online 32(2),* 505–9.

Streiner, D., Norman, G. (1995). *Health measurement scales. A practical guide to their development & use.* (2nd ed.) New York: Oxford University Press.

van der Vleuten, C.P.M., & Schuwirth, L.W.T. (2005). Assessing professional competence: From methods to programmes. *Medical Education, 39,* 309–17.

Waugh, C.K., & Gronlund, N.E. (2012). *Assessment of student achievement.* 10th ed. New Jersey: Pearson.

FURTHER READING

Black, P., & Wiliam, D. (1998). Assessment & classroom learning. *Assessment in Education, 5,* 7–74.

Dent, J.A., Harden, R.M. & Hunt, D. (2017). *A practical guide for medical teachers.* (5th ed.), Edinburgh, Elsevier.

Epstein, R.M., & Hundert, E.M. (2002). Defining & assessing professional competence. *Journal of American Medical Association, 287,* 226–35.

Fredriksen, N. (1984). Influences of testing on teaching & learning. *American Psychologist, 39,*193–202.

Gibbs, G., & Simpson, C. (2004) Conditions under which assessment supports student learning. *Learning & Teaching in Higher Education.* 1, 3–31.

Hawkins, R.E., & Holmboe, E.S. (2008). *Practical guide to the evaluation of clinical competence.* Philadelphia: Mosby-Elsevier.

Jackson, N., Jamieson, A., & Khan, A. (2007). *Assessment in medical education & training: A practical guide.* New York: CRC Press.

Miller, G.E. (1976). Continuous assessment. *Medical Education, 10,* 611–21.

Norcini, J. (2003). Setting standard in educational tests. *Medical Education, 37,*464-69.

Singh, T., Gupta, P., & Singh, D. (2021). *Principles of Medical Education.* (5th ed.) New Delhi: Jaypee Brothers Medical Publishers.

Singh, T., Anshu & Modi, J.N. (2012). The Quarter Model: A proposed approach to in-training assessment for undergraduate students in Indian Medical Schools. *Indian Pediatrics, 49,* 871–6.

Swanwick, T., Forrest, K., & O'Brien, B.C. (Ed.) (2019). *Understanding medical education: evidence, theory & practice.* (3rd ed.) West Sussex: Wiley-Blackwell.

Wass, V., Bowden, R., & Jackson, N. (2007). Principles of assessment design. In Jackson, N., Jamieson, A., Khan, A. (Eds.). *Assessment in medical education & training: A practical guide.* (1st ed.) Oxford: Radcliffe Publishing.

Chapter 2

Assessment of Clinical Competence: A Curtain Raiser

Tejinder Singh, Jyoti N Modi, Rita Sood

KEY POINTS

- Clinical competence is a multidimensional construct, requiring multiple tools for its assessment.
- Assessment tools should be chosen according to described frameworks.
- Assessment should improve learning and have a positive educational impact.
- Feedback improves the outcome of assessment and learning.
- Moving up the Miller pyramid brings professional authenticity to assessment.

Clinical competence is a complex and multidimensional construct that evades easy explanation. It encompasses all that goes into the making of a good doctor. A simple approach to understanding it would be by enlisting all the qualities one would want to see in one's own physician consistently. Further, these qualities are not watertight compartments, but they depend on, and influence each other in a complex manner, e.g., a doctor with suboptimal communication skills may not be able to gather clinical information adequately from patients despite a sound theoretical knowledge about what to ask. This is only one aspect of the complexity of clinical competence. The context, place and settings also have some bearing on the components of clinical competence.

It is of prime importance that the concept of clinical competence is well understood by teachers (and students, as key stakeholders) before embarking upon the task of planning and implementing assessment practices. Assessment must be then aligned to this concept. It would be appropriate to say that 'clinical competence' is 'professional competence' as applied to medical profession. Therefore, use of the word 'clinical' must not mislead into thinking that it only pertains to the clinical skills. Earlier descriptions of the term have emphasized mainly on the diagnostic and therapeutic abilities (Burg, Lloyd, & Templeton, 1982). There have been many views and debates on defining the term clinical competence (Neufield & Norman, 1985). Clinical skills

TABLE 2.1: Description of an ideal doctor, and outcome product of graduate medical education by various agencies globally

WHO: Five Star Doctor (1996)	ACGME Outcomes Project, USA (Batalden et al., 2002)	CanMEDS Project, Canada (1996)	Tomorrow's Doctors, GMC, UK (1993, 2009)	Indian Medical Graduate (IMG), MCI (2019)
❖ Care provider ❖ Decision-maker ❖ Communicator ❖ Community leader ❖ Manager	❖ Medical knowledge ❖ Patient Care ❖ Practice-based learning and improvement ❖ Interpersonal and Communication skills ❖ Professionalism ❖ System-based practice	❖ Medical Expert/ clinical decision maker ❖ Communicator ❖ Collaborator ❖ Manager ❖ Health advocate ❖ Scholar ❖ Professional	❖ The doctor as scholar and scientist ❖ The doctor as a practitioner (includes communication as a subhead) ❖ The doctor as a professional	❖ Clinician ❖ Leader and member of healthcare team ❖ Communicator ❖ Lifelong learner ❖ Professional

are an essential core component of clinical competence, and there are several other components that make the picture complete.

A consensus on the term has gradually evolved, as is obvious by the commonalities in the description of an ideal doctor in various countries as shown in **Table 2.1**. Thus, clinical competence is no longer seen as being limited to diagnostic and therapeutic ability. Various agencies have described the qualities of an ideal doctor, and defined them as desired outcomes either as roles or core competencies. The Accreditation Council for Graduate Medical Education (ACGME) in the United States defines them as core competencies (Swing, 2007), while Canada's CanMEDS project identifies the roles of a doctor (The Royal College of Physicians and Surgeons of Canada CanMEDS 2000 Project Societal Needs Working Group, 1996). These qualities were described as outcomes by the General Medical Council (2009, first published in 1993) in the United Kingdom.

Similarly, the Medical Council of India (2019) has proposed five different roles of the Indian Medical Graduate (IMG), namely, clinician, leader, professional, life-long learner, and communicator.

Since these frameworks define the outcome product of graduate medical education, they imply a mandate for assessment of these attributes before a doctor can practice in the society. Some of these attributes can be easy to define and measure, while others are not amenable to easy description or measurement.

Assessment of clinical competence must therefore be multi-dimensional, unlike traditional assessment that focused on easily measurable attributes alone (Sood & Singh, 2012). Like clinical competence, it would be appropriate to view assessment as a complex construct. There are three perspectives on how assessment can drive learning, and these influence whether the assessment predominantly

has a pre-learning effect, a post-learning effect, or a pure learning effect. These perspectives are:
- Assessment *of* learning (Segers et al., 2003)
- Assessment *for* learning (Black & William, 2009)
- Assessment *as* learning (Clark, 2010)

These contribute to the multidimensional nature of assessment. Vleuten et al., (2017) further elucidate the various principles and frameworks that help translate these perspectives into actual assessment practices.

Assessment *of* Learning

This is the classical and most utilized perspective on assessment. Its focus is on measuring what has been learnt, or as a measure of learning. It emphasizes the decision-making function of assessment and is hence called *summative assessment*. However, it is not a passive exercise in assessing learning. It has the potential to modulate and guide learning. It is well accepted that what is not assessed is not learnt. So, by designing the assessment appropriately, the students can be guided towards learning the desired. This is an example of *pre-learning* effect where the nature of assessment alters the prior learning behavior of the student.

The key considerations: here are the assessment methods, the framework for choosing the appropriate method, key principles that guide the use of methods, psychometric properties of various methods, blueprinting (content and context representation, and areas which deserve emphasis), the testing time, pre- and post-learning effects.

Framework for Choosing Assessment Methods

In the past, much emphasis was placed on testing the skills in a domain-specific manner, and the choice of assessment method was guided by it. Nothing could be less authentic and farther from truth than isolated testing of cognitive, affective, and psychomotor skills in a compartmentalized manner. With the adoption of competency-based education globally, it is the whole tasks performed in real settings, that must be assessed. Every professional activity involves a judicious and integrative use of more than one domain (Holmboe et al, 2016).

The conceptual framework of competence proposed by Miller (1990) is almost a universally used framework now. He conceptualized competence as having various hierarchical levels, within which assessment could be planned. The four layers are distinguished as *knows, knows how, shows how,* and *does* (**Fig. 2.1**). Each layer contributes to the development of clinical competence. The model is represented in the shape of a pyramid and has some important implications for assessment. The lower three levels represent discrete or isolated competence of knowledge or skills whereas the topmost layer represents the collective competence.

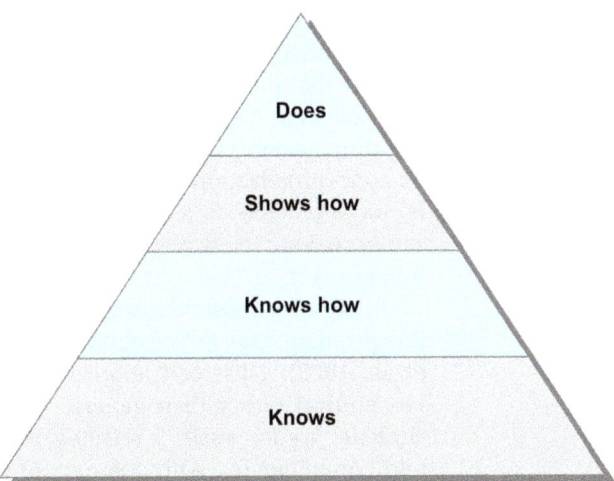

Fig. 2.1: Miller pyramid of clinical competence (Miller, 1990).

The base of the pyramid is formed by knowledge, while the top denotes action in the actual field. The transition from knowing to doing includes ability to use the knowledge in complex situations and ability to demonstrate skills required to effectively function (Wass et al, 2001). Knowledge has a very high degree of correlation with performance (Glaser, 1984). However, the hierarchical nature of the layers is suspect because a task can be learned and performed even with tacit knowledge. Based on these, it has also been suggested to distinguish between competence (ability to perform something) and performance (actually performing) (Senior, 1976). This is like the ability of a car to run at 180 km/hour under test conditions (*competence*), whereas in real conditions, it may only run at 80 km/hour only (*performance*), indicating that performance is affected by many factors other than competence.

Some key implications of using this model as a framework are:

- Performance measurement is essential to assess clinical competence.
- Move beyond assessing only 'knows' and 'knows how' and build authenticity even at these levels by using real life situations/case vignettes to test higher cognitive levels such as problem solving. However, a word of caution here is that the knowledge forms the base of the pyramid and lower levels must not be presumed to have been achieved just because the trainee is able to demonstrate competence at higher levels. The appropriate contextual testing of knowledge is still required.
- A combination of assessment methods and tests may have to be used for a satisfactory assessment. This calls for using more than the traditional essay or MCQ tests and practical examination that have been used for several decades.

It is not uncommon for some people to suggest that a single sample would suffice to assess clinical competence, drawing an analogy from the fact that only a few grains of rice are adequate to assess if it has been cooked. It would have been true if clinical competence was a uni-dimensional concept consisting of only knowledge/skills but with its conceptualization as a multi-dimensional construct, this analogy is not applicable to assessment of clinical competence (to use the same analogy, clinical competence is like *biryani*, rather than like boiled rice!).

It has been observed that a doctor, who is 'good' in diagnosing one problem, may not be equally good in diagnosing another (Elstein et al., 1978). This realization of 'content' and 'context' specificity, i.e., clinical rather than generic, brought a sea change in the way students are assessed. It resulted in emphasis on multiple contexts and competencies, with a variety of tools for such assessment. The concept of *assessment toolbox* (ACGME and American Board of Medical Specialties, 2000) has originated from this perspective and allows the assessors to select the right tool for the right task.

Assessing 'Knows' and 'Knows How'

This is the base of Miller pyramid. Conventionally, essay questions, short answer questions, MCQs and viva-voce have been used for assessing at this level. Unfortunately, often the questions test only factual recall. It is possible to design these questions to assess the students at the higher levels of learning such as application, synthesis, and problem solving. Newer varieties of MCQs, such as extended matching and script concordance tests are extensively used for such purpose. Scenario based MCQs are another option, and they help to build authenticity.

Most of the time, the emphasis when setting the questions, is on their 'format' (e.g. short answers and MCQs). However, research has shown that it is the stimulus format which is more effective. In other words, what is asked is more important than how it is asked (Vleuten et al., 2017).

Assessing 'Shows'

'Shows' assesses the competence of the students. It is the ability to perform under controlled conditions. Long cases, short cases, and OSCEs are the common tools used for this purpose. Long case, though with real patients, is limited in utility by its content specificity issues. The OSCE has a major advantage of sampling of a wider content area and clinical contexts. But it also fragments the clinical competence into small areas, stacking of which may or may not result in overall competence, i.e., the sum of parts may not add up to the whole. Moreover, as given in the car example above, competence may not always transform into performance.

Assessing 'Does'

This is the performance level and at this level the assessment happens at the actual workplace. Direct observation is the key here. Workplace Based Assessment (WPBA) tools such as mini-Clinical Evaluation Exercise (mini-CEX), Direct Observation of Procedural Skills (DOPS), Multisource Feedback (MSF), etc. are used for this purpose. Portfolios are used to document the progress of the student. This type of assessment is more useful for postgraduate students, who are directly in-charge of patient care. Some of these are also being adapted for assessing undergraduate students, especially DOPS. The role of expert subjective judgment in performance assessment in real settings cannot be overemphasized (ten Cate & Regher, 2019). The effort at highly objectivizing such assessments may be detrimental.

Assessing the Affective Domain

Much-needed importance is now being accorded to assessment of non-cognitive abilities, such as professionalism, communication, teamwork, and ethics. There is a growing realization that these attributes are responsible for success (or failure!) in the market, more than knowledge and skills. Many of these are not assessable by using the traditional objective and standardized methods but may need subjective judgments. The same is true for higher-order clinical decision making, which does not lend itself to checklist-based assessment. Further, these attributes cannot be assessed during a certification or in the final examination, and hence must be assessed during training.

Principles and Psychometric Considerations

Certain key principles apply to assessment irrespective of the method used. Competence assessment requires sampling of many elements to derive reliable inferences since competence is context-specific (Vleuten et al., 2017). This calls for use of multiple methods in multiple contexts. The assessment must be valid (precise; measures what is supposed to measure), reliable (consistent), acceptable, feasible, and with a positive educational impact. These attributes of assessment were discussed in depth in Chapter 1. A conceptual model of assessment that regards utility of assessment as a notional product of multiplication of these five attributes (Vleuten, 1996; Vleuten & Schuwirth, 2005) has also been proposed. This implies that an assessment method that scores low on certain attributes e.g., reliability, may still be useful by virtue of having a high educational impact. The choice of method depends on the purpose for which it is being used, and which of the attributes is more relevant for that purpose. Further, the psychometric properties of one method may complement those of another method, and a judicious combination of methods is recommended. Use of a single method of assessment for a high-stake decision is strongly discouraged. In fact, it is suggested that instead of evaluating individual assessment methods, it is more meaningful to evaluate the psychometric properties of the combination of methods or the entire assessment program (Vleuten & Schuwirth, 2005).

Validity, rather than being an inherent quality of the assessment method or instrument, is user-dependent and can be enhanced by the way the instrument is used and interpreted. An authentic testing environment at the 'performance' level of Miller pyramid contributes in a significant manner to validity of assessment. At lower levels, authenticity can be enhanced by using case scenario based written tests, or tasks.

An important consideration in competence assessment especially at performance level is the use of expert subjective judgment that has been erroneously equated with bias. Increasing the number of examiners can minimize this alleged bias (Virk et al., 2020). Subjective expert opinion is a necessity in performance assessment since it takes place in real settings, and a global rather than reductionist approach is important. The utility of subjective assessments has been discussed in Chapter 26.

Another consideration is the testing time, which contributes to validity and reliability of the assessment. The desirable testing time is about 3–4 hours (or longer depending on the method and feasibility) for enhancing the reliability of the observations made (Vleuten & Schuwirth, 2005).

Blueprinting and Standard Setting

Blueprinting and standard setting remain two extremely useful tools, which are often not put to optimum use. Blueprinting involves creation of a grid, also called a 'table of specifications' that specifies the weightage given to various content areas and the competency being tested. It works as a guide to the teachers while choosing the assessment tool, ensuring wide sampling of content areas. It also conveys the relative importance accorded to various content areas to the students. This is discussed in detail in Chapter 6. A blueprint of the entire assessment program may also be created for the longitudinal temporal arrangement of assessments, the combination of methods used at various stages of training, the relative distribution of marks, and the modality of final decision making.

Standard setting is guided by the purpose for which the assessment is being carried out. It could be norm-referenced or criterion-referenced. Norm-referenced refers to scoring of students relative to other students. However, a cut off still needs to be defined. Criterion-referenced refers to attainment of specific level of performance (prior agreed upon and defined) by a student irrespective of the level of performance by other students. In competency-based education, the latter, i.e., criterion-referenced assessment is essential, since competency can be said to be attained only when an acceptable level of performance for that stage of training is demonstrated by the student.

Assessment *for* Learning

This perspective on assessment emphasizes how assessment can be utilized for improving and modulating learning. It can also be viewed as the *post-learning* effect of assessment. This is possible by way of providing feedback to the learner after the assessment. The powerful effect of feedback on learning has been well established and accepted.

The best use of assessment for learning is during training, or during the learning process, and so sometimes it is the *formative assessment*. However, it is more appropriate to refer to it as the formative function of assessment. After an assessment, the teachers provide feedback to the learners with suggestions to improve further (*feed forward*). It is crucial that such practice is made routine, a conducive environment for continued and frequent student-teacher dialogue is created, a culture of feedback is nurtured, and teachers as well as students are sensitized to giving and receiving feedback.

It would be erroneous to think that only providing the feedback is enough for learning (Hattie & Timperley, 2007). For the feedback to translate into learner improvement, it is essential that the learner reflects on the feedback and feels motivated to follow a plan of self-improvement. A mentor can effectively catalyze this process of translation into action for improvement. Faculty development in giving effective feedback, and mentoring go a long way in tapping this potential of assessment. Students sensitized to the culture of frequent assessment with feedback will be able to best utilize this effect. Self-assessment, and peer-assessment with reflective practice are other ways students can work towards improvement. However, self-assessment must be combined with other methods since self-assessment is not usually accurate.

With competency assessment, this perspective on assessment, i.e., use of *assessment for learning* is at the core. This is because competency attainment is developmental. In other words, competency is gradually acquired by progressing through various levels of competence, such as the novice, competent, proficient, expert and master (Dreyfus & Dreyfus, 1986). It is crucial therefore that the student learning is closely monitored and guided to keep the students on the right course of learning progression and competency attainment (Holmboe et al., 2016)

A more detailed discussion on *Assessment for Learning* can be found in Chapter 16.

Assessment as Learning

In this perspective, the boundaries between assessment and learning are blurred. Assessment and learning happen simultaneously, and the assessment methods potentially can be utilized as learning modalities. High quality feedback, continuous ongoing assessment (often observation-based), feedback as a culture and students as feedback-seekers form the cornerstone of this perspective (Vleuten et al., 2017). The distinction between summative and formative is also dissolved in this perspective as all assessment is used for learner improvement.

The concept of *Programmatic assessment* proposed by Vleuten et al., presents a unified view of the three perspectives on assessment. It describes assessment as a program that is a judicious combination of various assessment methods (choice driven by purpose and stage of training) in the temporal frame of training program. Each individual method functions only as a low-stakes data point but does not contribute directly to the high-stakes or pass/fail decision. This allows for a relatively stress-free environment for learning on a scaffold of assessment (*of, for* and *as* learning).

There is a general agreement that the role of assessment as an aide to better learning is often neglected. It has been suggested that the major chunk of assessment of clinical competence should be formed by formative assessment and only a fraction should be left to the summative part. This is especially true of competency-based curricula. Formative assessment should be utilized for *reflections* and *feedback* as well as for *feed up* and *feed forward*. The aspect of using assessment to promote learning has been discussed in detail in Chapter 16. With this perspective, summative assessment should move over to become a tool of quality assurance.

At the beginning of this chapter, the complexity and multidimensional nature of clinical competence was discussed. Following the discussion on assessment, it is obvious that assessment too is a multidimensional and complex concept. A schematic representation of this is shown in **Figure 2.2**. Clinical competence is shown as a multidimensional pyramid with levels described by Miller (1990). The faces and a 3-dimensional design represent the various competencies. This pyramid of competence acquisition is set in an environment (the sphere) of assessment and learning. The choice and combination of assessment methods is based on the foundational principles. The overall assessment (or high-stakes decision) is made by taking a holistic view of the entire assessment and learning events. Additionally, a learning orientation is given to each assessment. The assessment itself should be subject to evaluation to maintain quality (Siddiqui, 2017).

It is further clear from this system that any change in the need, purpose or any element of the system must involve careful thought and complementary changes. Our experiences with student learning when MCQ-based selection tests were introduced are a testimony

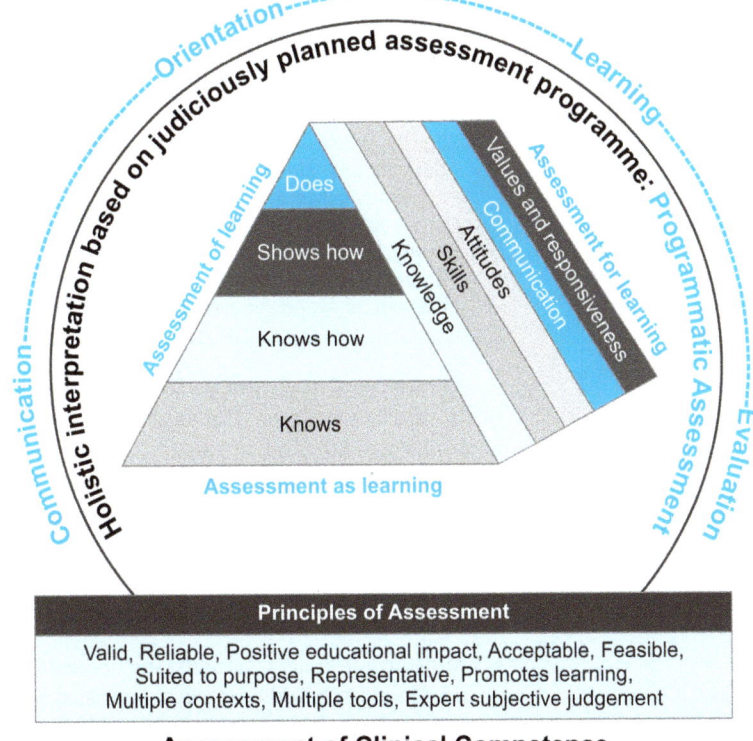

Assessment of Clinical Competence

Fig. 2.2: Clinical competence represented as multidimensional pyramid assessed by multidimensional assessment programme based on key principles of assessment.

(Compiled from Miller, 1990; Mahey & Burns, 2009; Siddiqui, 2017; Vleuten et al., 2017; Medical Council of India, 2018)

to this (Mahajan & Singh, 2017). The reasons are not difficult to guess-not following the systems approach of bringing changes in teaching-learning and increasing the stakes in assessment to highly distorted levels.

Assessment can be likened to a good meal. It should be prepared with careful thought to the ingredients, method of cooking and combination of dishes, etc. It should also be consumed in a balanced manner for best benefit. Eating only a single dish or ingredient, meal after meal is not desirable for health reasons. Specific situations may require a change in the meal plan or constitution. Similarly, assessment must be a carefully thought-out plan or program that utilizes several methods in judicious combination, and modify the assessment plan based on purpose, and/or students' needs.

Assessment derives from an idea important to educators – that of sitting down beside or together with the learner (Latin *as + sidere*). Some key considerations in assessment that will help the learner make the most of the assessment process are summarized in **Box 2.1**.

> **BOX 2.1:** Key considerations in using assessment for learning
> - Clear learning outcomes that are shared with students
> - Use variety of assessment procedures, guided judiciously by purpose and needs
> - Aligned to instruction; sometimes assessment as instructional method
> - Adequate and wide sample of student performance
> - Procedures fair to everyone
> - Criteria for judging success clear to all stake holders
> - Feedback to students
> - Comprehensive grading and reporting system: with due emphasis on observation, expert judgment, narrative comments

Assessment itself needs to be assessed in the form of program evaluation to ensure that it is serving its intended purpose. We have already alluded to the COLE framework in Chapter 1. In the chapters that follow, you will find an elaboration of these principles to help you select most useful strategy for assessment of clinical competence.

REFERENCES

ACGME Outcome Project. Accreditation Council for Graduate Medical Education & American Board of Medical Specialist. (2000). *Toolbox for assessment methods, version 1.1.* [online] Available from www.acgme.org/outcomes/assess/toolbox.pdf. [Last accessed July, 2020].

Batalden, P., & Lech, D., Swing, S., Dreyfus,H. & Dreyfus, S. (2002). General competencies & accreditation in graduate medical education. An antidote to over specification in the education of medical specialists. *Health Affairs, 21,* 103–11.

Black, P., William, D. (2009). Developing the theory of formative assessment. *Educational assessment, evaluation & accountability, 21(1),* 5–31.

Burg, F.D., Lloyd, J.S., & Templeton, B. (1982). Competence in Medicine. *Medical Teacher, 4(2),* 60–4.

Clark, I. (2010). Formative assessment: 'There is nothing so practical as a good theory'. *Australian Journal of Education, 54(3),* 341–52.

Dreyfus, H.L., & Dreyfus, S.E. (1986). *Mind over Machine: The Power of Human Intuition & Expertise in the Age of the Computer.* Oxford: Basil Blackwell.

Elstein, A.S., Shulman, L.S., & Sprafka, S.A., (1978). *Medical problem solving: an analysis of clinical reasoning.* London, Cambridge, Mass: Harvard University Press.

General Medical Council. (2009). *Tomorrow's doctors. Outcomes & standards for undergraduate medical education.* General Medical Council, Manchester, UK.

Glaser, R. (1984). Education & thinking: the role of knowledge. *American Psychologist, 39,* 93–104.

Hattie, J., & Timperley, H. (2007). The power of feedback. *Review of Educational Research, 77,* 81–112.

Holmboe, E.S., Edgar, L. & Hanstra, S. (2016). *A practical guide to evaluation of clinical competence.* Elsevier.

Mahajan, R., & Singh, T. (2017) The national licentiate examination: pros & cons. *National Medical Journal of India, 30,* 275–8.

Medical Council of India. (2019). *Competency based Undergraduate curriculum for the Indian Medical Graduate*. pp. 14–20.

Mehay, R., & Burns, R. (Eds.) (2009). *The Essential handbook for GP training and education*. London. Radcliffe Publishing Limited

Miller, G.E. (1990). The assessment of clinical skills/competence/performance. *Academic Medicine*, 65(9 Suppl), S63–7.

Neufeld, V.R., & Norman, G. R. (1985). *Assessing Clinical Competence*. New York: Springer-Verlag.

Segers, M., Dochy, F., & Cascallar, E. (Eds.). (2003). *Optimizing new modes of assessment: In search for qualities & standards*. Dordrecht: Springer.

Senior, J.R. (1976). *Toward the measurement of competence in medicine*. Philadelphia: National Board of Medical Examiners.

Siddiqui, Z.S. (2017). An effective assessment: From Rocky Roads to Silk Route. *Pakistan Journal of Medical Sciences, 32(2)*, 505–9.

Sood, R., & Singh, T. (2012). Assessment of clinical competence: evolving perspectives & current trends. *National Medical Journal of India, 25*, 357–64.

Swing, S.R. (2007). The ACGME outcome project: retrospective & prospective. *Med Teach, 29*, 648–54.

ten Cate, O., & Regher, G. (2019). The power of subjectivity in the assessment of medical trainees. *Academic Medicine*, 94, 333–7.

The Royal College of Physicians & Surgeons of Canada CanMEDS 2000 Project Societal Needs Working Group. (1996). *Skills for the new millennium: report of the societal needs working group*. Ottawa: Royal College of Physicians & Surgeons of Canada.

van der Vleuten C.P.M. (1996). The assessment of professional competence: developments, research & practical implications. *Advances in Health Sciences Education*, 1, 41–67.

van der Vleuten, C.P.M., & Schuwirth, L.W.T. (2005). Assessment of professional competence: from methods to programs. *Medical Education, 39*, 309-317.

van der Vleuten, C.P.M., Sluijsmans, D. & Joosten-ten-Brinke, D. (2017). Competence assessment as learner support. *Competence-based Vocational & Professional Education. Technical & vocational education & training: Issues, concerns & prospects* 23, DOI 10.1007/978-3-319-41713-4_28.

Virk, A., Joshi, A., Mahajan, R., & Singh, T. (2020). The power of subjectivity in competency-based assessment. *J Postgrad Med, 66*, 200-205.

Wass, V., van der Vleuten, C., Shartzer, J., & Jones, R. (2001). Assessment of clinical competence. *The Lancet, 357*, 945-9.

World Health Organization. (1996). *Doctors for health: a WHO global strategy for changing medical education & medical practice for health for all*. World Health Organization. Geneva.

Chapter 3

Assessment of Knowledge: Free Response Type Questions

Anshu

KEY POINTS

- Knowledge forms the base of clinical competence and should be given due emphasis.
- What is asked is more important than how it is asked.
- Essay questions and their variants help in assessing knowledge beyond recall of facts.

Miller pyramid for assessing clinical competence (Miller, 1990) has already been discussed in Chapter 2. The base of the pyramid is formed by knowledge (*knows*) and understanding (*knows how*). As we move toward the top of the pyramid, we find that testing performance in controlled settings (shows how) and in realistic situations (does) take priority. In the last decade we have seen the traditional methods of assessment in medical education being replaced by more sophisticated strategies. There is a trend to move from assessment of knowledge toward assessment of clinical competence. Are knowledge and competence two watertight compartments, separate from each other? Are these terms mutually exclusive? Or are they interlinked? Can a student perform competently without knowledge of a subject?

There are some issues about assessment of competence that need to be clarified here. Miller's model is pyramidal in shape—which implies that a student needs to 'know', before he 'knows how'; and that he needs to 'know how', before he can 'show how' or actually perform in a real-life situation. However, what is more important here is that this relationship is non-linear. In other words, while it is difficult to climb up the pyramid without completing the lower step; attainment of a step does not mean that the lower step has been automatically completed. The implications for us are therefore clear. One, we cannot test clinical competence without assessing knowledge. And two, merely knowing will not guarantee application. It also follows that assessment of clinical competence needs to happen at each level. It is important to realize that knowledge forms the base or the foundation of the pyramid (*see* **Fig. 2.1**). If the foundation is weak, the upper levels cannot be strong. Testing knowledge is thus an important component of our teaching which cannot be ignored, for it is the very foundation on which clinical competence is based.

There is ample research evidence to suggest that assessment of knowledge is integral to assessing clinical competence. Knowledge has been shown to be the best predictor of clinical competence. In addition, it shows best correlation with acquisition of practical skills.

It may also be useful to clarify that knowledge can occur in various forms. Eraut (1985) has distinguished between Type A and Type B knowledge. Type A or *declarative* knowledge is the knowledge, which is from published sources, which can be verified and includes information on how to carry out skills (although it does not include actually performing those skills). Type B knowledge, which includes knowledge of processes and skills, comes out of personal experience and includes *procedural* and process knowledge. We see no conflict of this terminology with Miller pyramid. Type A knowledge can be equated with the 'knows' level of Miller, while type B knowledge can be equated with the 'knows how' and 'shows' levels. This further strengthens our original position that assessment of knowledge at any level is crucial to form valid interpretation about clinical competence.

This concept is also well illustrated by Newble's model for clinical competence (Newble, 1992). Clinical competence requires mastery of relevant knowledge, proficiency in skills (including interpersonal, technical, clinical and communication skills), development of the right attitudes, all of which are inter-related. All of these play a role in clinical performance and affect the quality of patient care. The components of clinical competence are illustrated in **Figure 3.1**.

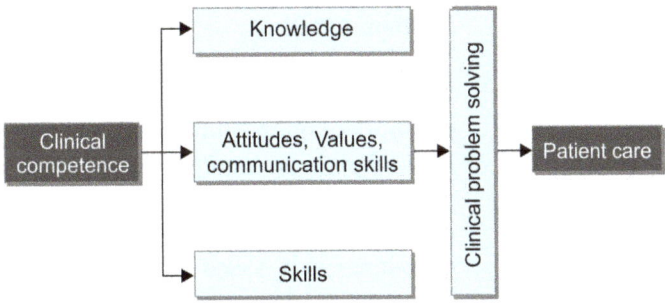

Fig. 3.1: Components of clinical competence.

Written Assessment Methods

We spend considerable time and effort in assessing knowledge using written assessment methods. Written assessment methods are popular because they are easy to conduct and cost-effective when many students must be tested.

The various written assessment tools are:
- Essay questions, structured essay questions, modified essay questions
- Short answer questions
- Multiple choice questions and their variants

Depending on the expected response format, written assessment methods can have either closed-ended or open-ended formats. The closed-ended questions provide a list of answers as options and are usually of the selection type. Closed-ended questions, i.e., multiple-choice questions will be discussed in Chapter 5. Open-ended questions require examinees to provide answers in their own words, and in this chapter, we will focus on the open-ended formats of written assessment.

Focus on the format of the answer often ignores the format of the stimulus, namely, what is it that the question expects the student to answer and this pertains to the content of the question. Depending on the stimulus format, questions can be context-rich or can be context-free (Schuwirth & Vleuten, 2004). In a context-free question, factual knowledge is usually tested, and the considerations are simple (yes/no type). When the question is directly related to a case and decisions are asked for, the thought processes invoked are entirely different from those evoked by context-free questions. In context-rich questions mainly propositional reasoning occurs, in that candidates weigh different units of information against each other when making a decision (Schuwirth et al., 2000). It is a myth that the format of the question determines the knowledge that is being tested. Research has shown that it is the content of the question, rather than the format which determines almost totally what the question tests (Schuwirth & Vleuten, 2004).

Each question type has its own advantages and disadvantages. Depending on the purpose of the assessment, one must select the most appropriate question type. The choice of question type will vary for high-stakes examinations and for formative assessment. Testing time is often a limiting factor which determines the type and number of questions that can be used. When using open-ended questions, fewer questions can be asked which means lesser content area which can be covered.

Assessment must always be conducted with the educational impact in sight as the students always prepare with examinations in mind. Examiners and question writers therefore must select topics of practical importance. Sadly, it is common practice to ambush the student by asking questions on rare and unusual topics. The intention is either to trip the unwary or to have a higher discrimination between the average and good students. This practice leads to deliberate omission of essential components of the curriculum.

Written assessment methods can be used to assess a student's comprehension and ability to analyze, synthesize, and organize information. Unfortunately, we often end up testing recall abilities and factual knowledge. Bloom taxonomy of educational objectives lists out different levels of knowledge which can be tested hierarchically.

Let us understand this with some examples in the **Table 3.1**:

As is seen from this example, instead of merely testing recall, it is possible to test higher levels of knowledge in most topics. We would like you to take a moment here to try and construct questions from higher levels of Bloom taxonomy for a topic that you have taught recently.

We hope that you will have noticed that using a bit of creativity and imagination can help in testing higher order of knowledge instead of

TABLE 3.1: Hierarchical assessment of knowledge

Bloom's levels of cognitive domain	Measures	Common verbs	Examples
Knowledge	Recall of information	Define, classify, describe, name, list	Define infective endocarditis.
Comprehension	Understanding and grasp of information	Explain, interpret, describe, summarize, differentiate, demonstrate	Explain the pathogenesis of infective endocarditis
Application	Use of learnt abstract information to solve a problem	Solve, illustrate, calculate, interpret, apply, demonstrate, put into practice, predict, show	Mr Sethi, a known case of rheumatic heart disease, presents with fever. How will you rule out infective endocarditis?
Analysis	Identification and appreciation of subject matters, most elemental ideas and relationships	Compare, contrast, analyze, discriminate, categorize, organize	Distinguish between acute and sub-acute infective endocarditis
Synthesis	Creating something new and advanced based on sound criteria	Design, hypothesize, support, plan, compose, create, develop	What advice will you give to prevent infective endocarditis in a patient of rheumatic heart disease with a prosthesis?
Evaluation	Judging the value of something for a particular purpose	Evaluate, estimate, judge, defend, appreciate, justify	Justify the use of antibiotics given to this patient with rheumatic heart disease (reports of blood culture and treatment attached)

framing questions which test rote knowledge. We will now briefly discuss the different types of questions routinely used in assessment of knowledge and learn how we can construct better questions.

Essay Questions

Essay questions are one of the most used formats for assessing knowledge. Here students are expected to write longer answers to broad topics and there is freedom to explore various facets of this topic. The essay question format has the potential to assess the breadth of a student's knowledge, depth of understanding, ability to organize thoughts, and critically analyze information.

Here is an example of the traditional way in which essay questions were posed:

> *Describe India's National Population Policy 2000.*

You will notice that this merely tests reproducibility of factual knowledge. While this kind of question is easy for examiners to construct, it hardly uses the opportunity to assess a student's reasoning capacity or any of the other potential strengths of essay questions listed above. A good essay question asks the student to process information rather than to reproduce it. If the same question is reframed, it gives an opportunity to test the student's higher order thinking.

> *Critically analyze India's National Population Policy 2000.*

The common criticism against essay questions is that the scores obtained are inconsistent and variable. Scoring is difficult to standardize when many examiners are involved in the assessment process and there is a great deal of inter-rater variability. It is hard to remove examiner bias due to the literary ability and handwriting of the student. While essay questions are easy to construct, scoring is rather tedious and time-consuming. Further, a very small sample of the whole content is tested, and this compromises *content validity*. Vaguely worded questions can confuse the student and making scoring difficult. Instead of using restricted response words ('what', 'when', 'list') or vague words ('describe' or 'discuss') in framing the questions it would be better to use words which explore the higher cognitive domains ('compare', 'distinguish between', 'critically analyze', etc.).

In testing knowledge using essay questions, it is important to maintain a balance between the higher cognitive skills being assessed and the consistency of scoring that can be achieved. Here the purpose of assessment must be kept in mind. When the purpose is primarily to assess higher cognition, the question format must allow the student to explore the topic fully and the expected response is unrestricted.

> *In view of the increasing cases of COVID-19 in this area, propose changes in the health education strategies being used by the national health agencies.*

However, in the quest to assess higher cognition, we have to pay a price in terms of reliability. The number of different essays that can be asked in an examination is limited. It is often difficult to construct an ideal model answer and achieve consistency of scoring.

On the other hand, if the examination format specifically requires reliability of scoring, a compromise is usually made with testing higher cognition. While all the problems associated with essay questions described above cannot be eliminated, they can be reduced by using the *structured essay questions*. Here, a question can have several short questions which restrict the responses to a limited range. A well-constructed model answer or key which gives details of expected answers, all possible alternative answers, and the scoring system is needed.

Look at this example:

> *Describe the etiopathogenesis, diagnostic criteria, sequelae, and complications of rheumatic fever.*

This question clearly tells the student exactly what is expected of him, and when a key or model answer is provided to the examiners, scoring is much more consistent. However, this type of question tests more of factual knowledge rather than problem-solving ability. Over-structuring can lead to trivialization of the process (Norman et al., 1991). Another way of improving reliability of scoring is by allowing one examiner to correct answers of all students of one essay each rather than assess the complete paper.

Modified Essay Questions

Of the three areas of cognitive ability (recall and recognition, interpretation of data, and problem solving), testing of problem-solving abilities is not only the most difficult, but also the most neglected aspect. Modified essay questions can help assess recall, comprehension, analysis, synthesis, and evaluation of knowledge.

In a modified essay question, a problem or case scenario is presented to the student and a context is set. The questions are then related to the context. Here is an example:

> *A 15-year-old girl presented with symptoms of joint pain in her right knee. She gives history of similar pain in her right elbow 10 days ago which has resolved on its own. She has a history of sore throat 2 weeks ago. On examination, she has a pericardial rub.*
> a. *What are the possible causes of this condition?*
> b. *What investigations will you do to arrive at a diagnosis?*
> c. *Describe the most expected gross and microscopic features of this patient's heart.*
> d. *If this patient is left untreated, what are the sequelae and complications that she is likely to develop?*

Here, the questions are framed sequentially in a real-life problem-solving approach. Common clinical situations are used, and the aim is to test information of practical importance. If required, additional information can be disclosed in the later questions. This variation in format helps in testing knowledge in a context and helps assess a student's ability to logically analyze and solve a problem.

The problems with framing these kinds of questions are that the latter questions may provide clues to the previous ones. Secondly, as the questions are sequentially connected to each other, the student may be continuously penalized for the same error. It is important that the questions are reasonably independent of each other.

Before deciding the construction and content distribution of the paper, it is necessary to come to an agreement about the marking pattern. The more specific and factual the questions are, the more concise the expected answers will be. While this makes marking more objective and consistent, these questions may not necessarily test the higher levels of cognition. The more one departs into constructing interpretation of data and problem-solving questions, the more "softer" becomes the marking pattern and it is more difficult to mark papers objectively (Irwin & Bamber, 1982). Here, the peer group of examiners must identify reasonable alternatives to answers beforehand. As an educational tool, the modified essay question has the potential of testing all of Bloom's levels. However in order to utilize its full potential, examiners must determine the balance between cognitive levels which they regard as appropriate and construct items which reflect this appropriate balance (Irwin & Bamber, 1982).

Short Answer Questions

Like modified essay questions, short answer questions (SAQs) evoke restricted responses. The expected answers are short and sequential, rather than discursive. SAQs are used in situations where reliability of scoring and objectivity is preferred. They are good at assessing specific content areas. They are usually used to test 'must know' areas. They are specific and should have unique single answers. SAQs should be used in those situations where spontaneous generation of the answer is an essential aspect of the stimulus (Schuwirth & Vleuten, 2004).

Short answer questions can be of several types:

a. **Completion type:** Here an important fact is tested by blocking out the key word. Here are some examples:

> ❖ *The microorganism responsible for COVID-19 is* _____
> ❖ *The dose of Vitamin A for prophylaxis in children above one year of age is* ____ *IU*
> ❖ *Body mass index (BMI) =* _____ / _____
> ❖ *Glycosuria normally occurs when blood glucose rises above* _____ *mg/dL.*
> ❖ _____ *crisis is caused in patients of sickle cell disease due to parvovirus infection.*

b. **Best response type:** Here specific responses are desired in the form of several facts or a labeled diagram:

> ❖ *What are the major modified Jones criteria?*
> ❖ *Draw a labeled diagram of a tubercular granuloma.*
> ❖ *Which of the following cardiac markers will be useful in diagnosis of myocardial infarction of a patient a week after the event has occurred and why? Myoglobin, LDH, CK-MB, Troponin I, Troponin C?*
> ❖ *A two-year-old girl presents with a triangular foamy white raised lesion over both conjunctivae.*
>   a. *What is the name given to the lesion in her eye?*
>   b. *What is the most probable cause for this lesion?*
>   c. *Name the drug and its dose that you will give to treat this condition?*

c. **Open SAQs:** Here are some examples of SAQs which allow a certain degree of flexibility in answers. It is important for the key to contain all possible answers to this type of question:

> ❖ *List four causes of macrocytic normochromic anemia.*
> ❖ *Enumerate two side effects of oral iron administration.*
> ❖ *List three complications of acute pyelonephritis.*
> ❖ *What are biochemical differences in cerebrospinal fluid between tubercular and viral meningitis?*

The testing time required for short answer questions is much lesser than what is needed with essay questions. They are less expensive to write and correct. And use of many pertinent SAQs can cover a greater proportion of the syllabus and several content areas in a small time.

Key Points in Framing Questions for Written Assessment

- All assessment methods have their own advantages and disadvantages. No single assessment type is intrinsically superior.
- A good examination will consist of a combination of assessment tools depending on the purpose of assessment.
- Question types should be selected depending upon their strengths and weaknesses.
- The content of the question is more important than the type or format of the question. The kind of thinking process or stimulus that the question will evoke in a student's mind is more important than the format of the question.
- Well-written questions are those which are clear, unambiguous, and can test higher order cognitive knowledge.
- It is important to have predetermined criteria and model answers to ensure consistency in scoring.

REFERENCES

Eraut, M. (1985). Knowledge creation and knowledge use in professional contexts. *Studies in Higher Education, 10(2)*, 117–33.

Irwin, W.G., & Bamber, J.H. (1982). The cognitive structure of the modified essay question. *Medical Education, 16(6)*, 326–1.

Miller, G.E. (1990). The assessment of clinical skills/competence/performance. *Acadamic Medciine, 65(9 Suppl)*, S63–7.

Newble, D.I. (1992). Assessing clinical competence at the undergraduate level. *Medical Educcaton, 26(6)*, 504–11.

Norman, G.R., Van der Vleuten, C.P.M., & De Graaff, E. (1991). Pitfalls in the pursuit of objectivity: issues of validity, efficiency and acceptability. *Medical Education, 25(2)*, 119–26.

Schuwirth, L., Verheggen, M., van der Vleuten, C.P.M., Boshuizen, H., & Dinant, G. (2000). Validation of short case-based testing using a cognitive psychological methodology. *Medical Education, 35*, 348–56.

Schuwirth, L.W., & van der Vleuten, C.P.M. (2004). Different written assessment methods: what can be said about their strengths and weaknesses? *Medical Education, 38(9)*, 974–9.

van der Vleuten, C.P.M. (1996). The assessment of professional competence: developments, research and practical implications. *Advances in Health Sciences Education, 1(1)*, 41–67.

Chapter 4

Assessment of Knowledge: Selection Type Questions

Ciraj AM

KEY POINTS
- Matching and extended matching questions can test higher levels of learning.
- Key feature questions are useful to assess decision-making skills.
- Extended matching questions do not give credit for partial knowledge.

A well-designed assessment will use different types of questions appropriate for the content being tested (Fowell *et al.*, 1999). The last decade witnessed a change in assessment strategies amongst medical teachers in India to accommodate some degree of objectivity in written assessment. Why did this happen? The reasons are many. Essay questions have the dubious distinction of low reliability due to the lack of agreement within a team of markers when each marked the same answers (Hamleton, 1996). The truth is that scores vary, even when marked by the same individual at different times. Hence these forms of written assessment, where examiners make individual judgments about the quality of a student answer, are termed as 'subjective'. Students also complain that scorers often get influenced by extraneous factors such as handwriting, color of ink, and even word spacing.

It was therefore felt that introducing more objective methods of assessment might help, and thus multiple-choice questions (MCQs) found a place in the medical teachers' assessment tool kit. The use of MCQs as a method of assessment is now common across most academic disciplines.

However, doubts are being expressed about the effectiveness of MCQs as they test recognition rather than recall and encourage or allow guessing during examinations (Fowell *et al.*, 2000). The nature of marking is objective as there are clear right and wrong answers. Other than the marking that is objective, they are prone to subjective errors as encountered with many forms of assessment (Burton, 2005).

Objective tests often motivate students to learn better than traditional examinations, but they carry the risks of encouraging superficial or test-directed learning; hence a careful design is warranted.

Selection Type Questions

As discussed previously, objective questions may either belong to the supply type where the correct answer needs to be supplied by the student or the selection type where a student needs to select the correct response from a list of options.

The most common selection types that are used in written assessment are listed below:

True–False Questions: This type of question consists of a statement which must be indicated true (T) or false (F) by the student. In their simplest form, the statement (or stem) contains only one idea, which the student rates either true or false. These questions can also be nested into a scenario.

> **Example:** *What treatment would you consider in a 3-year-old child who has recently been diagnosed with acute lymphoblastic leukemia?*
>
> | T | F | Allopurinol |
> | T | F | Cytosine arabinoside |
> | T | F | Cytarabine |
> | T | F | Methotrexate |

Such questions may also be presented in the form of a series, covering different aspects of the same topic.

Multiple-choice Questions

In these questions, the student is expected to 'choose one answer from a list' of possible answers. They are often referred to as one- best or single best answer type. These questions contain a problem, question or a statement called the 'stem' and 4–5 options for the answers. The correct answer is called the 'key' while the other options are called 'distractors'. MCQs may be 'context dependent' which require significant interpretation and analysis. Contexts can include case studies, scenarios, graphical, and tabulated data (Collins, 2006). We will discuss about MCQs in Chapter 5.

Multiple Response Questions

These are similar to MCQs but involve the selection of more than one answer from a list.

Ranking Questions

These require the student to relate items in a column to one another, and can be used to test the knowledge of sequences, order of events or level of gradation.

> Rank the following states in increasing order of their sex ratio (from lowest to highest)
> 1. Kerala
> 2. Haryana
> 3. Uttar Pradesh
> 4. Maharashtra
> 5. Bihar

Assertion–Reason Questions

These questions combine the elements of MCQs and true-false questions. Assertion-reason tests can be used to explore cause and effect and identify relationships. Items constructed in this category allow testing of more complicated issues that require a higher level of learning (Morrison & Free, 2008).

Assertion-reason questions may be regarded as variations of the true-false question form. Each item has an assertion linked to a reason. The student is required to decide whether the assertion and reason are individually correct or not, and if both are correct whether the reason is a valid explanation of the assertion. The answer is indicated by marking each item A, B, C, D or E according to a predetermined code. In other words, each item in an assertion-reason question consists of two items—an assertion and a reason that are linked together.

An example of an assertion-reason question is provided below:

	Assertion		Reason
Question	On staining with triphenyl tetrazolium chloride, the infarcted heart muscle takes up dark brown color	because	Dehydrogenases leak out of damaged cardiac cells

Indicate your answer from the alternatives below by circling the appropriate letter
A. Both assertion and reason are true, and reason is the correct explanation for assertion
B. Both assertion and reason are true, but reason is not the correct explanation for assertion
C. Assertion is true, but reason is false
D. Assertion is false, but reason is true
E. Both assertion and reason are false.

When framing assertion–reason questions, the following points must be considered:
- ❖ The reason should be a free-standing sentence so that it can be considered separately from the assertion.
- ❖ Avoid using trivial reasons. These can result in an ambiguous question.
- ❖ Options A–E must be repeated in full for each question

Also called K type questions, these are not recommended by most experts.

Matching Questions

Matching items consist of two lists of statements, words or symbols which must be matched with one another. The two lists contain different numbers of items, with those in the longer list that do not correspond to items in the shorter one serving as distractors (Nitko, 2004).

Two variants of such matching items are given below. The first example is a conventional matching item with the second list having the answers.

Against each of the morphological or biological properties listed in Column A, select the bacterium which has the corresponding property from Column C and write it in the appropriate place in Column B.

A. Properties	B. Bacteria	C. Options
Filamentous	-------	Salmonella
Capnophilic	-------	Coxiella
Coccobacilli	-------	Actinomycetes
Cell wall deficient	-------	Mycoplasma
Acid fast	-------	Mycobacteria
Anaerobic	-------	Brucella
		Acinetobacter
		Vibrio
		Bacteroides

Given below is a reversed matching item with the first list containing the answers.

Name of the bacteria		Properties
A. *Mycobacteria*	1............	Cell wall deficient
B. *Actinomycetes*	2............	Spirochaete
C. *Vibrio*	3............	Curved rods
D. *Treponema*	4............	Acid fast
E. *Mycoplasma*	5............	Branching filamentous

Extended Matching Questions

The key elements of extended matching questions are a list of options, a theme, 'lead-in' question, and some case descriptions or vignettes. It is a variation of an MCQ where the stem of the question takes the form of a small problem or a vignette with details (such as the patient's symptoms, the results of laboratory tests, etc.) provided and the student asked to arrive at a diagnosis. The scenario is followed by a long list of items each of which must be matched with a list of options. Students should understand that an option may be correct for more than one vignette, and some options may not apply to any of the vignettes. The idea is to minimize the recognition effect that occurs in standard MCQs because of the many possible combinations between vignettes and options. By using cases instead of facts, the items can be used to test application of knowledge or problem-solving ability. For the same reasons these question types are popular in medicine and if well-written can test higher level skills (Case & Swanson, 1993).

List of options
a. *Acinetobacter baumannii*
b. *Brucella melitensis*
c. *Haemophilus parainfluenzae*
d. *Helicobacter pylori*
e. *Klebsiella aerogenes*
f. *Pseudomonas aeruginosa*
g. *Salmonella enteritidis*
h. *Shigella sonnei*
i. *Stenotrophomonas maltophilia*
j. *Vibrio cholerae*

For each of the following clinical and laboratory scenarios, select the most likely organism from the list of options. Each option may be used once, more than once, or not at all.

Theme
1. Imipenem-resistant organism isolated from the sputum of a patient in the intensive care unit.
2. Gram-negative, oxidase positive bacilli grown in blood cultures of a patient with neutropenic sepsis.
3. Multidrug resistant, oxidase negative coccobacilli, isolated from the ICU environment.
4. Gram-negative nonmotile Bacillus, indole-negative and a late lactose fermenter isolated from a child with diarrhea in a play school.
5. Short Bacillus isolated from blood cultures after 5 days, from a patient being investigated for pyrexia of unknown origin.

Steps

The steps for writing extended matching questions (EMQs) are as follows:
- Identify the 'theme' (disease, drug, metabolite, organism)
- Write the 'lead-in', (i.e., For each patient described in the given scenario, select the most likely diagnosis).
- Prepare the list of 'options'. These should be single words or short phrases and should be in alphabetical order and they should all be of the same sort, i.e., disease, drug or organism as stated above. One list may be used for several question stems.
- Write the items. They should be broadly similar in structure.

This format retains many of the advantages of MCQ tests. Scoring of the answers is easy and could be done with a computer. The reliability of this format has been shown to be good (Beullens et al., 2002). EMQs transform the questions into items that can ask students to solve problems rather than recall isolated pieces of information. They can also help to prevent students answering by elimination rather than knowing the answer. EMQs are best used when large numbers of similar sorts of decisions need testing for different situations as in the case of reaching a diagnosis or ordering of laboratory tests.

The format of EMQs is still relatively unknown, so teachers need training and practice before they can write these questions. There is a risk of an under-representation of certain themes simply because they do not fit in this format.

Key-feature Questions

Key-feature questions are designed to assess reasoning and decision-making skills at every stage of a consultation process. This format helps in assessing the ability of a candidate to make critical decisions, e.g., choose essential and cost-effective investigations, arrive at a diagnosis, or to provide appropriate short- and long-term management of the patient's problems based on the data provided. These questions aim to measure problem solving ability validly without losing too much reliability (Page et al., 1995).

Students rate key-feature questions as one of the most difficult and discerning among objective assessments as it tests the highest level of learning, i.e., the evaluation and clinical reasoning (Schuwirth & Vleuten, 2003). However, the key-feature approach is rather new and therefore less well-known than the other approaches. And construction of these questions is time consuming.

A 4-year-old girl is in anaphylactic shock. She has audible upper airway noises, wheezing, cyanosis, and a decreasing level of consciousness.

What would be the most appropriate course of action?
a. Count her respiratory rate
b. Check for pulse
c. Establish an IV line for medication
d. Ready your intubation equipment.

What's New in the Arena?

Computer-based objective forms of assessment are emerging technologies, with great potential for improving the assessment in medical education. In addition to many practical advantages, computer-based testing can facilitate the development of more valid assessments (Scalise & Gifford, 2006; Collins & Duncan, 2007). Though popular with candidates due to efficient marking and delivery, the costs and expertise necessary to use this technology should not be underestimated.

A few among them are listed below:

i. **Graphical hotspot questions** involve selecting/choosing an area(s) of the screen, by moving a marker pointer to the required position. Advanced types of hotspot questions include labeling and building questions. These types of questions are likely to supplement if not replace cadavers, microscopes, and tissue sections in medical school laboratories.

ii. **Text/numerical questions** involve the input of text or numbers at the keyboard.

iii. **Sore finger questions** utilize one word, code or phrase that is unrelated to the rest of a passage. It could be presented as a "hot spot" or text input type of question. Similar ones are already practiced in medical education for formative purposes.

iv. **Sequencing questions** require the student to position the text or graphic objects in each predetermined sequence. These are particularly good for testing knowledge of pathways and methodology that frequently appear in various disciplines and will have an important role in the assessment of both basic science and the clinical curricula.

v. **Field simulation questions** offer simulations of real problems or exercises and would be of immense help in the assessment of virtual medicine.

Other forms of computer-assisted objective assessment at higher level require students to identify and/or manipulate images. Students may be asked to plot a graph, complete a matrix, or even build up an image.

Selection type questions have the advantage of being objective yet requiring more than simple recall from the students. Properly framed, and integrated with other forms of assessment, they can serve a very useful purpose to assess even higher levels of knowledge.

REFERENCES

Beullens, J., van Damme, B., Jaspaert, H., & Janssen, P.J. (2002). Are extended-matching multiple-choice items appropriate for a final test in medical education? *Medical Teacher, 24(4)*, 390–5.

Burton, R.F. (2005) Multiple-choice and true/false tests: myths and misapprehensions. *Assessment and Evaluation in Higher Education, 30(1),* 65–72.

Case, S.M., & Swanson, D.B. (1993). Extended-matching items: A practical alternative to free-response questions. *Teaching and Learning in Medicine, 5(2),* 107–15.

Collins, C., & Duncan, A. (2007). Re-designing computer-based assessment tests for use as a learning tool: profiling tacit learning processes instead of measuring learning outcomes. Assessment design for learner responsibility, 29-31 May 07. Available from http://www.reap.ac.uk [Last accessed August, 2020].

Collins, J. (2006). Education techniques for lifelong learning: writing multiple-choice questions for continuing medical education activities and self-assessment. *Radiographics, 26(2),* 543-51.

Fowell, S.L., Maudsley, G., Maguire, P., Leinster, S.J., & Bligh J.G. (2000). Report of findings: student assessment in undergraduate medical education in the United Kingdom. *Medical Education, 34(Suppl. 1),* 1–78.

Fowell, S.L., Southgate, L.J., & Bligh, J.G. (1999). Evaluating assessment: the missing link? *Medical Education, 33(4),* 276–81.

Hamleton, R.K. (1996). Advances in assessment models, methods, and practices. In: D.C. Berliner, R.C. Calfee (Eds.), *Handbook of Educational Psychology.* (pp. 899-925) New York: Simon & Schuster Macmillan.

Morrison, S., & Free, K. W. (2008). Writing multiple-choice test items that promote and measure critical thinking. *Journal of Nursing Education, 40 (1),* 17–24.

Nitko, A.J. (2004). *Educational assessment of students.* (4th ed.) Upper Saddle River, NJ: Merrill Prentice Hall.

Page, G., Bordage, G., & Allen, T. (1995). Developing key-feature problems and examinations to assess clinical decision-making skills. *Academic Medicine, 70(3),* 194–201.

Scalise, K., & Gifford, B. (2006). Computer-Based Assessment in E-Learning: A Framework for Constructing "Intermediate Constraint" Questions and Tasks for Technology Platforms. Journal of Technology, Learning, and Assessment, *4(6).* Retrieved from https://ejournals.bc.edu/index.php/jtla/article/view/1653/1495

Schuwirth, L.W.T., & van der Vleuten, C.P.M. (2003). ABC of learning and teaching in medicine: Written assessment. *British Medical Journal, 326,* 643–45.

Chapter 5

Assessment of Knowledge: Multiple Choice Questions

Ciraj AM

KEY POINTS

- Multiple choice questions (MCQs) can test various levels of knowledge including analysis and problem solving.
- Quality of MCQs depends on the quality of distractors.
- Writing good MCQs requires training and practice.
- Mathematical models are available to reduce guessing effect.

Now that we have learnt about most types of selection type questions, let us now discuss certain important aspects related to the single-best-answer question, the most common form of Multiple Choice Questions (MCQs) used in the Indian context.

Any form of assessment needs to be evaluated for its utility against five criteria: reliability, validity, educational impact, feasibility, and acceptability (Schuwirth & Vleuten, 2019). For a chosen content area, many MCQs can be developed. This would provide a broad coverage of concepts that can be tested consistently. That would enhance the test validity as well as reliability. If items are drawn from a representative sample of content areas that constitute the intended learning outcomes, they would ensure a high degree of validity. Educational impact is important because students tend to focus strongly on what they believe will appear in the examinations. Therefore, they will prepare strategically depending on the type of questions used. If carefully designed, this approach would stimulate higher levels of thinking, and enhance skills of critical thinking and decision-making based on evidence (University of Oregon website, 2002).

The MCQs are commonly used due to the logistical advantage of being able to test large number of candidates in a short period of time and with minimal human intervention. The acceptability of MCQs due to the reasons cited previously has made them a preferred tool for written assessment across most academic disciplines.

Strengths of MCQs

- With proper planning, the learning outcomes ranging from simple to complex can be measured.
- If designed well, highly structured and clear tasks can be provided.
- A wide range of issues can be tested in a short time.
- Items can be written such that students are required to discriminate among options that vary in degrees of correctness. It avoids the absolute judgments found in True-False tests.
- Marking is quick and easy using a computer, which also provides an easy access to item analysis.
- They may be used for quick revision.
- Future preparation time may be considerably reduced by construction of a question bank.
- Item analysis can reveal how difficult each item was and how well it discriminated between the strong and weaker students in the class.

Why is there Opposition to use of MCQs in Written Assessment?

Critics of MCQs feel that a different cognitive process is involved in proposing a solution versus selecting a solution from a set of alternatives, which takes the context out of real-world solutions. As the items focus only on recall of information, they believe that MCQs fail to test higher levels of cognitive thinking, which includes the students' problem-solving skills and ability to organize and express ideas. However, this criticism is more often attributable to flaws in the construction of the test items rather than to their inherent weakness. Appropriately constructed MCQs result in objective testing that can measure knowledge, comprehension, application, analysis, and synthesis. We shall demonstrate this in the later sections by providing appropriate examples. However, creativity cannot be tested using MCQs and they are certainly not the preferred tools of assessment for the psychomotor and affective domains.

In assessment terminology, each MCQ is called an Item.

Challenges with MCQs

- Constructing good items is a time-consuming process.
- Plausible distractors are difficult to construct especially in cases where higher-order cognitive skills are being tested.
- As the assessment process involves selection of alternatives alone, MCQs restrict students' ability to develop and organize ideas and present these in a coherent argument.

Chapter 5: Assessment of Knowledge: Multiple Choice Questions

- More than one 'correct' answer can create problems.
- Language and comprehension ability of the student can influence the scores.
- Cueing effect can result in guessing. The recognition of the correct answer when it is seen listed in a row of distractors is called the *cueing effect*. The recognition of right answer is enough to answer the question correctly.
- Feedback on individual thought processes is lacking. Hence it is difficult to comprehend as to why individual students selected incorrect responses.
- Students can sometimes read more into the question than what was intended.
- Attention to security is an issue if you are planning to reuse the items.

Why do you Need Good MCQs?

Faulty items interfere with accurate and meaningful interpretation of test scores. This can have an adverse impact on student pass rates. Therefore, to develop reliable and valid tests, items must be constructed that are free of such flaws.

Structure of an item

A traditional MCQ or item is one in which a student chooses one answer from several choices supplied. It is often referred to as the single best answer (SBA) question. A single-best-answer question has three major parts—the stem, the lead-in, and options.

Parts of an MCQ

- *Stem:* The text of the question is called stem.
- *Lead-in:* The stem may be followed by the lead-in which is generally short and precise and poses a single question.
- *Options:* The choices that follow the stem are called options.
- *Key:* The correct answer in the list of options is called the key.
- *Distractors:* These are the incorrect answers in the list of options.

An example illustrating these components is given below:

Stem: A previously fit 78-year-old man has a transurethral resection of the prostate (TURP) performed under general anesthesia taking 90 minutes to complete. Half an hour after arrival in the recovery room he has not regained consciousness. Respiratory effort is adequate and vital signs are stable.

Lead-in: Which of the following deranged investigations is most likely to account for his current clinical condition?

Options:

a. Hemoglobin: 7.1 g/dL   Distractor
b. PaCO$_2$: 7.4 kPa   Distractor
c. PaO$_2$: 8.9 kPa (FiO$_2$ = 0.35)   Distractor
d. Serum sodium: 114 mmol/L   Key

Construction of Good Items: A Challenge

Multiple choice examinations are commonly used to assess student learning. However, instructors often find it challenging to write good items that ask students to do more than memorize facts and details. Characteristics of effective MCQs can be described in terms of the overall item, the stem, and the options. Though there have been elaborate descriptions on constructing flawless items, Haladyna's guidelines and NBME series on "Constructing Written Test Questions for the Basic and Clinical Sciences" remain the most referred and preferred documents (Haladyna *et al.*, 2002; Case & Swanson, 2001).

In the sections that follow, we shall discuss the steps followed to create effective MCQs that test the listed learning objectives. These general guidelines listed may be applicable to other forms of objective assessment also.

Guidelines for Writing Flawless Items

Initial Focus

Before you begin constructing MCQs, you need to focus on these aspects:
- The standard and scope of the examination being conducted. The content area, the level of questions asked, and the scoring pattern will depend on this.
- The number of questions you wish to ask will depend on the time available for the examination.
- The source of your questions.

General Item Writing Guidelines

Plan Well in Advance

It takes time and creativity to write good items. Perhaps the best time to write them is as and when you teach the material. Doing so ensures the correctness and weightage of the content being asked and you are likely to get better ideas for construction, based on students' questions or responses.

Revisiting and Reflecting

The next step would be to revisit the questions you've written in a day or two with a fresh eye.

Peer Review

The items must then be peer-reviewed. This is also known as *pre-validation*. This may be easily achieved by passing on your questions to your colleagues in the department and finding their opinions on these items. Remember, the more critical they are, the more well-constructed items you gain.

Trial Run

After peer review it would be a good practice to administer your questions. Results generated thus would help us determine the Facility Value (FV) and Discrimination Index (DI) of each item. The use of FV and DI with the procedures adopted in calculating them will be discussed in Chapter 22.

Be certain to allocate enough time for editing and other types of item revisions.

Procedural Tips

Clear Instructions are Important

It is mandatory to clearly state what the student is expected to do in the process of marking their selection on the answer card/sheet; whether it is by blackening the bubble or by marking the appropriate box or by ringing the appropriate letter.

Choosing a Format

While framing your items you may resort to the single best answer format or correct answer format. Single best answer (SBA) format refers to a list of options that can all be correct, but one of them would be the best. In the correct answer format, there can be one and only one right answer. Many item writers prefer the latter one, as there is less scope for ambiguity and contention.

Include Items with Varying Levels of Difficulty

Be aware of the difficulty level of each question. Make sure that you have enough easy and challenging questions so that you will be able to distinguish a better student from a good one, and perhaps the best one from a group of better ones.

Well Begun is Half Done

A deliberate attempt to make the first few items relatively easy can help students settle down fatser so they can focus on the more challenging questions to come.

One at a Time

Do not attempt to test too many things in a single question. It reduces your ability to discriminate amongst students with differing levels of comprehension. Try to write more than one multiple choice question rather than test multiple concepts in a single item.

Vertical Formatting

Format the options vertically and not horizontally. Horizontal placement may be confusing for the students.

Frame Clear and Unambiguous Items

As much as possible, minimize examinee reading time in phrasing each item. Clarity of items in terms of content, grammar, punctuation, and spelling is strongly advocated as it can eliminate unwanted ambiguities and save valuable time.

Content-related Rules

- Each item framed should be based on an important learning objective of the course.
- Test for important or significant information.
- Focus on a single problem or idea for each test item.
- Use your items to assess higher-order thinking.
- Keep the vocabulary and usage of language consistent with the students' level of understanding of the subject matter. The items should probe knowledge of medicine and not their ability to understand linguistic nuances.

Rules-related to Construction of Stem

Select the Format

State the stem in either question form or completion form, but see that it has only relevant text. If you are using the completion format, do not leave a blank for completion in the beginning or middle of the stem.

Clarity is Important

Ensure that the directions and wordings in the stem are clear; the examinee should know exactly what is being asked for. Use only a single, clearly defined problem and include the main idea in the question.

Vignettes Offer Definite Advantages

The stem can be a short statement or outline of a clinical scenario. There are definite advantages of using a clinical scenario instead of a statement as the stem of an MCQ. If carefully designed, this approach would stimulate higher levels of thinking and enhance skills of critical thinking and decision-making based on evidence. As it matches with real-life situations, application of basic science knowledge in a clinical format would help integrating various disciplines.

Use Short Stems with Caution

Stems that are only one word usually need long options. This is not a problem, but there is a danger that the determinate response style of an MCQ can be weaselled into a set of five straight true/false questions, only faintly related to each other.

Use Negatives Sparingly

Negative stems may be appropriate in some instances, but they may be used selectively. Avoid negative phrasing such as 'not' or 'except.' If this cannot be avoided, the negative words should always be highlighted by underlining or capitalization. Beware—too much of negative phrasing portrays a negative mindset.

Do not put negative options following a negative stem. Such items may appear to perform adequately, but brighter students who naturally tend to get higher scores have an edge over an average student to cope with the logical complexity of double negatives.

No Window Dressing Please

Do not offer superfluous information as an introduction to a question. This approach probably represents a subconscious effort to continue teaching during assessment and is not likely to be appreciated by the students, who would prefer direct questions and less to read in the process of being assessed.

Developing the Options: The General Rules

- Place options in logical or numerical sequence.
- Use letters in front of options rather than numbers; numerical answers in numbered items may be confusing to students.
- Keep options independent; options should be mutually exclusive and not be overlapping.
- Keep all options homogeneous in content.
- Keep the length of options consistent.
- Phrase options positively as much as possible.

Rules for Developing the Key

One and Only One

Make sure that there is only one correct option especially if you follow the correct answer format. Leave no room for ambiguity.

Balance Your Key

Position the correct option in such a way it appears about the same number of times in each possible position for a set of items. Balance the placement of the correct answer. Vary the position of the key in a random manner so that the student fails to detect any clues by detecting a pattern of any sort. One could avoid this problem by listing the various options in alphabetical order or in the order of its length.

Rules for the Development of Distractors

Use Plausible Distractors

Distractors must be plausible; that is the cardinal rule in the construction of good MCQs. Since all the distractors in an MCQ must be plausible, one obvious rule is that the closer a distractor is placed to the correct answer, the more plausible it is. And the more plausible the distractor is, the more likely it is that the learner will choose it over the correct answer. In short, research your options properly; do not use random or very easy distractors. Implausible distractors deny chances to test a learner (Downing, 2003).

Do not Get too Close

A word of caution—do not get too close to the right answer, otherwise it won't be a good distractor because the learner will then be tested on precision (unless that is exactly what you want to test). This technique is straightforward: make the answer that is perceived as most obvious the correct answer. In other words, make the correct answer seem implausible.

Avoid (Also see Box 5.1)

- Cueing one item with another. Keep items independent of one another
- The use of over-specific knowledge
- Verbatim phrasing from textbook descriptions
- Issues that would invoke gender and cultural issues or questions which unfairly advantage or disadvantage groups
- Tricky items that mislead or deceive test takers into answering incorrectly
- Items based on assumptions
- Items that check trivial information
- Window dressings (excessive verbiage) in the stem
- Negative phrasing: As much as possible, word the stem positively.
- Providing clues by faulty grammatical construction
- Giving unintended cues, such as making the correct answer longer in length or precise than the distractors
- Specific determiners such as never or always
- The use of 'all of the above' as an option or use it sparingly
- The use of 'none of the above' as an option or use it sparingly

BOX 5.1: The Avoid Box

(This box provides you with examples of what is to be avoided while constructing items. You will agree that most of them are frequently encountered in MCQs)

What is to be avoided?	How do they appear?	Why is it to be avoided?
Using abbreviations, acronyms and eponyms	BP may be read as blood pressure, British pharmacopeia or boiling point.	The candidate may misinterpret your question.
Long distractors with pairs or triplets of reasons	M. tuberculosis is acid-fast because it gets decolorized by mineral acids due to the presence of mycolic acid in its cell wall.	This should not be used especially when one reason is correct but not others.
Double negatives as distractors	Which of the following drugs is least unlikely to work in a patient of drug-resistant tuberculosis?	May confuse students.
Undefined or imprecise terms	Use of words such as abundant, mild, moderate in the stem or distractors.	It is difficult to interpret the associated significance often misleading the candidate.
Grammatical clues and inconsistencies	Using 'always', 'never'. 'best', 'most/least likely' Use of :.... is example of an: it gives a clue that the correct answer should start with a vowel.	May provide clues to the candidate or distract them.

Nuances of AOTA and NOTA

Use of AOTA (all of the above) and NOTA (none of the above) deserves a special mention as they seem to be most used (abused!) in our MCQ papers.

AOTA: Use of AOTA is strongly discouraged, the reason being recognition of one wrong option eliminates "all of the above," and recognition of two right options identifies it as the answer, even if the other options are completely unknown to the student (Harasym *et al.,* 1998).

NOTA: You may ask NOTA but as a final option, especially if the answer requires some degree of calculation. NOTA if used will make the question harder and more discriminating, because the uncertain student cannot focus on a set of options that must contain the answer. NOTA cannot be used if the question requires selection of the best answer and should not be used following a negative stem (Dochy *et al.,* 2001).

Construction of Items Based on Bloom Taxonomy

Apart from the guidelines mentioned above, knowledge of Bloom taxonomy is certainly an added advantage for item writers. It can serve as a guide to construct more stimulating items. Assessment items developed using this framework will include a range of levels and thinking processes (Haladyna & Downing, 1989). Keep in mind that we want our students to think, make connections, question the information included in the problem, process the information, and reflect on their answers. Each category requires more complex thinking than the one preceding it and incorporates the preceding types of thought in order to proceed to the 'higher' levels.

Knowledge

Writing questions that test knowledge is a relatively straightforward task. These items test basic recall. A test at this level can easily become a "trivial pursuit" exercise!

> *Which one of the following gram-negative bacilli is an obligate anaerobe?*
> *a. Acinetobacter baumanii*
> *b. Bacteroides fragilis*
> *c. Escherichia coli*
> *d. Klebsiella pneumoniae*

Note that the responses are internally consistent—they are all the names of gram-negative bacilli, *Bacteroides fragilis* being the only obligate anaerobe in the list.

Let us examine this item:

> *Sterilization of carbohydrate solution is achieved by:*
> *a. Autoclaving*
> *b. Inspissation*
> *c. Tyndallization*
> *d. Radiation*
> *e. Filtration*

This also involves simple recall of the correct method. Internal consistency and plausibility are maintained in that all responses are actual sterilization practices. Look at another example:

> *Which one of the sequences shown below is correct in relation to steps followed in Polymerase Chain Reaction?*
> *a. Denaturation, annealing, extension*
> *b. Extension, annealing, denaturation*
> *c. Annealing, extension, denaturation*
> *d. Extension, denaturation, annealing*
> *e. Denaturation, extension, annealing.*

In this example, nothing more is required than the recall of the order of certain pieces of related information.

Comprehension

Comprehension questions test whether your students have understood the meaning of the knowledge they are recalling. At this level, knowledge of facts, theories, procedures, etc. is assumed, and one tests for understanding of this knowledge.

> *Your patient is 54-year-old male who looks weak and confused. You suspect that he is suffering from undiagnosed diabetes mellitus.*
>
> *Which of the following signs and symptoms would best serve to confirm your suspicion?*
> *a. Poor skin turgor with tenting*
> *b. Recent decrease in appetite*
> *c. Increased thirst and urination*
> *d. Unexplained bruising of the abdomen*

Application

The testing of application is achieved by providing the student with a novel scenario/case study and inviting her to apply her knowledge to the scenario. The scenario that you provide should be a new one that your student was not hitherto exposed to or there is a risk that you are still testing recall. In order to classify a question into this group, ask yourself if prior knowledge of the background to the question is assumed to be both known and understood and whether one is merely expected to apply this knowledge and understanding.

> *A 72-year-old man who has had several attacks of coronary disease is admitted to hospital for incipient gangrene of one leg and is found on admission to have symptoms of intestinal obstruction.*
>
> *What is the most probable cause of obstruction?*
> *a. Cancer of the colon*
> *b. Intussusception*
> *c. Mesenteric thrombosis*
> *d. Strangulated hernia*
> *e. Volvulus*

Analysis and Synthesis

Analysis and synthesis are harder to assess by objective testing but questions at these levels can be achieved by presenting students with data, diagrams, images, and multimedia that require analysis before a question can be answered.

A synthesis question might require students to compare two or more pieces of information. Questions in these categories could, for example, involve students in separating useful information from the irrelevant one.

> *Your patient is a stuporous 68-year-old female in obvious respiratory distress. A patent airway, labored respirations, and weak pulses are noticed. The skin appears cool and diaphoretic. The capillary refill time is significantly delayed. Vital signs:*
>
> *Pulse rate: 136 min*
>
> *Blood pressure: 60 mm Hg/palpation, Respirations: 32 min with bilateral crackles.*
>
> *Which type of shock is this patient suffering from?*
> a. Cardiogenic
> b. Neurogenic
> c. Hypovolemic
> d. Septic

Evaluation

Evaluation questions require the student to make a diagnosis or decision. A question that provides specific patient information along with pertinent clinical findings, imaging data and which asks the learner to choose the most appropriate strategy for management is an example of this category. This type of questions might ask the candidate to pass a judgment on the validity of an experimental procedure or interpretation of data. Key-feature questions and assertion-reason questions mentioned below are best examples under this category.

Introducing MCQ Formats in Written Assessment

How do you Prepare Your Students to Take an MCQ Test?

If your students are taking an MCQ test using computer-readable answer sheets for the first time, please ensure that they are adequately prepared for this. Show them in advance the answer sheet they will be required to use. This can be achieved by projecting a transparency of the answer sheet and indicating to students how they must record their personal details and answers.

Scoring, Guessing, and Negative Marking

Scoring: The hardware and software:
- Non-academics can be employed to assist with the marking of paper-based objective assessments.
- Computers can be used to scan and mark paper-based objective tests.

- Online objective assessments can be delivered, marked, and analyzed using computers.

Optical Mark Reading Scanner and Data Analysis Software

The answers to MCQs are recorded on a machine-readable answer sheet. These sheets are fed through an Optical Mark Reading Scanner (OMR). The OMR allows automated data entry that turns pencil marks into useable computer information. If two or more circles are filled in on the answer sheet, or the correct answer is carelessly marked, the question will be marked 'wrong'. Specially written software controls the test scoring and item analysis. This service provides a rapid turnaround time for results and a detailed analysis of multiple choice items. The analysis usually shows:

- Individual students' total scores
- The class distribution of scores
- The performance of individual test items to allow informed modifications to the test if necessary

Regular quality control checks to ensure the reliability of the system is mandatory.

Approaches to Scoring

Various approaches are adopted for scoring MCQs. Raw scores are usually tabulated by calculating the total number of correct responses. This refers to right scoring in which nothing is deducted for omission and incorrect responses (Bar-Hillel *et al.*, 2005).

Guessing was thought to have resulted in inflated student scores. Alternative approaches to marking have been developed because of concerns of guessing. Critics of MCQs say that the answer to an MCQ can always be guessed with approximately 20–25% chance of getting the correct answer without knowing anything about the subject matter. This led to the introduction of approaches that discouraged random guessing. They include the ones listed below (Ben-Simon *et al*, 1997):

Approaches to reduce guessing:

i. **Rewarding partial knowledge:** This approach allows students to choose more than one possibly correct response and awards partial mark provided one of the responses chosen is the item key.
ii. **Not sure:** Choosing a 'Not sure' option for which the candidate is awarded 0.2 of a mark.
iii. **Negative marking:** Another commonly used method to discourage guessing is the 'negative marking' which means that some marks are deducted from the overall test score for each wrong answer. They come in different forms:
   a. *Simple negative marking schemes*: Equal numbers of marks added and subtracted for right and wrong answers. Here

omitted answers or selection of a 'No answer' option have a neutral impact on marks.
b. *Formula marking*: Marks are rescaled according to a mathematical formula which takes account of the number of distractors offered. A suggested negative marking approach is to penalize a wrong answer for an MCQ with a negative mark that equals the correct mark divided by the number of incorrect options, (*e.g.*, an MCQ with 5 options, one correct answer awarded a correct mark of 4, each of the four incorrect options is awarded a -1 mark). This means that a student randomly guessing answers to all questions would get an overall mark of approximately zero. However, the assessment literature generally does not support the use of formula to correct for guessing when marking MCQs.
c. *Confidence-based assessment*: A student's rating of his/her confidence in an answer is considered in the marking of the answer. Not all scales used for confidence-based assessment involve negative marking.

Why is Negative Marking a Contentious Issue?

Although many argue in favor of negative marking, this practice is now a contentious issue among medical educators (Goldik, 2008). There are valid reasons for this position.

Purely Mathematical Reasons

Firstly, let us examine the cumulative probability of guessing correctly over many items. With five options to choose from, the probability of guessing the correct option (if the student really is guessing blindly) is 0.2 (20%). The probability of correctly guessing the answers to two items is $(0.2)^2$, or 0.04 (4%); and the probability of correctly guessing the answers to three items is $(0.2)^3$ or 0.008 (0.8%). If the student really knows little about the subject matter and randomly selects answers, the likelihood of correctly guessing answers for more than one item is very small.

A Necessary Skill Neglected

Informed guessing is one's ability to decide based on some understanding and information. This is a necessary skill in everyday life. It is an element of problem solving which is a generic skill advocated in medicine. In most disciplines people rarely have full information on which to base their decisions. Students who are not certain of the correct answer but have partial knowledge are likely to make intelligent guesses based on the knowledge they possess. Some feel that by implementing negative marking we discourage students from making intelligent guesses based on good partial knowledge.

More a Personality Issue

It is known that the tendency to guess or not to guess when in doubt is influenced by personality factors. Some students are more likely to be adversely affected in this game of guessing. Thus the examination may end up assessing an element of their traits rather than their knowledge, inducing Construct Irrelevance Variance.

Who is the Best?

Imagine two candidates who achieve the same final score in a negatively marked examination. One candidate attempts only a part of the paper, completely avoiding the questions to which she might end up losing a few marks for her wrong answers. The other answers almost the entire paper, getting far more correct, but also getting several wrong and having marks deducted due to negative marking. In this situation how do you judge as to which student knows more about the subject that was assessed?

Extension of Theoretical Range

The use of negative marking extends the theoretical range of marks for the examination. For example, if one mark is awarded for every correct answer and one deducted for each wrong answer, the theoretical range of the exam is - 100 to +100%. However, this is not usually considered when performing the statistical analysis of the examination and, therefore, the performance indicators may be wrong. It also raises the question of what the examination has been testing in the case of a candidate whose final mark is less than zero.

These examples provide enough evidence to comment that negative marking has too many adverse characteristics. Instead of continuing the quest for a negative-marking system that works, MCQ examinations can be improved by reducing omissions to a point where confidence differences have no real distorting effect on the estimation of achievement or ability. There is evidence that this approach works.

MCQs for Integration

Most of the Indian medical schools follow the conventional discipline-based approach. An attempt to rope in horizontal and vertical integration in certain corners is a laudable effort. It is a welcome sign that our medical teachers have started debating and discussing problem-based learning (PBL) and competency-based learning strategies; some even daring to implement them. However, these strategies are often demanding in terms of infrastructure and logistics. Instead, one may consider using MCQs to integrate across various disciplines. Carefully constructed MCQs can cut across disciplines and probe the critical thinking and reasoning skills of the students examined (Azer, 2003). The Extended Matching Questions (EMQs) and assertion-reason types are better strategies in this context. These have been discussed in Chapter 4.

Using MCQs in an integrated format where a conventional discipline-based curriculum is followed should be done with proper planning and extra caution. It will be wise enough to address these issues before you embark on this daunting task.

Philosophy and Spirit of Integration

Ensure that your team is aware of the structure, design, and the philosophy of integration and assessment in this context.

Discuss areas to be covered in MCQs and allocate roles of various disciplines in the integrated format. It is necessary to have clear-cut guidelines regarding the different components of assessment, i.e., the types of MCQs that are going to be used or what should be the extent of contribution from each discipline? For example, a question on tuberculosis can be framed to elicit responses pertaining to microbiological, pathological, pharmacological, and preventive medicine aspects of the disease.

Standard Setting

There is no single recommended approach to setting standards for MCQs. If you are using it for classroom assessment or certification purposes, a criterion-referenced standard is preferred to a norm-referenced (fixed pass rate) or holistic model (arbitrary pass mark at, say, 50%). It is said so because the level of performance required for passing should depend on the knowledge and skills necessary for acceptable performance and should not be adjusted to regulate the number of candidates passing the test.

The purpose of a criterion-referenced standard is to determine 'how much is enough' to be considered as an acceptable performance. The validity of the pass or fail inference depends on whether the standard for passing makes a valid distinction between acceptable and unacceptable performance. These standards suggest that an absolute expectation for passing should be established prior to the examination based on the examination content (McCoubrie, 2004).

For multiple choice examinations, popular methods of establishing a criterion-referenced standard are content-based procedures (*e.g.*, the modified Angoff procedure) or a compromise model (*e.g.*, Hofstee). Content-based procedures are relatively simple, but compromise models are less time-consuming and probably equally reliable (Bandaranayake, 2008). These will be discussed in Chapter 23.

The outcomes of a standard setting exercise may be different when different methods, experts, or items are used in the process. Thus, there is error associated with the criterion-referenced standard setting process as it depends, in part, on the subjective judgments of experts. Therefore, adjusting for the error of measurement surrounding the pass point when setting the criterion standard, is legitimate and provides confidence that only candidates who should pass, will pass.

Once the criterion-referenced standard is established, test-equating methods allow it to be carried forward to subsequent tests, so that candidates are required to meet the same standard to pass regardless of when they take the examination.

Role of the Feedback

Feedback from the candidates about the questions can be very informative. An explanation about the reasons why an option is correct or incorrect can be a powerful learning tool for students, if it is correctly constructed (Harden, 1975). However, feedback responses are difficult and time-consuming to write. Because of the extra time needed, collecting feedback is not possible in qualifying examinations, where conditions are to be strictly controlled. However, if you are using MCQs for formative assessment, a blank sheet may be provided, and an extra 10 minutes allowed for candidates to provide their feedback. It is unlikely that this will stop candidates complaining, but at least they will know you care.

Bottom-line

Contrary to the notion that MCQ tests dumb-down higher order learning ideals, in many instances, the literature strongly supports the fact that they can provide information about students' higher levels of understanding. If items are correctly designed these tests are no way inferior in assessing the depth and breadth of students' knowledge. Medical teachers cannot abstain from objective forms of assessment. The only way out is to frame good items, evaluate them, and appreciate their place in the field of written assessment.

REFERENCES

Azer, S.A. (2003). Assessment in a problem-based learning course: Twelve tips for constructing multiple choice questions that test students' cognitive skills. *Biochemistry & Molecular Biology Education, 31(6),* 428–34.

Bandaranayake, R.C. (2008). Setting & maintaining standards in multiple choice examinations: AMEE Guide No. 37, *Medical Teacher, 30(9),* 836–45.

Bar-Hillel, M., Budescu, D., & Attali, Y. (2005). Scoring & keying multiple-choice tests: A case study in irrationality. *Mind & Society, 4,* 3–12.

Ben-Simon, A., Budescu, D., & Nevo, B. (1997). A comparative study of measures of partial knowledge in multiple-choice tests. *Applied Psychological Measurement, 21(1),* 65–88.

Case, S.M., & Swanson, D.B. (2001). *Constructing written test questions for basic & clinical sciences.* 3rd edn. National Board of Medical Examiners (NBME), Philadelphia, USA. Accessed from *http://www.nbme.org/pdf/ itemwriting_2003/2003iwgwhole.pdf.*

Dochy, F., Moerkerke, G., De Corte, E., & Segers, M. (2001). The assessment of quantitative problem-solving skills with "None of the Above" items (NOTA Items). *European Journal of Psychology of Education, 16(2)*, 163–77.

Downing, S.M. (2003). The effects of violating standard item writing principles on tests & students: The consequences of using flawed test items on achievement examinations in medical education. *Advances in Health Sciences Education, 10*, 133–143.

Goldik, Z. (2008). Abandoning negative marking. *Eur J Anaesthesiol, 25*, 349–51.

Haladyna, T.M., & Downing, S.M., (1989). A taxonomy of multiple-choice-item writing rules. *Applied Measurement in Education, 2(1)*, 37–50.

Haladyna, T.M., Downing, S.M., & Rodriquez, M.C. (2002). A review of multiple-choice item-writing guidelines for classroom assessment. *Applied Measurement in Education, 15(3)*, 309–33.

Harasym, P.H., Leong, E.J., Violato, C., Brant, R., & Lorscheider, F.L. (1998) Cueing effect of "all of the above" on the reliability & validity of multiple- choice test items. *Evaluation & the Health Professions, 21*, 120–33.

Harden, R.M. (1975). Student feedback from MCQ examinations, *Medical Education, 9(2)*, 102–5.

McBeath, R.J. (Ed.). (1992). *Instructing & Evaluating Higher Education: A Guidebook for Planning Learning Outcomes.* New Jersey: ETP.

McCoubrie, P. (2004). Improving the fairness of multiple-choice questions: a literature review. *Medical Teacher, 26(8)*, 709–12.

Schuwirth, L.W.T., & van der Vleuten, C.P.M. (2019). How to design a useful test: The principles of assessment. In: Swanwick, T., Forrest, K., O'Brien, B.C. (Ed.) *Understanding medical education: evidence, theory and practice.* West Sussex: Wiley-Blackwell

Writing multiple-choice questions that demand critical thinking. (2002). Retrieved March 10, 2010 from the University of Oregon, Teaching Effectiveness Program: *http://tep.uoregon.edu/resources/assessment/multiplechoicequestions/mc4critthink.html*

FURTHER READING

Burton, R.F. (2005). Multiple choice & true/false tests: myths & misapprehensions. *Assessment & Evaluation in Higher Education, 30*, 65–72.

Ozuru, Y., Briner, S., Kurby, C.A., & McNamara, D.S. (2018). Comparing comprehension measured by MCQs and open ended questions. *Canad J Exp Psychol, 67*, 215–227.

Przymuszala, P., Piotrowska, K., Lipski, D., & Marsiniak, R.(2020) Guidelines on writing multiple choice questions. *SAGE Open, 3*, 1–12.

Pugh, D., Champlain, A.D., & Touchie, C. (2019). Making a continued case for the use of MCQs in medical Education. *Medical Teacher, 41*, 559–577,

Royale, K.D., & Hedgepeth, M. (2017). The prevalence of item construction flaws in medical school examinations. *EMJ Innov, 1*, 1-66.

Tarrant, M., & Ware, J. (2008). Impact of item writing flaws in multiple choice questions on student achievement in high stakes nursing examinations. *Medical Education, 42*, 198–206.

Zaidi, N.L.B., Grob, K.L., Monrad, S.M. et al (2018) Pushing Critical Thinking Skills With Multiple-Choice Questions: Does Bloom's Taxonomy Work? *Academic Medicine, 93*, 856–859,

Chapter 6

Question Paper Setting

BV Adkoli, KK Deepak, KA Narayan

KEY POINTS
- Setting an effective question paper lies at the heart of written assessment
- It drives student learning, directs teaching efforts, brings transparency, and credibility to the assessment system
- The systematic process of setting a question paper involves designing the outline of a question paper, preparing a blueprint, writing questions along with a marking scheme, editing, review, and moderation of the paper
- Training of the faculty and commitment to enforce a robust examination system are the *sine qua non* for effective assessment

'Assessment drives student learning' is a *mantra* chanted by every educationist; however, what indeed drives assessment is the question paper! The way a question paper is designed can make or mark the prospects of passing an examination for a student. A well-designed question paper can very effectively complement skills assessment in ensuring that only competent graduates pass out from medical colleges. On the other hands, if the job of question paper setting is given in wrong hands, it can be disastrous to both students community as well as the civil society which trusts the quality of graduate outcomes. Knowing how to set a good question paper is, therefore, a vital skill for individual teachers. It an equally important issue for an educational institute or examining body to bring credibility to its functioning. Ultimately, it is one of the foremost tools to ensure quality assurance.

In this chapter, we will take you through the various steps involved in setting a question paper.

Existing Practices in India

The assessment system in most medical colleges in India is largely governed by the practices adopted by the universities to which they are affiliated. Broad guidelines in terms of examination subjects and total number of marks allotted to a paper are provided by the regulatory body, the Medical Council of India. However, these guidelines are not always adequate either for the students or the paper setters. The actual pattern of question paper varies from one university to other, depending upon their policies, convention, and standards which they wish to maintain.

The limitations of the existing system of setting question paper along with their impact on quality of assessment have been outlined in **Table 6.1**.

TABLE 6.1: Limitations of conventional practices of question paper setting

Problems and pitfalls	Implications on the quality of assessment
Lack of clear policy guidelines about what type of questions should be asked and how they should be assessed*	Paper setters set questions according to what *they* think is important. Teachers teach according to what *they* think is important. Students have no clue about what is expected of them. When the examiners are different from paper setters, the communication gap gets wider. Communication gap among paper setters, teachers, students, and examiners leads to poor assessment and mis-alignment with the curricular goals.
Lack of content validity	Questions are often set according to the whims and fancies of paper setters. There is often poor sampling of the content. This prompts the students to pursue selective study. This is unfair to a student who has taken pains to study the whole syllabus. Interpretations from such assessments are bound to be flawed
Ambiguity in formulating questions	Good students suffer when questions are poorly written, ambiguous, and vague. Even after knowing the correct answer, students will not be able to do well. For example: If the questions such as *Write what you know about mutation* or *Write a short note on HIV/AIDS* are asked, the student becomes clueless about what is expected and loses marks. Similarly, when too complex language is used to frame questions, the examination becomes a test of the student's comprehension of the language rather than a test of knowledge (Construct Irrelevance).
Unclear directions	Sometimes, the instructions given to the candidates are misleading. For example, if the MCQ part is to be submitted within first 30 min but it is not mentioned there. This creates an unnecessary confusion in the mind of the students.
Too difficult or too easy paper	Both are detrimental as they fail to get an accurate assessment of a student's understanding of the subject. Too difficult a paper causes trauma or fear of failure. Too easy a paper leads undeserving students to pass. Too difficult a paper may prove unfair even to good students.
Effect of extraneous factors	Factors such as handwriting of the student can bias the examiner and vitiate scoring accuracy. Even testing conditions, if not congenial, can cause problems.

Contd...

Contd...

Problems and pitfalls	Implications on the quality of assessment
Lack of clear marking scheme	Absence of a clear scheme leads to subjective interpretation and affects the inter-examiner reliability of the assessment. Students are also unable to make a judgment of how much is expected to be written for each question.
Faulty policies regarding appointment of paper setter; Absence of training of paper setters	Often, seniority rather than competence in assessment forms the basis of appointment of examiners in our settings. The paper setters are not trained, and still asked to set papers. This leads to the repetition of outdated questions and dominance of recall type of questions rather than questions that test higher cognitive levels.

*These details are now provided in the 2019 MCI Module on Assessment for Competency-based undergraduate medical education

Vleuten and Schuwirth (2005) proposed a notional concept of utility of assessment as a product of validity, reliability, feasibility, acceptability and educational impact. Absence of judicious sampling of contents affects validity and therefore utility. It also leads to selective examination-oriented reading habits which hampers the educational impact.

Another issue is that the conventional system relies heavily on manual processing which is expensive compared to electronic methods of paper setting or marking. The only point in favor of the conventional system is the acceptability of the system, mainly due to absence of alternatives. Increasing number of complaints and allegations against valuation require a shift to use of digital technologies that are relatively more transparent and resource effective.

Steps for Effective Question Paper Setting

STEP 1: Lay down rules of the game: Prepare a design of the question paper
STEP 2: Prepare a blueprint
STEP 3: Prepare questions and plan the marking scheme
STEP 4: Edit the question paper
STEP 5: Review and moderate the question paper

The first and the second steps, viz., designing the question paper and preparing the blueprint are closely interrelated and can even be combined in to one step. The key issue here is the allocation of weightage which we have further amplified at the end of the chapter (*see* Appendix).

STEP 1: Lay down Rules of the Game: Prepare a Design of the Question Paper

The design of the question paper is a policy statement laid down by the examining agency which indicates the weightage to be given in the question paper to:

- Various content areas or topics specified in the syllabus
- Different types of questions: Long-Answer Questions (LAQ), Short-Answer Questions (SAQ), and Multiple-Choice Questions (MCQs)
- Different categories of the curriculum: 'must know', 'desirable to know' and 'nice to know' or 'core' and 'non-core' areas as designated in the competency-based model, and
- Varying difficulty level: difficult, average, and easy questions.

The design of the question paper sets the rules of the game. It is not a confidential document. On the contrary, it should be widely publicized amongst students, faculty, and external examiners to bring transparency into the system. This also results in 'buy-in' from all the stakeholders and prevents litigations. Once the design is approved, it should be mandatory for the examining agency to follow the prescribed pattern for at least three years to ensure uniform standard of assessment. Thereafter, it should be reviewed and realigned with the curricular revisions which are likely to take place as a result of new developments in the field and obsolescence of some concepts.

Determining Weightage to be Allocated to Various Topics

Allocation of weightage to different topics is a critical issue. The general considerations for deciding the weightage are as follows:

- Exclude topics which involve elements such as skills, attitudes or communication, which can be better tested by practical, oral or other formats of assessment.
- Allocate higher weightage to the topics which students 'must know' rather than topics which are 'desirable to know'. Nice to know topics can be left for self- learning.

There are two approaches used in deciding the weightage distribution to various topics. The first approach is related to the medical curriculum which considers a combination of *frequency of a disease* (health problem) and its *impact* on the population. The second approach is common in health science universities which follow the credit system for running their programmes and courses. The details of both these approaches are provided in the Appendix at the end of this chapter. The common principle underlying both the approaches is that the weightage allocation should be commensurate with the importance or emphasis given to the topic and the teaching-learning time given to that topic. Obviously, a consensus is needed in making such policies.

An example of allocation of weightage to various topics of Community Medicine in MBBS (Part I) examination has been given in the **Table 6.2**. In this example, there are two theory papers each carrying 100 marks. Thus, total marks for the subject will be 200.

TABLE 6.2: Example of allocation of weightage to various content areas in two theory papers of Community Medicine Paper I and Paper II

Topics/content area of the subject			Weightage	Percentage
Paper I: Basic Sciences Related to Community Health				
a.	Behavioral aspects		20	10
	i. Sociology	(8)		
	ii. Health Education	(6)		
	III. AETCOM	(6)		
b.	Biostatistics Demography		14	7
c.	Concepts of Health		20	10
d.	General Epidemiology, screening		24	12
e.	Environmental Sanitation		8	4
f.	Nutrition		8	4
g.	Entomology		6	3
Total of Paper I			100 Marks	50%
Paper II: Healthcare Organization and Epidemiology of Specific Diseases				
a.	Specific Epidemiology			
	I. Communicable diseases	(24)	36	18
	II. Non-communicable	(12)		
b.	Health care of special groups			
	I. Occupational Health	(7)	14	7
	II. Geriatrics, Genetics, and Mental Health	(4)		
	III. School Health	(3)		
c.	Maternal and Child Health and Family Welfare		20	10
d.	Health care of the community, Health programs, Planning and management, International Health		24	12
e.	Miscellaneous (Health legislation, ethics, disasters, genetics)		6	3
Total of Paper II			100	50%
Grand Total of Paper I and Paper II			200	100%

*Illustrative example only. The actual weightage to be worked out based on competencies as per the MCI document and corresponding content areas.

The allocation of weightage in the above example has been decided as a consensus after discussions held in the department.

Epidemiology appears in both the papers. The general epidemiology is placed in the first paper (weightage 24) and specific aspects are dealt in the second paper to attain a balance (weightage 36). This is further divided into communicable disease (weightage 24) and non-communicable diseases (weightage 12). This shows that the papers are not water-tight compartments. Questions can be framed in a manner that concepts of epidemiology can be explained with examples of specific diseases and epidemiological principles such as rates, ratios, screening could be highlighted while describing a disease. Similarly, small topics such as occupational health, geriatrics, genetics and mental health, and school health have been combined to allocate 14 marks.

Distribution of Weightage to Question Types

It has been established that no single type of question can effectively measure all learning outcomes. We need to have a combination of different types. While MCQs can help in assessing a wide range of content area in a short time, SAQs can test higher abilities such as interpretation, analysis, and application. Essay questions are needed to assess highest level of cognition, i.e., synthesis, evaluation, and creation.

However, the problem arises when we combine marks of MCQs and SAQs/LAQs to arrive at a final score. The standard error of measurement for MCQs and SAQs are different. Moreover, unless crafted very well, they test different levels of knowledge. We therefore tend to argue in favor of having a separate paper on MCQs rather than allocating 20% to MCQs. The practice of adding MCQ marks to other types may boost the pass percentage, but it does not add to the quality of assessment. Moreover, as the practice of using optical mark reading sheets has become more popular in conducting effective and efficient assessment, the three issues, viz., MCQs, item analysis and question banking have assumed a great significance in the overall assessment scheme.

Deciding Weightage to the Difficulty Level of Questions

The actual difficulty level of a question can be determined only after the examination, by conducting item analysis. However, it is possible to conduct pre-validation of questions preferably by a team of experts. The difficulty level can be estimated on a three-point scale such as: difficult (A), average (B), and easy (C). Since an item with average difficulty (B) can discriminate effectively between high and low achievers, it is advisable to include many average items (60–70%) in a paper. About 10–20% difficult questions can be included to provide a challenge to high achievers. About the same proportion of easy questions can be included to motivate low achievers.

STEP 2: Prepare the Blueprint of the Question Paper

Once the design of the question paper is in place, the next step is the preparation of a blueprint. Just as an architect prepares a blueprint to guide a construction, the examining agency should prepare a test blueprint to guide the paper setter in framing the right type of questions in the right proportion. A blueprint is a *table of specifications*. It assumes two dimensions when the table indicates (a) weightage to content areas and (b) types of questions. When it also includes weightage allotted to the objectives, like recall, interpretation and problem solving, it assumes three dimensions.

We have illustrated a blueprint of two question papers in Physiology meant for I MBBS summative assessment in **Table 6.3**.

*TABLE 6.3: Blueprint for physiology assessment
Theory examination for MBBS (first professional summative assessment)

Sl. No.	Topics	Weightage	Marks allotted	
			Essays/SAQs	MCQs
	Question paper I			
1	General & NM Physiology	8	14	2
2	Cardiovascular System	10	16	4
3	Respiratory System	8	12	4
4	GIT & Metabolism	7	12	2
5	Blood and Immunity	7	10	4
6	Environmental Physiology	5	8	2
7	Nutritional Physiology	5	8	2
		50	80	20
	Question paper II			
8	Central Nervous System	18	33	3
9	Special senses	10	16	4
10	Endocrine Physiology	8	12	4
11	Yogic Physiology	3	4	2
12	Reproductive Physiology	4	5	3
13	Renal Physiology	7	10	4
		50	80	20
	Total	100	160	40
	Weightage	—	80%	20%

*Illustrative example only. The actual weightage to be worked based on competencies as per MCI document and corresponding content areas.

MCQs should be contextual and assess the ability to interpret data. The area assessed by essays/MCQs should not overlap. SAQs should not be recall type and should present clear tasks to the student.

One can derive several blueprints from a design of the question paper. However, it may be wiser to stick to a blueprint for at least three years for the sake of uniformity in assessment.

One can also prepare several question papers based on a blueprint. In case the examining agency decides to go for a computerized question bank, it is easily possible to generate many question papers which can be administered manually or online.

Several authors have listed the advantages of preparing a test blueprint. The aim of blueprinting is to reduce two major validity threats (Hamdy, 2006):

a. *Construct under-representation*, which means under-sampling of a course content, e.g., too little weightage for a topic of national health importance.
b. *Construct irrelevance variance*, which means inclusion of flawed item formats, too easy or too difficult questions, or examiner bias (tendency to test favorite, or 'hot', or trivial topics).

The advantages of preparing a blueprint with respect to the students, paper setters, teachers, and curriculum planners have been outlined in **Table 6.4**.

TABLE 6.4: Advantages of blueprinting to various stakeholders

Stakeholders	*Advantages of blueprinting*
Students	Blueprinting brings fairness and transparency to assessment. Expectations become clear. It discourages selective learning habits and encourages study of the whole curriculum
Paper setter	Avoids under-sampling of course content (*Construct under representation*) Reduces chances of litigation and disputes arising from flawed items, too easy or too difficult paper, or examiner bias in choosing the topic (*Construct irrelevance variance*)
Teachers	Helps teachers in aligning teaching strategies with expected outcomes Facilitates judicious allocation of time for teaching various topics;
Curriculum planners	Helps in aligning assessment with curriculum

Thus, the design of the question paper combined with a blueprint makes assessment clear, explicit, and transparent to everyone involved in the process of education: the curriculum planners, teachers, examiners, and students.

STEP 3: Prepare Questions and Marking Scheme

The preparation of individual questions demands not only in-depth knowledge of the content, but also skill in framing questions in a clear and unambiguous manner. The instructions for framing various types of questions have been explained in their respective chapters. However, we would like to emphasize the need to visualize the probable answer and to refine the question in such a way that it elicits the expected answer from students. Should the question be written first or the answer? This is like finding out whether egg comes first or the chicken! Many believe that the framing of a question and the answer expected should be done simultaneously, to ensure validity of the assessment.

It is advisable to prepare *question cards* or *item card* (a term preferred for MCQs) for individual questions. An item card, apart from stating the actual question and the marking scheme, contains valuable information on the content/topic addressed, type of question, objective/outcome tested, marks allocated, estimated difficulty level, and the time required for answering the question.

We have illustrated two specimens of Item Cards related to Physiology **(Box 6.1)** and Community Medicine **(Box 6.2)**.

Please note that the *item card* in physiology is a part of question bank in physiology which shows the details of the item analysis conducted and the results thereof, which facilitates the paper setter in picking a suitable question from the bank, subject to a security system developed by the examining agency. Also, the marking scheme indicates how the answer is to be assessed by the examiner, which improves reliability in marking.

In case the question bank is computerized, it is possible to include the parameters of item analysis, i.e., the difficulty index (sometimes called facility value), discrimination index, and distractor effectiveness along with the year/date of administration. Based on the actual findings the questions are either continued, modified or deleted.

Every examiner should be conversant with the marking scheme. All cases of dissent or disagreement should be discussed and resolved before marking. A typographical error in the scoring key of MCQ can be disastrous, especially when the items are marked electronically. Many experts advise that in case of MCQs, it is better to mention a standard source based on which the 'key' has been prepared in order to avoid dispute.

STEP 4: Edit the Question Paper

Editing of the question paper deals with issues such as, stating general instructions to be given to candidates, grouping or sequencing of the questions, besides enhancement of the esthetics and achieving overall user-friendliness of the paper. It may be good idea to pilot the test on a small group of candidates, like the target group to ensure language compatibility and length of the test vis-a-vis time allocated.

The questions can be grouped according to content areas or types of questions used. While it is more convenient to group questions according to the question types for the sake of easy

BOX 6.1: Specimen item card from a question bank in Physiology

Front page of item analysis card

DEPARTMENT OF PHYSIOLOGY

XXXXXX

QUESTION BANK ITEM				
		TIME FOR ANSWERING	PREPARED BY	DATE
		1 min	XXX	XXX

REF NO.	SYSTEM	TOPIC
xx.xx.xx	RESPIRATORY	Hypoxia

QUESTION ITEM

When carbon dioxide and hypoxia act together, the increased ventilation is:
a. A sum of the effect of each
b. The same as the effect of either acting alone.
c. More than the sum of the effects of each.
d. Less than the sum of the effects of each.

Key – (c)

Reverse page of Item analysis card

S. No.	Class	Exam.	Exam date	No. Examined Gp size	Sub. Gp	No. of Responses A	B	C	D	E	Blank	Difficulty Index*	Discrimination index**	Interpretation Difficulty	Discrimination	Remarks
1.	MBBS	End Sem	Dec 1985	T-51	H-14	2	0	11	1	-	0	53.5	0.5	Moderate, Acceptable	Excellent	Accept, excellent
					L-14	3	1	4	1	-	5					
2.	MBBS	1st Prof	July 1987	T-55	H-15	-	-	13	2	-	-	56.6	0.6	Moderate, Acceptable	Excellent	Accept, excellent
					L-15	2	1	4	3	-	5					
3.				T	H											
					L											
4.				T	H											
					L											
5.				T	H											
					L											
6.				T	H											
					L											

*For Difficulty Index: 0–10 Extremely difficult, 10–20 Very difficult, 20–30 Difficult, 30–70 Acceptable, 70–80 Easy, 80–90 Very easy, 90–100 Extremely easy.
** For Discrimination Index: < 0–0.15 Poor (discard), 0.15–0.25 Marginal (revise), 0.25–0.35 Good, >0.35 Excellent
Abbreviations used: Gp. - Group; T- Total number of students drawn for item analysis; H- Number of correct responses in high group; L - Number of correct answers in low group(ranking); Please refer to the procedure relating to item analysis in other chapters

BOX 6.2: Specimen of item card from Community Medicine

Target Group: MBBS Final	Content/Topic: General epidemiology – Study designs		Estimated difficulty level: Average
Objective tested: Application	Question: Select a suitable epidemiological study and describe the study design to study the risk factors for colon cancer. Discuss the common bias in epidemiological research.		Estimated time (in min.): 15 minutes
Type of question: LAQ	Points of Answer or Scoring Key: a. Case-control design, rationale for selecting – rarity of disease, cost and time. b. Description of case control design c. Common types of bias, reasons for the same, bias in case control studies. Total Marks: 10		Marks for each point: 2+5+3
Reference for scoring key			
Reference	Date of Administration: 14 June 2019	Date of Administration:	Date of Administration:
Difficulty index:	0.58		
Discrimination index:	0.39		

Comments: Item can be continued/needs modification/may be deleted
Item can be continued. Colon cancer has low incidence in India. The more common cancer could be used as the topic for description.
Abbreviation used: LAQ – Long-answer question

marking, it may be difficult for the candidates to switch their thought process from one topic to the other. If the questions are grouped according to topics, students can recall concepts more easily. The initial questions of the paper should be easy questions so that students feel comfortable and settle down quickly. A thumb rule is to begin with MCQs (often as a separate section), followed by SAQs and LAQs.

Editing of the paper involves polishing of the questions, defining their scope, and improving readability. Some deletions may be warranted to avoid repetition of questions. Attention should be paid to the proper layout of the question paper, numbering of the questions, and sub-questions, font size, spacing and margins, to enhance readability.

STEP 5: Review and Moderation of the Question Paper

While editing of the question paper is done by the paper setter, the review and moderation is done by an independent moderator. It is a vital step for removing the flaws and enriching the quality of the paper. In fact, a joint moderation by a panel can be more effective, especially when multiple sets of question papers are drawn. But within the constraints of time and resources, individual review is the most practiced step. **Table 6.5** is a checklist of 10 questions to ask before finalizing a question paper.

TABLE 6.5: Ten questions to ask before finalizing a question paper

1.	Is the question paper in conformity with the design and blueprint declared by the examining agency?	☑
2.	Does the question paper cover the full syllabus?	☑
3.	Does the question paper test a wide range of abilities/outcomes (various levels of cognitive domain)?	☑
4.	Does it make judicious use of various types of questions?	☑
5.	Is the question paper of appropriate difficulty level? (Neither too difficult, nor too easy)	☑
6.	Does the question paper have the ability to discriminate good students from poor students?	☑
7.	Can the paper be answered within the stipulated time by an average student?	☑
8.	Is the language of questions, well understood even by poor learners?	☑
9.	Are the options given, if any, balanced in all respects?	☑
10.	Does the question paper avoid repetition of questions from previous examination?	☑

Should the question paper be set by the internal or external examiner? Who should review and moderate the paper? These are tricky issues addressed by the examining agencies in different ways depending upon their policies. In fact, a panel approach may lead to more authenticity. In some universities while the paper is set by external examiner, it is got vetted by the internal examiner to better align with the teaching that has happened. However, this should not be used as a ploy to boost the pass percentage. If a robust blueprint is in place, the question of external or internal hardly matters.

Conclusion

The future directions in assessment are likely to emphasize assessment as an educational process rather than a psychometric tool. Multiple tools administered by multiple observers on multiple occasions are likely to supplement the end of the course 'one-time' assessment. Nevertheless, the question paper will continue to play a key role in high-stake examinations. An attempt to systematize the process of question paper setting is bound to yield rich dividends in terms of an examination with better credibility, and hence it ensures quality assurance to the process of assessment. It also promotes radical changes in the way teachers teach and the way the students learn. What is required is simply an orientation of the faculty in this exercise, and leadership and commitment on part of the examination agency to translate this into action. The earlier the policy makers realize this secret, the better it is for ensuring quality control in medical education, which in the ultimate analysis, is an instrument for the attainment of health objectives.

REFERENCES

Abdellatif, H., & Al-Shahrani, A.M. (2019). Effect of blueprinting methods on test difficulty, discrimination, and reliability indices: cross sectional study in an integrated learning program. *Advances in Medical Education and Practice, 10*, 23–30.

Adkoli, B. (1995). Attributes of a good question paper. In Sood R. (Ed.). *Assessment in Medical Education: Trends and tools*. New Delhi: KL Wig Centre for Medical Education and Technology, AIIMS. pp. 67–82.

Bhat, B.V. (2000). Mechanics of question paper setting. In: Ananthakrishnan N, Sethuraman KR, Santhosh Kumar (Eds). *Medical Education: Principles and Practice.* (2nd ed.) Pondicherry: National Teacher Training Centre; JIPMER, Pondicherry. pp. 113–8.

Biggs, J. (Ed.). (1999). *Teaching for quality learning at University*. Buckingham: SRHE and Open University Press.

Coderre, S., Woloschuk, W., & McLaughlin, K. (2009). Twelve tips for blueprinting. *Medical Teacher, 31*, 322–4.

Downing, S.M., Haladyna, T.M., & Yudkowsky, R. (2009) Validity and its threats. In *Assessment in Health Professions Education*. New York: Routledge. pp. 21–56

Epstein, R. (2007). Assessment in Medical Education. *New England Journal of Medicine, 356,* 387–95.

Goyal, S.K., Kumar, N., Badyal, D., Kainth, A., & Singh, T. (2017). Feedback of students to aligned teaching-learning and assessment. *Indian Journal of Psychiatry, 59(4),* 516–7.

Hamdy, H. (2006). Blueprinting for the assessment of health care professionals. *The Clinical Teacher, 3,* 175–9.

Hopkins, K. (1998). *Educational and Psychological Measurement and Evaluation*. Needham Heights: Allyn and Bacon.

Miller, GE. (1990). The assessment of clinical skills/competence/performance. *Academic Medicine, 65(9 Suppl),* S63–7.

Patel, T., Saurabh, M.K., & Patel, P. (2016). Perceptions of the use of blueprinting in a formative theory assessment in Pharmacology education. *Sultan Qaboos University Medical Journal, 16(4),* e475–81.

Patil, S.Y, Manasi Gosavi, M., Bannur, H.B., & Ratnakar, A. (2015). Blueprinting in assessment: A tool to increase the validity of undergraduate written examinations in pathology. *International Journal of Applied and Basic Medical Research, 5(Suppl 1),* S76–9.

Schuwirth, L., & van der Vleuten, C.P.M. (2010). How to design a useful test: the principles of assessment. In: Swanwick, T. (Ed.). *Understanding Medical Education: Evidence, Theory and Practice*. ASME: Churchill Livingstone. pp. 195–207.

van der Vleuten, C.P.M., & Schuwirth, L. (2005). Assessing professional competence: from methods to programs. *Medical Education, 39,* 309–17.

Appendix

Notes on determination of weightage in designing question paper

A. Approach based on perceived impact and frequency of disease

In this approach, the weightage to a topic is decided based on a combination of two factors. The weightage is a product of:
1. The perceived impact/importance of a topic in terms of its impact on health (I).
2. The frequency of occurrence of a disease or health problem (F) (Coderre et al., 2009).

Thus, the following formula can be used:
$W = I \times F$ where
W = Weightage
I = Impact
F = Frequency of occurrence of the disease in the community
T = Sum of the products of I and F

Steps:

Assign scores for Impact and Frequency as follows **(Table A6.1)**.

TABLE A6.1: Calculation of impact factor and frequency factor to decide weightage to the topics in a question paper

Impact factor (I)	Score	Frequency factor (F)	Score
Topic of high impact/life threatening condition	3	Very frequently seen	3
Moderate impact	2	Somewhat frequent	2
Little or no impact	1	Rarely seen/encountered	1

A topic which has little impact (non-urgent condition) and which is somewhat frequently seen will have a weightage of $1 \times 2 = 2$. A life-threatening condition which is also common, should carry a weightage of $3 \times 3 = 9$.

In case of basic sciences, the impact may be replaced by clinical application potential (highest—3 and lowest—1) and frequency may be replaced by volume of the topic (largest topic—3 and smallest topic—1).

Once the impact and frequency scores are decided, calculate the product ($I \times F$); and divide by total possible scores to get an index. This index should be multiplied by total number of items to be included in the test, which gives the weightage for the topic **(Table A6.2)**.

TABLE A6.2: Table showing method of calculating weightage to be given to various topics

Topic No	Impact (I)	Frequency (F)	Product (I × F)	(I × F)/T	Weightage for the topic* [(I × F)/T] × 60 Rounded off
1	2	2	4	4/21=0.19	11
2	2	3	6	6/21=0.28	17
3	1	2	2	2/21=0.09	06
4	3	3	9	9/21=0.42	26
			21		Total = 60**

*The last column figures (weightages) are rounded off to nearest integer
** A minimum of 60 items with DI of 0.35 are required to achieve an acceptable reliability (Hopkins, 1998).

B. Approach based on the credit system

A major reform being launched in higher education system in India is the adoption of choice-based credit system (CBCS). CBCS deals with the allocation of certain credits to each unit of study. This unit can be considered as a learning module or topic. Several topics constitute a course (sometimes called as Paper). Several courses put together constitute a program. The essence of the credit system lies in combining the following information:

a. Credit hours earned by the student (decided based on requirement of attendance, completion of assignments, projects, etc.)
b. Credit points derived from the performance of students in the examination.

Steps for Designing and Blueprinting:

- For each topic calculate the credit hours: For the direct contact sessions one credit is equivalent to 16 hours; For practical, tutorial etc. 32 hours of engagement is needed for awarding 1 credit. For example, Topic No 1 shown in the **Table A6.3** fits in to this and gets 2 credits.
- Convert the credits into percentage of marks fixed for the paper. For example, Topic 1 which has 2 credits in a 10-credit course requires a weightage of 20% in the paper.
- Assign weightage for various types objectives, for example, recall, understanding and application.
- Assign weightage for various types of questions: MCQs, short answer and long answer questions.

Method of estimating weightage to the topics in a credit-based system has been illustrated below by taking an example of a 10-credit course (Course A) which has say four topics. See the breakup of theory and practical teaching hours which have been converted into credits. **(Table A6.3).**

Table A6.3: Estimation of weightage for the topics of course A, based on credit system

Topic number	Theory direct Contact hours And credit	Practical/ Self-directed learning contact hours and credit	Total credit hours assigned to the topic	Weightage Allocation for a 100 Marks paper
Topic 1	16 (1.00)	32 (1.00)	2	20%
Topic 2	12 (0.75)	40 (1.25)	2	20%
Topic 3	24 (1.50)	48 (1.50)	3	30%
Topic 4	20 (1.25)	56 (1.75)	3	30%
TOTAL	72 Hours	176 Hours	10	100%

Let us assume the weightage to be given to various Objectives as follows:

Knowledge	Understanding	Application	Total
25%	35%	40%	100%

Let us also assume the weightage to be given to various types of questions as follows:

Long answer question (LAQ)	Short answer question (SAQ)	MCQs	Total
20%	60%	20%	100%

Using the three sources of information, we can arrive at a following blueprint of the question paper as given in **Table A6.4.**

TABLE A6.4: Blueprint of the question paper of Course A

Topic and credits	Knowledge 25%			Understanding 35%			Application 40%			Total %
	LAQ	SAQ	MCQ	LAQ	SAQ	MCQ	LAQ	SAQ	MCQ	
Topic 1 Credit 2	—	2 (1)	2 (2)	—	5 (1)	2 (2)	—	7 (2)	2 (2)	20
Topic 2 Credit 2	—	2 (1)	2 (2)	—	6 (2)	2 (2)	—	6 (2)	2 (2)	20
Topic 3 Credit 3	10 (1)	3 (1)	1 (1)	—	—	3 (3)	—	9 (2)	4 (4)	30
Topic 4 Credit 3	—	3 (1)	—	—	17 (4)	—	10 (1)	—	—	30
Total Credits 10	10 (1)	10 (4)	5 (5)	28 (7)	7 (7)	10 (1)	22 (6)	8 (8)		100%

Note: Figures within the bracket indicate the number of questions to be prepared and the figures outside indicate the weightage.

Chapter 7

The Long Case

Tejinder Singh

KEY POINTS

- Despite its low generalizability, the long case provides useful information about clinical competence.
- Observing the trainee during history taking and physical examination is a useful strategy to improve the value of long case.
- Tools like objective structured long examination record (OSLER) can be used to structure the long case and provide feedback to the student, thereby increasing its educational value.

The long case was introduced by the University of Cambridge in 1842 as an assessment tool for the University's clinicians (Jolly & Grant, 1997). Despite a number of newer and apparently more reliable assessment tools coming in over the last many years, the long case has retained its position as a major tool for assessment of clinical competence, especially at the undergraduate level. Some of the perceived advantages of the long case could be related to its requirement for students to take a history and perform physical examination that will enable them to integrate information, synthesize, and verbally present their clinical findings to the examiner. This, to some extent, replicates the skills required when presenting a patient after admission on a ward round during routine clinical work. Since long case uses real patients, it has authenticity and views the problems of the patient comprehensively. It promotes direct contact between the student and the examiner. It is on this basis that the long case is regarded both as a valid and educationally valuable assessment tool (Wass & Jolly, 2001; Wass et al., 2001).

Process

For many years, the long case has been the mainstay of assessment of clinical competence around the world. Although, in many countries, educationists have moved away from the long case as a means of summative assessment, it is likely to stay put in Indian medical schools for a long time to come. There have been many variations in the format of the long case, including the time allotted for this (for example, semilong or short cases) but in essence, it entails asking the student to take an *unobserved* history and perform physical examination of a patient over 30–45 minutes. At the end of this period, the student presents the history, findings, and management plan to one or two examiners. The examiners ask clarifying questions, and may ask the student to demonstrate certain physical findings and critique his management protocol.

In our country (and many other countries), the long case involves a real patient and that can be considered as one of its strengths. It allows the student to work in unstructured complex settings, which are so common in real-life situation. A wide variety of clinical problems or settings can be assessed using long case—though sometimes, examiners may insist on at least one of the cases being a central nervous system (CNS) case in medical specialties. Nevertheless, compared to say the objective structured clinical examination (OSCE), long case focuses on the entire clinical problem rather than on an isolated part of it.

Assessment Issues

The major problem with using the long case as an assessment tool is the limited sample that can be assessed, given the time involved. In a lighter vein, long case can be compared to an essay type questions, which can test only limited content, compared to multiple-choice questions (MCQs). This limits the generalizability of the results (Norman, 2002). It is wrong to presume that a student who presents a CNS case well will be able to present a case of anemia equally well. Often examiners try to camouflage this by arguing that they are looking at the 'process' rather than on the 'content' of the case. This argument is unfounded because even the process of approaching a case is context specific and not generic. We have already discussed in Chapter 1 and provided literature support to show that a major reason for low reliability in assessment is the case- or context-specificty (Norman et al., 1985). While we do not have such data from India, American experience indicates that using two cases, both marked by two examiners gave a reproducibility of only 0.39, indicating that students' ability accounted for only 39% of the marks, the remaining 61% being due to extraneous factors. If only one case was used, the reproducibility dropped to 0.24 (Norcini, 2002).

Inter-examiner variations: These can also account for low reliability of the long case. Examiners' own thought process, prior experience, setting of the examination, students' way of presentation, gender, etc., can all influence the ratings. The major reason related to examiners, however, may be a lack of agreement on what is being assessed (Norcini, 2002). The competencies assessed are not clearly defined based on the level of the students, settings, and purpose of the examination. Since this is not done, it is possible that examiners are not clear about the objectives of assessment of a long case.

Context specificity: Inter-rater reliability does not seem to be a major problem with long case—the problem rather is of intercase reliability (Wass & Vleuten, 2004). A good performance on a single case will not predict good performance on another case. Dugdale (1996) rightly drove the point home by stating that "if a student failed to diagnose my (hypothetical) prostatic carcinoma, it would be little consolation to know that he had done brilliantly on a case of multiple sclerosis". In fact, in our setting, it may not be wrong to say that "if a student fails to diagnose anemia, it may be little consolation that he did brilliantly on a case of tubercular meningitis". This is probably the reason, why no amount of measurement intervention will improve reliability of a long case (Norcini, 2001) to an acceptable level for summative assessment. The problem lies elsewhere—*inadequate sampling* and that is where all interventions have to be directed. However, in view of the logistics involved, especially for undergraduates, it is unlikely that the process will change.

While OSCE provided an immediate solution to the problem by providing a wider sample of clinical competence, the time available for each competency shrinks (Wass & Vleuten, 2004) and it has been rightly pointed out by these authors that "depth of assessment has been sacrificed to gain breadth". The reported benefits of OSCE do not stem from standardization or structuring. It is the *wider sampling* of cases that does the trick. On the same note, making drastic changes to what the examiners do at one case is likely to be less fruitful than increasing the number of cases. You will find a more detailed discussion on this in Chapter 26.

Building on the Positives

Various strategies have been suggested in the literature to improve the value of the long case. Most of them focus on the major recognized shortcomings, viz. lack of observation, lack of structure, and small sample of clinical problems.

Observation of the process: Since the long case utilizes a relatively long time of contact between the examiner and the student, it could have advantages in terms of validity and reliability—however, the unfortunate part is that most of this time is used in presentation rather than in observing the student. Unobserved time, element of luck (easy or difficult case, uncooperative patient, 'dove' or 'hawk' examiner), unstructured assessment, and lack of clear consensus on what is being observed take their toll on validity despite of it being a real-life situation. *Observing the student* during the process of history taking or performing physical examination may be a useful strategy. Observation of history taking provides a useful and distinctive component of competency assessment over and above that provided by presentation (Wass & Jolly, 2001). Observation provides the opportunity to reconcile the multiple interactions happening between the content and constructs measured in assessment (Dare et al., 2008). It provides students with an opportunity to receive feedback on history taking and diagnostic skills.

The long case still finds its way in the recommended program for assessment of undergraduate medical students in many universities (Dare et al., 2008) because of its validity and resemblance to 'real-life' patient encounters. However, an observing examiner is added during the history taking and physical examination to improve reliability. Observation is recommended in order to directly assess the student-patient interaction, directly assess the hypothetico-deductive approach taken by the student and provide *valid feedback* to students based on their approach to the process in order to improve future performance. It has also been suggested that considering the fact that the long case can provide useful inputs about the interviewing skills of the students, it can be used as a screening tool, and students with severe problems can take other forms of examination like OSCE (Norcini, 2001).

Increasing sample size: It has been demonstrated that using multiple short cases, where a student is asked to demonstrate a physical finding or interpret data is likely to predict the outcome better (Hijazi et al., 2002). The key feature of this intervention will again be the *direct observation* of the student. Some authors have proposed use of sequential 'shorter' long cases (McKinley et al., 2005), standardizing the patient group, increasing the number of long case assessments (a minimum of eight assessments may be required to achieve a reliability of at least 0.8, or 'moderate reliability', with a single examiner), and introducing an observing examiner into the history taking and physical examination part of the assessment (Dare et al., 2008).

Standardizing and structuring: Assessing a long case using a structured grid has not been shown to have any addition to its reliability (Ponnamperuna et al., 2009). No difference in the perception of students or assessors regarding fairness was however noticed for examiners who used structured questions and those who did not. Rather, students felt (Oslon et al., 2000) that they were scoring fewer marks where examiners were using a structured grid. Wass and Jolly (2001) found global ratings to give a better reliability than checklist-based ratings. In this study, the reliability of history taking part was higher than the presentation part. However, in line with the thinking that content-specificity is more of a threat to reliability, it has been suggested that a better option for improving reliability will still be increasing the number of cases rather than structuring observation. However, if the long case is being used as a tool for providing formative feedback, then structuring will help to make such feedback more explicit.

Another intervention (McKinley et al., 2000) of using a structured and observed six student-patient encounters for formative assessment helped to attain a reliability of 0.94 in making a pass/fail decision. However, as the authors pointed out, this method had its validity demonstrated by identifying 39 competencies which physicians are likely to face in general practice and using a suitable sample of this to test the students. It was also ensured that the case mix given to the students was classified as appropriate for a general practice scenario. The authors were also able to demonstrate a positive educational impact of the assessment as evidenced by feedback from the students. Reliability of long case with two pairs of examiners was reported to be similar to that of OSCE (Wass et al., 2001). It was estimated that using two examiners to observe history taking on 10 long cases will give a reliability of 0.8. If the time is equal, the long case is considered better than OSCE in terms of reliability (Norman, 2002) but this is not feasible, at least in our settings for the time being.

Objective Structured Long Examination Record (OSLER)

With a view to overcome some of the problems associated with long case, Gleeson (1997) suggested using an OSLER. It aims at improving the shortcomings of the long case related to objectivity, validity, and reliability. In essence, OSLER is a 10-item structured record, where the examiners can identify the case difficulty and agree beforehand on what is to be examined. All students are examined on the same points. The process of taking history, product of history, and communication skills are some of the aspects included. It can be incorporated in the usual examination procedure, without requiring any special preparations. A brief description of OSLER follows.

Generally, a time of 30 minutes is allowed per student to assess 10 items—which include 4 on history, 3 on physical examination, and another 3 on other aspects of patient care. Since different students are likely to get different cases, examiners establish case difficulty beforehand. Examiners individually mark the students on each of the 10 items as P+, P, and P–. P+ denotes excellent or very good, P denotes pass or borderline performance while P– denotes not attaining the pass grade in that item. After all the items have been individually marked, examiners decide overall marks from a designated list of overall marks. It may be a good idea to go through the detailed description of the method (Gleeson, 1997). A sample format for OSLER is available at *http://medind.nic.in/jac/t01/i4/jact01i4p251.pdf.*

Educational consequences of testing are an important consideration in deciding the mode of assessment. OSLER provides a good means to provide good educational feedback to the student. Despite being weak in measurement, it can be used for formative assessment in a big way. This will not make the long case better as a tool for summative assessment however due to content specificity.

Implications: To improve the utility of long case as an assessment tool, we will also need to work on the following:
1. *Increasing the number of cases* so that the process of generalizability can be improved. However, since a long case takes at least 60–90 minutes for workup and presentation, there is a limit to the number of cases that can be included. Theoretical calculations suggest that for an acceptable reliability, we will need to have 480 minutes of testing for the long case, which seems impossible considering the number of students and faculty at our disposal.
2. *Increasing the number of examiners* is another useful strategy. However, some clarity may be needed here. The choice that often needs to be made is having four examiners for one case or four cases for four examiners. Experts suggest that despite bringing some inter-rater variation, four cases for four examiners is a better strategy as it gives better inter-case reliability. This will take care of content specificity of the cases and allow a (slightly) bigger sample of cases.
3. *Training the examiners* for assessment, encouraging pre-examination discussions on what is being assessed and acceptable standards of performance are some other interventions which can help to improve the value of the long case.

If we look at what has been discussed above, the following points emerge. Being closer to real-life settings, the long case presents a real problem to the student but this also works as a disadvantage of using this method as the generalizability of the results becomes less. We also note that it is not the inter-rater variation as much as it is the inter-case variation which is the main cause of low reliability. Lack of clarity about what is being assessed (*clif. construct irrelevance*) lowers the validity. Structuring the assessment of the long case is not likely to result in significant gains in reliability due to the problem of context specificity. Increasing number of cases might be a better option than increasing the precision of measurement. Observing the students during the process brings another construct of history taking into picture and is likely to add to validity. An important use of observation is to generate educationally useful feedback for the student.

What Lessons can we Draw?

The first and foremost is to increase the number of cases (4–6) and ensure that these are representative of the tasks that the students are likely to encounter in later years. In addition, the examiners and the students need to be clear before the examination regarding what is being assessed. In effect, this would mean that long case assessment should no longer be an opportunistic matter—rather it has to be meticulously planned to include cases considered important for that level of students. A fallout of this argument is to get away from the notion to have 'at least one CNS case' (or something similar for surgical branches) for every level of examination.

The second important issue is to appropriately use the time spent on a long case in a productive way. Presuming that the student spends 45 minutes on working up and another 45 minutes on presentation, the first 45 minutes do not contribute to the assessment process. By observing the student during that time, a significant improvement in reliability can be obtained (as it doubles the testing time). It helps to improve validity as well (Dare et al., 2008). We will like to emphasize it here that all such observations need not be checklist based or structured—even global ratings from subject experts can provide a fairly reliable assessment of many of the competencies. It also needs to be kept in mind that observation will lead to only a small increase in the reliability of assessment due to case specificity problem (Norcini, 2001).

Do we retain the long case as a means of summative assessment? Strictly speaking, in view of its low reliability, it should not be used for this purpose. However, keeping the logistics and facilities at our disposal, it stands to reason that the long case needs to stay, but must be supplemented by other tools, especially at postgraduate level. However, the long case offers wonderful opportunities for providing educationally useful feedback to the students as part of formative assessment.

REFERENCES

Dare, A.J., Cardinal, A., Kolbe, J., & Bagg, W. (2008). What can the history tell us? An argument for observed history taking in the trainee intern long case assessment. *New Zealand Medical Journal, 121(1282)*, 51–7.

Dugdale, A. (1996). The long-case clinical examinations. *Lancet, 347(9011)*, 1335.

Gleeson, F. (1997). Assessment of clinical competence using the objective structured long examination record (OSLER). *Medical Teacher, 19*, 7–14.

Hijazi, Z., Premadasa I.G., & Moussa M.A. (2002). Performance of students in the final examination in paediatrics: importance of the "short cases". *Archives Diseases Childhood, 86(1)*, 57–8.

Jolly, B., & Grant, J. (1997). *The good assessment guide.* London: Joint Centre for Education in Medicine.

McKinley, R.K., Fraser, R.C., van der Vleuten, C., & Hastings, A.M. (2000). Formative assessment of the consultation performance of medical students in the setting of general practice using a modified version of Leicester assessment package. *Medical Education, 34(7)*, 573–9.

Mckinley, R., Hastings, S., & Petersen, S. (2005). The long case revisited. *Medical Education, 39(5)*, 442–3.

Norcini, J.J. (2001). The validity of long cases. *Medical Education, 35(8)*, 720–1.

Norcini, J.J. (2002). The death of the long case? *British Medical Journal, 324(7334)*, 408–9.

Norman, G.R., Tugwell, P., Feightner, J.W., Muzzin, L.J., & Jacoby, L.L. (1985). Knowledge and clinical problem-solving. *Medical Education, 19(5)*, 344–56.

Norman, G. (2002). The long case versus objective structured clinical examinations. *British Medical Journal, 324(7340)*, 748–9.

Oslon, L.G., Coughlan, J., Rolfe, I., & Hensley, M.J. (2000). The effect of a structured question grid on the validity and perceived fairness of a medical long case assessment. *Medical Education, 34(1)*, 46–52.

Ponnamperuna, G.G., Karunathilake, I.M., McAleer, S., & Davis, M. (2009). The long case and its modifications: a literature review. *Medical Education, 43(10)*, 936–41.

Rethans, J.J., Sturmans, F., Drop, R., van der Vleuten, C., & Hobus, P. (1991). Does competence of general practitioners predict their performance? Comparison between examination setting and actual practice. *British Medical Journal, 303(6814)*, 1377–80.

Sidhu, R.S., Hatala, R., Baron, S., & Gordon, P. (2009). Reliability and acceptance of the mini-clinical evaluation exercise as a performance assessment of practicing physicians. *Academic Medicine, 84(10 Suppl)*, S113–5.

Sood, R. (2001). Long case examination: can it be improved? *Journal Indian Academy of Clinical Medicine, 2(4)*, 251–5.

Wass, V., & Jolly, B. (2001). Does observation add to the validity of the long case? *Medical Education, 35(8)*, 729–31.

Wass, V., Jones, R., & van der Vleuten, C.P.M. (2001). Standardized or real patients to test clinical competence? The long case revisited. *Medical Education, 35(4)*, 321–5.

Wass, V., & van der Vleuten, C.P.M. (2004). The long case. *Medical Education, 38(11)*, 1176–80.

Chapter 8

Objective Structured Clinical Examination

Piyush Gupta, Pooja Dewan, Tejinder Singh

KEY POINTS

- ☞ Objective structured clinical examination (OSCE) can assess several skills and competencies.
- ☞ Advantages of OSCE accrue from its wider sampling of content than to its objectivity.
- ☞ It is better to move away from one 'competency-one station model' and design stations which test competencies in an integrated manner.
- ☞ Examiner training improves the utility of OSCE.

That learning is driven by assessment is a well-known fact. This is also referred to as the *steering effect of examinations.* To foster actual learning, assessment should be educative and formative. Medical education aims at the production of competent doctors with sound clinical skills. Professional competence encompasses six inter-related domains as developed by the Accreditation Council for Graduate Medical Education (ACGME): (1) knowledge, (2) patient care, (3) professionalism, (4) communication and interpersonal skills, (5) practice-based learning and improvement, and (6) systems-based practice (ACGME, 2002). Various other frameworks of professional competence including the concept of the Indian Medical Graduate have been earlier discussed in Chapter 2. Epstein and Hundert (2002) have defined competence of a physician as "the habitual and judicious use of communication, knowledge, technical skills, clinical reasoning, emotions, values and reflection in daily practice for the benefit of the individuals and the community being served". The community needs to be protected from incompetent physicians; and thus, there is a need for summative component in the assessment of medical graduates.

■ Looking Beyond the Traditional Assessment Tools

The traditional tools for assessment of medical students have mainly consisted of written examinations (essay type, multiple choice, and short-answer type questions), bedside viva and clinical case presentation. These have focused on the 'knows' and 'knows how' aspects, i.e., the focus has been on the base of the Miller pyramid of competence **(Fig. 8.1)**. These methods of assessment however have drawn a lot of criticism over the years because of their inability to assess the top levels of the pyramid of clinical competence.

Some of the common flaws associated with traditional assessments include:

- The sample size of the problems assessed is generally too small, impacting both validity and reliability.
- They test only the factual knowledge and problem-solving skills of students, which may be appropriate only in the early stages of the medical curriculum. These methods do not assess the clinical competence of students. Important aspects like performing a specific physical examination (shows how), clinical manoeuvres, and communication skills are not tested. Only the result is tested and not the process of arriving at a result.
- The students are tested on different patients (*case variability*). Each student is adjudged by only one or two examiners, thereby leaving a scope for marked variation in the marking by different examiners (*examiner variability*). These factors increase the subjectivity of assessment.
- There is often a lack of clarity on what is being tested *(lack of validity)*. Assessment is usually global and not specific competency based. Students are not examined systematically on core competencies.
- There is *no systematic feedback* for the students from teachers.

To obviate the drawbacks of conventional clinical evaluation, OSCE was first introduced in 1975, as a more objective tool of assessment (Harden et al., 1975). In an ideal OSCE, all domains of learning are tested, specially the process part; the examination is organized to assess all students on identical content by the same examiners using predetermined guidelines, and a systematic feedback is obtained from both students and the teachers **(Box 8.1)**. OSCE is meant to test the 'shows how' level of the Miller pyramid (Harden & Gleeson, 1979).

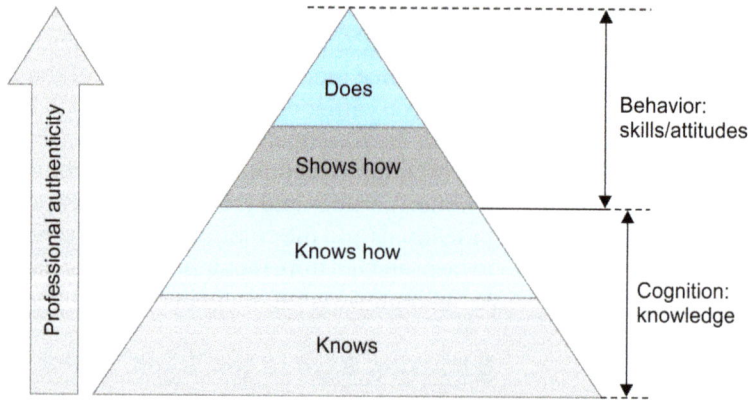

Fig. 8.1: Miller (1990) pyramid.

> **BOX 8.1:** Key features of Objective Structured Clinical Examination (OSCE)
> 1. Assessment of predetermined competencies at 'shows how' level.
> 2. Each competency is broken into components including knowledge, skills, attitudes, and communication required for performance.
> 3. Every student is assessed on the same tasks.
> 4. Each component is observed and assessed using a checklist or global rating.
> 5. Immediate feedback is provided to the student based on direct observation.

What is an Objective Structured Clinical Examination?

Objective structured clinical examination (OSCE) consists of a circuit of stations which are usually connected in series **(Fig. 8.2)**. Each station is devoted to assessment of one specific competency. The student is asked to perform a specific task at each station. These stations assess practical, communication, technical and data interpretation skills and there is a predetermined decision on what is to be tested. Students rotate around the complete circuit of stations and keep on performing the tasks at each of the stations. All students move from one station to another in the same sequence. The performance of students is assessed independently on each station, using a standardized checklist. Thus, all the candidates are presented with the same test, and are assessed by the same or equivalent examiners. Students are marked on a checklist (Gupta & Bisht, 2001) or on the global rating by the examiner.

Types of Objective Structured Clinical Examination Stations

The hallmark of OSCE is a chain of *stations*. These stations are categorized as *procedure stations* or *question stations*. Procedure stations are observed (by the examiner) while question stations are

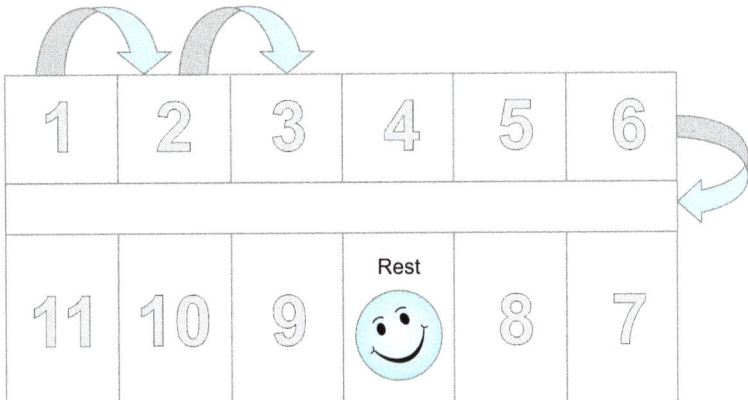

Fig. 8.2: Station map.

unobserved (only a written answer is required). Student performance on a procedure station is marked there and then only, while the question stations can be assessed later.

Procedure Station

At the procedure station, the student is asked to carry out a task in front of an observer who rates the examinee using a checklist. The tasks can be taking a history, performing an examination, counseling, or demonstrating a procedure.

Tables 8.1 to 8.3 (hand wash, resuscitation, history/examination) depict the design of three observed stations specifying the task to be done and the item-wise checklist for each of them. Marks in the checklist are given for each itemized component and these may not be necessarily equal for all items. Items considered to have been performed adequately are awarded full marks; those performed inadequately/poorly or not at all receive zero marks.

Certain procedure stations which assess the student's ability to perform a crucial skill can be designated as *critical.* These are awarded more marks and it is usually mandatory to get pass-marks on these stations to clear the examination.

Role of the Examiners

The examiner restricts herself to marking the provided checklist and refrains from interacting with the student and converting it into a viva voce. The examiner(s) do not interfere with the station setup, simulated patient's role, or the marking scheme. Teaching points are delivered after the examination, during the feedback session.

Question Stations

The student works independently and is not observed by any examiner. Response to certain questions is anticipated, either based on the previous procedure station or chosen to evaluate areas of knowledge, interpretation, problem solving, etc. These may be in the form of simulated patient problems, case histories, laboratory or field data, radiographs, specimens, equipment, clinical photographs, etc. The stations are so designed that the student is unable to answer the questions correctly without using the data provided. The completed answer sheets are evaluated later by comparing with model answers and a key containing the distribution of marks.

Procedure stations and question stations can also be used together. Candidates are given a task to perform in station 1 (which is observed and assessed by an examiner) and the questions are presented later (in station 2). Questions in station 2 are related to station 1 only. This has two advantages: (1) different domains of learning can be assessed by them and (2) the effect of cueing is minimized. An example is given here:

> **Station 1**
> Task: Examine the eyes of this patient.
>
> **Station 2**
> Task: Mark the statements as true or false based on your findings in station 1.
> 1. There is ptosis of left eye.
> 2. There is palsy of the left abducens nerve.
> 3. Direct and consensual light reflexes are absent in the left eye.
> 4. The left optic disk is chalky white on fundoscopy.

You will appreciate that if these questions would have been presented to the learner at station 1 itself, she would not have examined the right eye of the patient.

TABLE 8.1: Example of an observed station related to handwashing

The first part delineates the task to be performed, while the second component provides a candidate's checklist including the mark sheet. The tasks to be performed are broken item-wise and scored accordingly by the observer. A separate checklist is used for each student. The observer is instructed to mark only one response out of two, i.e., adequate or inadequate, for each item respectively.

OSCE Station No.|_____| Max Marks 10|_____| Student Roll No.|_____|

Task: Demonstrate proper technique of handwashing and dressing prior to entering the operation theater.

The Checklist

Items	Max. marks	Adequate	Inadequate
Bares hands up to elbows and removes watch/jewellery	½		
Uses soap/solution and makes lather/foam	½		
Lather			
Cleans/scrubs			
Palms and fingers	½		
Interdigital clefts	½		
Back of hands and knuckles	1		
Thumb	1		
Finger tips	1		
Forearm up to elbow	½		
Scrubs vigorously for 2 minutes	1		
Rinses properly (hand to wrist)	½		
Dries hands	1		
Wears gown and mask correctly	1		
Performs fluently	1		
Grand total	10		

TABLE 8.2: Example of an observed station related to resuscitation

The first part delineates the task to be performed while, the second component provides a candidate's checklist including the mark sheet. The tasks to be performed are broken item-wise and scored accordingly by the observer. A separate checklist is used for each student. The observer is instructed to mark only one response out of two, i.e., adequate or inadequate, for each item respectively.

OSCE Station No.|_____| Max Marks 15|_____| Student Roll No.|_____|

Task: A term baby is born by normal vaginal delivery to a second gravida mother. Amniotic fluid is not stained with meconium. The baby is limp and is not crying. Go ahead with the process of resuscitation with provided mannequin and equipment. You are free to ask for vital signs of the baby from the observer, wherever appropriate.

The Checklist

Items	Max. marks	Adequate	Inadequate
Check supplies	1		
Calls for help and assigns team leader	1		
Performs all basic steps in correct order within 30 seconds	2		
Evaluates/asks for vitals and decides for bag and mask ventilation	1		
*Does not evaluate/skips bag and mask ventilation	–1		
Positions baby and himself correctly	1		
Selects proper size mask	1		
Attaches sPO$_2$ monitor to the baby's palm	1		
Appropriate ventilation (rate and rise)	1		
Evaluates/asks for heart rate after 30 seconds	1		
Takes ventilation corrective steps and decides for chest compression	1		
*Does not evaluate/skips chest compression	–1		
Locates compression area correctly	1		
Uses right method of compression	1		
Compresses consistently at appropriate rate	1		
Connects oxygen and reservoir	1		
Evaluates/asks for heart rate after 45–60 seconds	1		
Takes ventilation corrective steps and decides for medication	1		
*Does not evaluate/skips medications	–1		
Overall conduct of resuscitation is fluent and is able to complete entire process in given time	1		
Grand total	**15**		

*Mark as "yes" or "no" in place of "adequate" or "inadequate" respectively.

TABLE 8.3: Example of an observed station related to examination techniques and etiquette

The first part delineates the task to be performed while, the second component provides a candidate's checklist including the mark sheet. The tasks to be performed are broken item-wise and scored accordingly by the observer. A separate checklist is used for each student. The observer is instructed to mark only one response out of two, i.e., adequate or inadequate, for each item respectively.

OSCE Station No.|_____| Max Marks 15|_____| Student Roll No.|_____|

Task: Examine the scrotal swelling of this 45-year old male.

The checklist

Items	Max. marks	Adequate	Inadequate
Explains to the patient what he is going to do	1		
Seek patient's permission before examining him	1		
Ensures privacy of the patient by using a screen	1		
Asks the patient to expose his whole abdomen and genitalia	1		
Warm hands before examination/ does not cause discomfort to the patient during examination	1		
Examines both sides of scrotum	½ + ½		
Palpates the spermatic cord	1		
Palpates the abdomen	1		
Examines the supraclavicular nodes on both sides	½ + ½		
Thanks the patient before leaving	1		

Rest Stations

It is advisable to incorporate a rest station for every 30–40 minutes into the examination. These stations are included to give the students, observers, and patients a break. They also allow time, if required, to substitute patients at a clinical station or to complete the written leftover task from the previous stations. The rest stations can be designed imaginatively; these may be planned with the intent to relax the examinee and highlighted with some slogan or thought for the student to ponder over.

Objective Structured Clinical Examination Setup: Traditional Design

The number of stations can vary from 12 to 30, though usually 20 stations suffice. The duration of a station is usually determined by the task involved. The usual time allotted is 5 minutes for each station; this includes time for performance as well as execution. The ACGME, however, recommends allocation of 10-15 minutes for each station. The given task may involve history taking, physical examination, and counseling on real or simulated patients, besides procedure demonstration on mannequins, etc. All students begin simultaneously. The number of students appearing in the examination should not exceed the number of stations. Plan two or parallel sessions of OSCE if the number of students exceeds the number of stations. These circuits can be run concurrently, or one after the other, depending on the availability of space, examiners, and other logistics. The entire examination is usually completed within 60-150 minutes.

Preparing for Objective Structured Clinical Examination

For smooth running of OSCE, it is important to make all practical arrangements well ahead of the scheduled examination. The following aspects need consideration.

Venue: Preparing the Station Map

Conduct of OSCE requires a considerable amount of floor space. Stations for clinical examination require a larger space to accommodate the patient and the observer, in addition to the student. Ideally, the OSCE should be conducted in a large single room; a floor area of 2 m^2 is needed to accommodate each station. Large halls with soundproof partitions (to ensure privacy for both patient and the candidates) or several adjacent rooms in the outpatient block or wards, each room housing an OSCE station, can be used. Procedure stations require more floor space compared to response stations. Additional space is needed to brief the examinees and allow patients to rest in between examinations. The transition time from one station to another must be incorporated into the 5 minutes allotted for a station. The position of a station is decided based upon the availability of floor space and finally a *station map* is prepared. A station map serves as the most important tool and reference material for all further preparations **(Fig. 8.2)**.

Equipment and Supplies

Once a station map has been constructed, the next step is to draw up a detailed list of all the equipment and manpower required **(Table 8.4)**. Ensure that the required number of tables and chairs and examination couches with mattresses are procured at least 2-3 days before the examination. Supply of clean and ironed tablecloths, towels, and linen should be ensured. All specimens and equipment

TABLE 8.4: List of materials needed for the conduct of objective structured clinical examination (OSCE)

General
1. Venue: Suitable spacious hall with soundproof partitions, or multiple adjacent rooms, waiting rooms for backup patients, rest rooms, refreshment area, briefing room
2. Furniture: Tables, chairs (for patient, examiner and examinee at each station), beds or examination couches, patient screen, signages, room heater or cooler
3. Timing Device: Stopwatch or bell
4. Stationery: Score sheets, checklists, answer scripts, pens/pencils
5. Manpower: Nurses, orderlies, simulated/real patients, helpers/marshals
6. Catering: Drinking water and food (snacks and lunch)

Station-specific

Station No.	Station description	Basic equipment	Specific needs	Patient requirement
1.	Data interpretation	Table, 1 chair	Calculator	-
2.	Clinical examination of CNS	Patient screen, examination couch/warmer, 2 chairs, heater/blower, handrub, paper napkins	Patellar hammer, cotton wisps, tuning fork	Four simulated patients
3.	Equipment: Phototherapy	Writing desk, 1 chair	Phototherapy equipment with duly labeled parts/components	-
4.	Rest station	Table, 1 chair	A tray with biscuits, napkins	-
5.	Clinical photographs	Mounting board, writing desk, 1 chair	A chart with affixed and labeled photographs	-

should be labeled and/or flagged as per the requirements of the task to be performed at least a day before the examination. Electrical connections, gadgets, and mannequins should be checked to be in good working order. Care should be taken that the disposables used are not thrown after the examination; these can be stored and recycled in subsequent OSCEs.

Clear signage indicating the station numbers, rooms for resting of patients and students, and washrooms help in the smooth conduct of the examination. A timing device—bell or stopwatch—is needed. Refreshments must be available for all examinees, examiners, patients, and staff assisting in conduct of examination.

All the station tasks are printed in big bold letters on at least A4 size paper in clear and unambiguous terms. Similarly, all the checklists for observed stations should be readied and printed in excess of that required. Surplus can always be used later. A copy of each of the tasks, as well as the checklist is kept with two senior persons; in case, any one of them fails to show up on the exact date and time of examination.

Recruitment of Examiners

Conducting an OSCE requires several examiners. This is often considered the strength of this form of assessment where each candidate is assessed by several examiners. At the same time, the reliability and fairness of this examination can be questioned as there may be inconsistency between different examiners. To improve the reliability, all examiners must undergo a structured examiner training to acquaint them with the basic principles of OSCE. This training includes using marked videoed OSCE stations and live OSCE stations, where the group members enact the roles of examinee, examiner, and patient. The process of sensitization starts a month prior to the examination and includes several brief sessions on the overview of the modern assessment techniques with special reference to clinical examination. At the end of these sessions, the participants should be able to define OSCE, design OSCE based on teaching-learning objectives, appreciate the usefulness of OSCE in formative and summative assessment and be conversant of the difficulties, advantages and limitations of this method as compared to the traditional clinical evaluation. A day before the examination, each examiner is finally allotted her station and provided the specific details of that station. They are also shown the checklists for their respective stations and the format of marking is discussed. They are instructed to be objective observers and maintain only the appropriate interaction with the student relevant to the concerned task.

Patient Selection

The use of patients for clinical examination stations is regarded as crucial to ensure authenticity and to build validity (Boursicot & Roberts, 2005). Only those patients who can withstand examination by multiple students for the duration of OSCE (usually 2 hours) should be selected. Child patients should be accompanied by their caregivers. It is important to have an extra patient available for each of the clinical stations. Duplicate patients should have similar clinical presentation so that they can be substituted when the original patient needs a break. The patients should be kept well briefed, warm, and comfortable. They should also be provided with medicines and food during the examination. Patients should be selected and recruited at least a day before. Maintenance of asepsis and temperature is of utmost importance while dealing with clinical examination of the newborns.

Recruitment of Simulated Patients

While real patients add to the validity of OSCE, it may not be appropriate to use real patients in certain situations like testing of communication skills. In such situations, simulated patients are needed. Real patients, when used in the examination, are prone to fatigue, and their cooperation can vary from student to student and it may be advantageous to use simulated patients in such situations. Once the blueprint of the OSCE is ready, simulated patients must be listed. Simulated patients may be actors or trained clinicians (residents, staff nurse, or other paramedic staff). It is may be useful to prepare a database of such actors and clinicians and they can be contacted to ensure their availability for the OSCE. Simulated patients should be trained for their role prior to the examination and given an outline of the proposed role and a draft script. They can be supervised by communication skills teacher or an experienced clinician to ensure a suitable standard. After the OSCE, the simulated patient is debriefed and criticism of the station is invited, which helps with future restructuring of station.

Blueprinting: Preparing the Stations

Once the consensus is reached on the number and type of stations to be included, the next task is to formulate the questions, model keys, and checklists for each station. When planning an OSCE, the learning objectives of the course and the candidates' level of learning need to be kept in mind. The test content needs to be carefully planned against the learning objectives—this is referred to as 'blueprinting' (Wass & Vleuten, 2004). Blueprinting ensures a representative sample of what the student is expected to have achieved. Blueprinting, in practice, consists of preparing a two-dimensional matrix: one axis represents the competencies to be tested (e.g., counseling, procedure, history taking, clinical examination) and the second axis represents the system or problems on which these competencies are to be demonstrated (e.g., cardiovascular system, nutritional assessment, managing cardiac arrest, etc.) (Newble, 2004).

Blueprinting is essential for a higher construct validity of OSCE by defining the problem which the student will encounter and the task within the problem which he is expected to perform. By laying down the competencies to be tested in a grid, the correct balance between different domains to be tested can be obtained **(Table 8.5)**.

Clinical skills (including psychomotor skills and certain affective skills) should be primarily identified and included in the OSCE setup. OSCE can test a wide range of skills ranging from data gathering to problem solving (Harden & Gleeson, 1979). OSCE is not very suitable for evaluating the cognitive domain of learning, and certain behaviors like work ethics, professional conduct, and teamwork skills. For these objectives, it is appropriate to use other modes of assessment. Feasibility of the task is equally important. Real patients are more suited for assessing the learner's examination skills, while simulated patients are more suited to evaluate the communication skills of the learner.

TABLE 8.5: Grid showing the OSCE blueprint for final year medical students*

	History	Examination	Procedure/Data interpretation
Cardiovascular system (CVS)	Chest pain	CVS	ECG interpretation; blood pressure
Chest	Fast breathing and cough	Respiratory system	Chest physiotherapy/ Peak flow
Abdomen	Abdominal distention	Abdomen examination	Ascitic tap
Central nervous system (CNS)	Headache	Nervous system/Eyes	Fundoscopy
Cardiac arrest			Cardiopulmonary resuscitation (CPR)

* Representative example only

Much effort and resources are needed to prepare an OSCE station. Each station needs to be written in advance of scheduled dates and enough time should be made available for pretesting the station before the actual assessment. Blueprint of an OSCE station must be detailed and the following components must be included:

* *Instructions to the examinees* indicating the exact task to be performed at the station.
* *Instructions to the examiners* specifying the exact skill to be assessed. The examiner is provided a checklist to score the student's performance. The contents of these checklists have been decided upon by a panel of examiners in advance.
* *Examiner score sheets* are to be prepared in advance and in sufficient number keeping the number of candidates in mind.
* *List of equipment* needed at each station must be prepared in advance, e.g., equipment like infantometer, weighing scale, and measuring tape must be available at a station where the examinee is needed to perform anthropometric examination.
* *Real and simulated patients* needed in the OSCE must be listed beforehand including details like age, sex, ethnicity, and the role to be played by the patient.
* *Duration of each OSCE station* must be specified. The usual duration of a station is 5 minutes and may be 10 minutes at some stations.

Conducting the Objective Structured Clinical Examination

All the stations are set up on the day of examination, though the furniture and station identification numbers are arranged a day before. The examiners should reach the venue of examination 2 hours prior to start of the examination. The students are called in 1 hour before the

OSCE is scheduled to start. If possible, students are rotated through the examination setup, before the questions are pasted. This will familiarize them with the flow of stations. The tasks/questions are pasted on the respective stations 30 minutes before ringing the first bell. Examiners are also handed over the checklists simultaneously.

Students' briefing: Students are briefed on the methodology of the examination. Each one of them is handed over a station map **(Fig. 8.2)** along with an answer book to record their answers on unobserved stations. The first station for each student is marked on his/her respective station map. If the students had not encountered this mode of examination in the past, they are instructed on how to move between stations with the help of the map. The students are also informed about the type of stations and reminded about the rest station. They are asked to display their roll numbers prominently on the lapels of their coats/aprons for ease of marking by the observer on procedure stations. The candidates are then escorted to the examination area. As the first bell sounds, the students disperse to their respective allocated first stations. The timekeeper rings the bell loud and clear enough to be heard at all stations. This should be prechecked. The bell is sounded at intervals of 5 minutes and a record of the elapsed time and the number of bells sounded is maintained.

Feedback

After the OSCE, the group of students is taken around all the stations and a feedback is provided to them with a breakdown of how they have performed at each station by the respective observer. Feedback is also given on the unobserved stations and model answers provided. The theme and aims of individual stations are outlined, correct response and/or procedure is informed and common mistakes committed by the students are emphasized. Lastly, the candidates are asked to provide a structured feedback on the entire exercise. The feedback should include their observations, suggestions for improvement, and future expectations.

Setting Standards

A major impediment in the success of OSCE remains setting the pass mark. OSCEs assess the clinical competence, so the standards for passing OSCE can be either relative (based on norm-referencing) or absolute (based on criterion-referencing).

Norm-referencing

Angoff approach and borderline approach are commonly used to set relative standards for OSCE. In the former, expert judges determine Angoff pass marks based on their estimates of the probability that a borderline examinee will succeed on each item in a test (Angoff, 1971). A major drawback of this method is that the overall performance of a candidate is not judged. Also, the estimates are based keeping a hypothetical candidate in mind and therefore may be incorrect. This way different pass marks will be set across different medical institutions (Boursicot et al., 2007). In addition, this is a time-consuming process and requires greater commitment from the examiners. A minimum of 10 judges are required to obtain reliable results (Kaufman et al., 2000).

The borderline approach (Dauphinee et al., 1997) is a simpler and more commonly accepted method for setting the pass marks. In this method, the expert judges score examinees at each station according to a standardized checklist and then give a global rating of each student's overall performance. The student can be rated as pass, borderline, fail, or above expected standard. The mean of examinees rated as borderline becomes the pass mark for the station and the sum of the means becomes the overall pass mark (Smee & Blackmore, 2001). To increase the reliability of this method, all the expert judges should be physicians and several examiners should examine at each station. The Otago study (Wilkinson et al., 2001) showed that 6 examiners per station and 180 examinees are needed to produce valid and reliable pass marks. This method has gained wider acceptance because the pass marks set are actually an average of differences in opinion of examiners unlike the *Angoff marks* which are obtained by arguing out the differences in opinion of the examiners.

Wass et al. (2004) state that "norm-referencing is clearly unacceptable for clinical competency licensing tests, which aim to ensure that candidates are safe to practice. A clear standard needs to be defined, below which a doctor would not be judged fit to practice. Such standards are set by criterion-referencing."

Criterion-referencing

An absolute clear-cut minimum accepted cutoff is decided beforehand (Cusimano, 1996). For example, the Medical Council of India (MCI) recommends 50% as the minimum pass marks for all summative examinations in medical specialties. The National Board of Examination (NBE), India also accepts overall 50% marks as minimum acceptable for passing in its OSCE examinations. A problem with using the overall pass mark as a benchmark for competence may not be acceptable as exceptional performance in a few stations would compensate for poor performance in other stations. It would be more appropriate to decide upon a minimum total score and a defined proportion of stations which the examinee must pass in order to pass the OSCE (Smee & Blackmore, 2001). Certain institutions also make it mandatory to pass the critical stations. *However, till date there is no consensus regarding use of criterion-referenced or norm-referenced assessment.* The purpose of the test guides the choice of an approach.

Checklists versus Global Rating

Checklists were designed and incorporated into OSCE to increase the objectivity and reliability of marking by different examiners. However, scoring against a checklist may not be as effective as it was thought to be (Reznick et al., 1998). Evidence is accumulating that global rating by an experienced physician is as reliable as the standardized checklist. Regehr et al. (1998) compared the psychometric properties of checklists and global rating scales for assessing competencies on an OSCE format examination and concluded that global rating scales scored by experts showed higher inter-station reliability, better construct validity, and better concurrent validity than did checklists. These results suggest that global rating scales administered by experts are a more appropriate summative measure when assessing candidates on performance-based assessment. However, there is still no consensus on the gold standard for the same. A balanced approach is suggested by Newble (2004) wherein checklists may be used for practical and technical skills stations and global rating scales are employed for stations pertaining to communication skills and diagnostic tasks. An example of global rating format is shown in **Table 8.6**.

TABLE 8.6: Example of a global rating scale for assessing communication skills

Task: *This 35 years old mother is HIV positive. Counsel her about feeding her newborn baby.*
The student is rated on a scale of 1–5. The examiner score sheet would read as follows:

1. Exceptional
2. Good
3. Average
4. Borderline
5. Poor/Fail

Note: A checklist can be provided to assist the examiner in making her judgment of the student's performance, though no marks are decided for each item on the checklist. Using a checklist for a global rating can enhance the validity and reliability of OSCE.

For example, in the above task, the examiner can look for the following points:
1. Makes the mother feel comfortable/greets the mother
2. Makes eye-to-eye contact with the mother by sitting down by her side before communicating with her
3. Asks open questions
4. Praises the mother
5. Emphasizes
6. Offers relevant information
7. Provides the mother an opportunity to choose the feeding option
8. Plans a follow-up visit
9. Thanks the mother before leaving

Concerns

Objective structured clinical examination, now into fourth decade since it was first used in 1975 to assess medical students' clinical competence, has had its share of bouquets and brickbats. Despite controversies, it has stood the test of the time and has come to be recognized as a standard tool for assessment of clinical competence. OSCE has been used for both formative and summative assessment at the graduate and postgraduate levels, across the globe.

However, there is a Mr Hyde side to this Dr Jekyll. **Table 8.7** outlines the factors that can affect the generalizability, validity, reliability, and practicality of OSCE. OSCE remains a toothless exercise if these factors are not taken care of. Unfortunately, that is what is happening at most of the places where OSCE is now being introduced. A detailed discussion follows:

TABLE 8.7: Factors affecting the utility of OSCE

Factor	Limitation
Number of stations	Requires a minimum of 14–18 stations. Lesser the number, lesser the reliability, and lesser the validity
Time for assessment	Lesser the time-lesser the reliability. A 10-minute station is more reliable as compared to a 5-minute station
Improperly standardized patients	Limits reliability and validity
Individualized way of scoring	Limits reliability
Assessing only one component at a time	Limits validity
Lack of item analysis	Affects reliability
Skill of the person preparing the checklist	May hamper objectivity; limits validity and reliability
Number of procedure stations	Lesser the number, lesser the number of clinical competencies that can be tested. Content specificity of stations limits reliability
Problematic stations	Decrease reliability
Improper checklists	May not exactly replicate an actual clinical encounter, limits validity
Blueprinting	Increases validity
Limitations to what can be assessed	Not useful for assessing the learning behavior, dedication to patients, and longitudinal care of patients
Expensive and labour-intensive	Limits practicality and feasibility

Feasibility and Practicality

It is agreed that the exercise is very resource-intensive in terms of manpower, labour, time, and money; requires very careful organization;

and meticulous planning (Harden & Gleeson, 1979). Training of examiners and patients, and preparation of stations and their checklists are a time-consuming affair. Cost is high both, in human resource needs and money spent in terms of patient (actor) payment, trainer payment, building rental or utilities, personnel payment, student time, case development, patient training, people to monitor and videotaping. Most OSCEs are administered in outpatient facilities of medical centers. A separate room or cubicle is needed for each station and this may be difficult to administer in smaller setups.

The problem is more acute in developing countries and resource-poor settings where a medical teacher must assume the role of a consultant, service provider, researcher, and administrator. This way, there is not much time the educator can spend on planning, preparing and executing an OSCE. This results in an OSCE which is more of hype and less of true assessment.

Objectivity

The objectivity of OSCE is determined by the skill of the experts who prepare the OSCE stations and checklists. Over the years, however, enthusiasm in developing detailed checklists (for increasing the objectivity) has led to another problem, i.e., 'trivialization'. The task is fragmented into too many small components and all of them may not be clinically relevant for managing a patient. Higher objectivity also does not imply that global ratings (which are by and large subjective) are an inferior tool for assessment, especially in the hands of expert. Global ratings are generally better for skills like communication and professionalism.

Validity

Content validity can only be ensured by proper blueprinting (Newble, 2004). Following this, each task must be standardized and there must be itemization of its components using appropriate scoring checklists. Blueprinting also ensures creation of multi-modality OSCE stations that increases the validity (Walters et al., 2005).

Objective structured clinical examination is not suited to assess the competencies like longitudinal care of patients, sincerity and dedication of the examinee to patient care, and long-term learning habits (Barman, 2005; Vleuten & Schuwirth, 2005).

Mavis et al. (1996) have questioned the validity of OSCE by arguing that "observing a student perform a physical examination in OSCE is not a performance-based assessment, unless data from this task is used to generate a master problem list or management strategy". Brown et al. (1987) have questioned the predictive and concurrent validity of OSCE by observing that the correlation between the students' result on OSCE and other assessment tools is low.

It would be appropriate to use OSCE to assess specific clinical skills and combine it with other methods to judge the overall competency. Verma and Singh (1993) concluded that OSCE needs to be combined with clinical case presentation for a comprehensive assessment. Panzarella and Manyon (2007) have recently suggested a model for integrated assessment of clinical competence studded with supportive features of OSCE (ISPE: Integrated Standardized Patient Examination) to increase the overall validity.

Improving Reliability

Reliability refers to the reproducibility and consistency of a set of measurements over time and using different samples of items. The factors can make OSCE an unreliable method of assessment like fewer stations, time constraints, lack of standardized patients, trainer inconsistency, and student fatigue due to lengthy OSCEs. A lot of variation has been reported when different raters have observed a station, and also between performance from one station to another. Larger the number of stations, greater is the inter-rater reliability.

High levels of reliability can be achieved only with a longer OSCE session (of 4–8 hours) (Walters et al., 2005). The reliability of a one- and two-hour session is as low as 0.54 and 0.69, respectively, which can be increased to 0.82 and 0.9 in a four- or eight-hour session, respectively (Vleuten & Schuwirth, 2005). However, it is impractical to conduct an OSCE of more than three hours duration. Newble and Swanson (1988) were able to increase the reliability of a 90-minute OSCE from 0.6 to 0.8 by combining it with a 90-minute free-response item written test, covering the problems included in the OSCE.

Item analysis of OSCE station and exclusion of problem stations is a useful exercise to improve the reliability of total OSCE scores (Auewarakul et al., 2005). Reliability can be improved by ensuring content validity and by increasing the number of stations so that enough items can be sampled.

Integrating Competencies

The OSCE model suggested by Harden et al., (1975) revolves around the basic principle of 'one competency-one task-one station'. Skills were assessed in an isolated manner within a short time span. This does not happen in the real-life scenario where the student must perform all his skills in an integrated manner with an ultimate aim to benefit the individual and the community. The contemporary educational theory also stipulates that integration of tasks facilitates learning (Vleuten & Schuwirth, 2005). It is imperative thus that the OSCE moves to integrated assessment. For example, dietary history taking, and nutritional counseling can be integrated at one Station; similarly, chest examination and advising chest physiotherapy (based on the physical findings) can be integrated.

Indian Experiences with Objective Structured Clinical Examination

The OSCE has by and large been used as an assessment tool for formative assessment of undergraduate medical students at a few centers (Verma & Singh, 1993; Mathews et al., 2004). Many of the faculty are not oriented to its use, and not many universities have incorporated it in their summative assessment plan for the undergraduates. Another main reason for hesitancy, we feel, is the lack of training and time required on the part of the faculty to initiate and sustain a quality OSCE. A good number of teachers continue to use OSCE as a test of theory rather than as a test of skills.

Modifications and Innovations

The current format of OSCE has been modified in order to provide direct feedback to students based on observations of their skills. This helps students to work upon improving their doctor-patient relationship skills, and ability to perform a focused history and physical examination. This form of active teaching-learning has been used for both undergraduate and postgraduate medical students. The various modifications of OSCE include:

1. **Group Objective Structured Clinical Examination (GOSCE):** The GOSCE assesses students in a group setting wherein students rotate in groups of 4-8, and one student is selected randomly to perform at each station. The performing student is observed by the remaining students of the group and the observer faculty, who provide feedback. It has been used as a self-assessment and learning tool in both undergraduate and postgraduate medical education, especially in resource-poor settings. It is particularly effective in formative assessment and has the benefit of providing peer feedback. It has been found to be particularly useful in teaching communication skills and developing clinical reasoning (Konopasek et al., 2014).
2. **Team Objective Structured Clinical Examination (TOSCE):** Healthcare involves collaborative working between medicine and allied branches like midwives, paramedical health professions, nursing staff, physiotherapists, dietitians, social workers, etc. However, lack of teamwork, adequate communication between team members, rigid hierarchical framework in healthcare and the use of different approaches by team members can be a major impediment in healthcare. TOSCE has been developed as a teaching aid to develop interprofessional competence (Symonds et al., 2003). A team of 3-6 members can rotate between the stations as a group and are assessed by an observer (faculty) while they perform tasks turn-wise (Singleton et al., 1999). The team comprises of students of allied specialties and each member is encouraged to swap roles. For

example, at a resuscitation station, a group of medical student(s), nursing student(s), and social worker(s) are expected to perform resuscitation on a patient and communicate to the relatives of the patient. The social worker and nursing student could be assigned the role of a nurse and physician respectively, while the medical student could be asked to communicate the event to the relatives. The observer would assess the competency of each student and provide individual feedback at the end. Role swapping in TOSCE helps to promote understanding role of other disciplines, shared decision-making, problem-solving, handling unexpected events (emergency care), giving feedback and closure. TOSCE helps students realize the importance and challenges faced by other disciplines, developing effective communication, understanding the need for role delineation and developing leadership skills and assuming complementary roles.

3. **Remote Objective Structured Clinical Examination (ReOSCE)/ Web-based Objective Structured Clinical Examination/ Telemedicine Objective Structured Clinical Examination (TeleOSCE):** It is a distance learning tool wherein the examiner can be in a remote location, trainees can be in a far-away location, or even remote standardized patients can be used. The TeleOSCE format has been shown to be a useful method to centrally administer clinical skills examinations for assessment of distance medical students (Palmer et al., 2015) in a cost-effective way. It is also an effective e-learning method in medical education.

4. **Computer Assisted Objective Structured Clinical Examination (CA-OSCE):** One of the major disadvantages of the traditional OSCE is the need for many patients and their cooperation which can be a task. Other problems with traditional OSCE include observer fatigue, need for large number of observers/faculty, and the time and effort needed for setting up several stations. These problems can be circumvented to some extent with the use of CA-OSCE (Brazeau et al., 2002). In contrast to the conventional OSCE where real patients are used, CA-OSCE makes use of virtual patients. A major limitation of this format is that the actual interaction with the standardized patient is not graded and hence the affective domain is not assessed. Also, it is not useful for assessing the psychomotor

---

BOX 8.2: Key points

- Properly designed objective structured clinical examination (OSCE) can test a variety of competencies.
- It is better to move away from the 'one competency-one station' model and design stations to test competencies in an integrated way.
- Advantages of OSCE accrue from wider sampling rather than objectivity.
- OSCE can be modified to serve as not only an assessment tool but also for active teaching and self-assessment.

domain of learning. However, it may be useful to incorporate this modality for assessment in resource-poor countries and for medical specialties like dermatology where the use of simulators is very limited. It may be used to design hybrid OSCE wherein CA-OSCE is used as an adjunct to the traditional OSCE (limited station OSCE).

5. **Admission OSCE: Multiple Mini-Interview (MMI):** It is a type of OSCE which assesses the student at the time of her entry in a medical course. While interviews rely solely on a student's academic excellence and cognitive ability, the MMI has the advantage of also assessing other skills, such as communication, professionalism, and aptitude to determine her suitability to join the medical profession (Eva et al., 2004). It can comprise of about 10–12 short OSCE-style stations, in which students can be presented with scenarios that require them to display their communication skills, discuss a health-related issue with an interviewer, or answer the conventional interview questions. It has been discussed in more details in Chapter 10.

Conclusion

All said and done, it is generally agreed that OSCE tests competency in fragments and is not entirely replicable in real-life scenarios. OSCE is useful for formative assessment and can be continued for this purpose. However, on its own, it cannot be relied upon to fulfill the three necessary prerequisites for a summative assessment as laid down by Epstein (2007), i.e., promote future learning, protect the public by identifying incompetent physicians, and choosing candidates for further training. Limited generalizability, weak linkages to curriculum, and little opportunity provided for improvement in examinees' skill have been cited as the reasons for replacing OSCE with alternative methods in certain medical schools (Mavis et al., 1996).

On a closer look, there are gaps with respect to objectivity, validity, and reliability of this tool, especially in resource-poor settings. It is costly and time-consuming. It does not measure the essential professional competencies including ability to work in a team, professional ethical behavior, and ability to reflect on own performance (self-appraisal). At best, it can be considered as a supplementary tool to other methods of assessment in the final examination. For a summative assessment, OSCE should not constitute more than one-third of the total assessment scheme.

REFERENCES

Accreditation Council for Graduate Medical Education (ACGME). (2002). *Outcome project*. [online] Available from http://www.acgme.org/Outcome/ [Last accessed August, 2020].

Angoff, W.H. (1971). Scales, norms, and equivalent scores. In: Thorndike, R.L. (Ed). *Educational measurement*. (pp. 508–600). Washington, DC: American Council on Education.

Auewarakul, C., Downing, S.M., Praditsuwan, R., & Jaturatamrong, U. (2005). Item analysis to improve reliability for an internal medicine undergraduate OSCE. *Advances in Health Sciences Education, 10,* 105–13.

Barman, A. (2005). Critiques on the objective structured clinical examination. *Annals, & Academy of Medicine, Singapore, 34(8),* 478–82.

Boursicot, K., & Roberts, T. (2005). How to set up an OSCE. *Clinical Teacher, 2(1),* 16–20.

Boursicot, K.A., Roberts, T.E., & Pell, G. (2007). Using borderline methods to compare passing standards for OSCEs at graduation across three medical schools. *Medical Education, 41,* 1024–31.

Brazeau, C., Boyd, L., & Crosson, J. (2002). Changing an existing OSCE to a teaching tool: the making of a teaching OSCE. *Academic Medicine, 77(9),* 932.

Brown, B., Roberts, J., Rankin, J., Stevens, B., Tompkins, C., & Patton, D. (1987). Further developments in assessing clinical competence. In: Hart, I.R., Harden R.M. and Walton H.J. (Eds). *Further developments in assessing clinical competence.* Montreal: Canadian Health Publications. pp. 563–71.

Cusimano, M.D. (1996). Standard setting in medical education. *Academic Medicine, 71(Suppl 10),* S112–20.

Dauphinee, W.D., Blackmore, D.E., Smee, S.M., Rothman, A.I., & Reznick, R.K. (1997). Using the judgements of physician examiners in setting the standards for a national multi-center high stakes OSCE. *Advances in Health Sciences Education: Theory and Practice, 2(3),* 201–11.

Epstein, R.M., & Hundert, E.M. (2002). Defining and assessing professional competence. *Journal of the American Medical Association, 287(2),* 226–35.

Epstein, R.M. (2007). Assessment in medical education. *New England Journal of Medicine, 356(4),* 387–96.

Eva, K.W., Rosenfeld, J., Reiter, H.I., & Norman, G.R. (2004). An admission OSCE: the multiple mini-interview. *Medical Education, 38(3),* 314–26.

Gupta, P., & Bisht, H.J. (2001). Practical approach to running an objective structured clinical examination in neonatology for the formative assessment of medical undergraduates. *Indian Pediatrics, 38(5),* 500–13.

Harden, R.M., & Gleeson, F.A. (1979). Assessment of clinical competence using objective structure clinical examination (OSCE). *Medical Education, 13(1),* 41–54.

Harden, R.M., Stevenson, W., Downie, W.W., & Wilson, G.M. (1975). Assessment of clinical competence using an objective structured clinical examination. *British Medical Journal, 1,* 447–51.

Kaufman, D.M., Mann, K.V., Muijtjens, A.M., & van der Vleuten, C. (2000). A comparison of standard setting procedures for an OSCE in undergraduate medical education. *Academic Medicine, 75(3),* 267–71.

Konopasek, L., Kelly, K.V., Bylund, C.L., Wenderoth, S., & Storey-Johnson, C. (2014). The group objective structured clinical experience: building communication skills in the clinical reasoning context. *Patient Education and Counseling, 96(1),* 79–85.

Mathews, L., Menon, J., & Mani, N.S. (2004). Micro-OSCE for assessment of undergraduates. *Indian Pediatrics, 41(2),* 159–63.

Harden, R.M., & Gleeson, F.A. (1979). Assessment of clinical competence using objective structure clinical examination (OSCE). *Medical Education, 13(1),* 41–54.

Harden, R.M., Stevenson, M., Downie, W.W., & Wilson, G.M. (1975). Assessment of clinical competence using objective structured examination. *British Medical Journal,* 1(5955), 447–51.

Mavis, B.E., Henry, R.C., Ogle, K.S., & Hoppe, R.B. (1996). The Emperor's new clothes: OSCE reassessed. *Academic Medicine, 71(5)*, 447–53.

Newble, D., & Swanson, D. (1988). Psychometric characteristics of the objective structured clinical examination. *Medical Education, 22(4)*, 325–34.

Newble, D. (2004). Techniques of measuring clinical competence: objective structured clinical examination. *Medical Education, 38(2)*, 199–203.

Palmer, R.T., Biagioli, F.E., Mujcic, J., Schneider, B.N., Spires, L., & Dodson, L.G. (2015). The feasibility and acceptability of administering a telemedicine objective structured clinical exam as a solution for providing equivalent education to remote and rural learners. *Rural and Remote Health, 15(4)*, 3399.

Panzarella, K.J., & Manyon, A.T. (2007). A model for integrated assessment of clinical competence. *Journal of Allied Health, 36(3)*, 157–64.

Regehr, G., MacRae, H., Reznick, R.K., & Szalay, D. (1998). Comparing the psychometric properties of checklists and global rating scales for assessing performance on an OSCE-format examination. *Academic Medicine, 73(9)*, 993–7.

Reznick, R.K., Regehr, G., Yee, G., Rothman, A., Blackmore, D., & Dauphinee, D. (1998). Process-rating forms versus task-specific checklists in an OSCE for medical licensure. *Academic Medicine, 73*, S97–9.

Singleton, A., Smith, F., Harris, T., Ross-Harper, R., & Hilton, S. (1999). An evaluation of the team objective structured clinical examination (TOSCE). *Medical Education, 33(1)*, 34–41.

Smee, S.M., & Blackmore, D.E. (2001). Setting standards for an objective structured clinical examination: the borderline group method gains ground on Angoff. *Medical Education, 35(11)*, 1009–10.

Symonds, I., Cullen, L., & Fraser, D. (2003). Evaluation of a formative interprofessional team objective structured clinical examination (ITOSCE): a method of shared learning in maternity education. *Medical Teacher, 25(1)*, 38–41.

Van der Vleuten, C.P.M., & Schuwirth, L.W. (2005). Assessing professional competence: from methods to programmes. *Medical Education, 39*, 309–17.

Verma, M., & Singh, T. (1993). Attitudes of medical students towards objective structured clinical examination (OSCE) in pediatrics. *Indian Pediatrics, 30(10)*, 1259–61.

Wass, V., & van der Vleuten, C.P.M. (2004). The long case. *Medical Education, 38(11)*, 1176–80.

Walters, K., Osborn, D., & Raven, P. (2005). The development, validity and reliability of a multimodality objective structured clinical examination in psychiatry. *Medical Education, 39(3)*, 292–8.

Wilkinson, T.J., Newble, D.I., & Frampton, C.M. (2001). Standard setting in an objective structured clinical examination: use of global ratings of borderline performance to determine the passing score. *Medical Education, 35*, 1043–9.

Chapter 9

Direct Observation-based Assessment of Clinical Skills

Jyoti N Modi, Tejinder Singh

KEY POINTS

- Direct observation-based assessments provide an opportunity to assess the process as well as the product.
- They help to make the feedback authentic by basing it on directly observed behavior.
- They help to improve the learning of clinical and analytical skills.
- Competencies like communication, empathy, and professionalism can be assessed during direct observation.
- These methods are mostly useful for workplace-based assessment.

The practice of medicine involves complex integration of knowledge, psychomotor skills, attitudes, communication skills, reasoning, and judgment; hence a holistic assessment of these in authentic or real settings is most representative of what a trainee will do in future professional life. 'Seeing is believing' is an age-old proverb and it is not difficult to imagine that assessing by directly observing the trainee would give the trainers (faculty) a high degree of confidence in their decision about the abilities of the trainee. With an increasing emphasis on competency-base d training, it is crucial to assess the abilities (competencies) of the student comprehensively rather than as assessment of individual component skills (Modi et al., 2015).

Skills and competencies develop in stages over a period of time implying that there are intermediate stages that eventually lead to a competent trainee who can function independently (Epstein, 2007). Therefore, the assessment plan during the course of training must also be developmental, i.e., assessed by using methods suitable for each stage of training (Holmboe et al., 2010).

As already discussed in Chapter 2, the conceptual framework of Miller pyramid is essential to planning the assessment during various stages of training (Miller, 1990). The bottom two levels of the pyramid, i.e., 'knows' and 'knows how' form the cognitive base and are more readily amenable to assessment by written tests. The next level 'shows how' refers to the practical demonstration of the acquired skills, attitudes, behaviors, and clinical judgment in a controlled environment or in examination settings. The importance of this level of assessment cannot be overemphasized since it provides a 'safe' setting for testing of competencies without undue risks to the patient. This also provides a relatively non-threatening environment for the student to practice clinical skills. The highest level of the pyramid is the 'does' level and it refers to the actual performance by the trainee in real and authentic clinical settings, e.g., in the outpatient clinics, in the ward or while doing an actual procedure. At the top two levels of pyramid, the assessment is based on direct observation of the trainee by the trainers (and sometimes also by peers, co-workers or even patients). This, however, does not imply compartmentalization of assessment methods since while assessing at 'shows how' and 'does' levels, there is a built-in component of assessment of knowledge and its application.

Skills, attitudes, behaviors, and soft skills such as communication are best tested by observation. Direct observation also augments the effectiveness of developmental feedback. The role of feedback as the most powerful influence on learners' progress is well established. Immediate feedback on an observed behavior is best integrated in the assessment tool itself.

Some of the commonly used observation-based assessment methods are mentioned in **Table 9.1**.

TABLE 9.1: Direct observation-based assessment methods

Setting	Tools
Controlled testing environment: examination hall, special designated area for testing, computer laboratories, simulation laboratories.	❖ Objective structured clinical examination (OSCE) ❖ Standardized patients (SP) ❖ Simulations or virtual reality-based assessment ❖ Objective structured long examination record (OSLER)
Real, clinical settings such as the outpatient clinic, wards, procedure rooms, etc., while actual working.	❖ Mini-clinical evaluation exercise (mini-CEX) ❖ Direct observation of procedural skills (DOPS) ❖ Acute care assessment tool (ACAT) ❖ Professionalism mini-evaluation exercise (P-MEX) ❖ Multisource feedback (MSF)/360° assessment/mini-peer assessment tool (mini-PAT)

In this chapter, we will discuss some of the commonly used methods for direct observation-based assessment of clinical skills. You will find detailed discussion of some other methods in Chapters 13.

Objective Structured Clinical Examination

The Objective Structured Clinical Examination (OSCE) was introduced as an improvement over the traditional long case for assessment of clinical competence. First proposed by Harden et al. (1975), its purpose was to make assessment objective by structuring, and standardizing it so that all trainees are tested in the same clinical contexts and on uniform parameters by direct observation of tasks performed by them. In OSCE, trainees rotate through a series of task stations spending about 5-10 minutes at each station. Usually, there are 15-20 stations and the time taken is about 2-4 hours. The tasks at these stations could be history taking, clinical examination, interpretation of clinical or laboratory data, performing procedures, communicating or counseling. This allows testing for a wider range of clinical or practical skills and more clinical contexts rather than just 1-2 cases. Multiple examiners and a structured pattern of marking are expected to reduce the influence of examiner bias. With an increasing experience and a better understanding of the utility of the method, OSCE has undergone several modifications and has evolved as a richer and more versatile tool than was perhaps originally envisaged. The details of setting up an OSCE and its psychometrics are discussed in Chapter 8. Some salient points that highlight the evolution of OSCE to its present form are as below:

- **Type of stations:** Originally, two types of stations were described—a history/examination/procedure station where the trainee was observed and marked by an examiner, followed by a question station that was based on the data gathered by the trainee in the earlier station. Subsequently stations such as data interpretation, problem solving, and counseling stations have also been developed.
- **'One station-one task-one competency' model to 'one station-multiple domains-multiple competencies' model:** Tasks are designed such that they test the ability of the trainee to integrate knowledge, clinical or procedural skills and relevant communication skills rather than testing of a single skill (Vleuten & Schuwirth, 2005). The marking for the task includes credit for multiple domains as well as for overall performance at the said station.
- **Checklists to global ratings:** Initially, standardized and itemized checklists were used for marking by the observer/examiner to ensure objectivity and uniformity in marking. Over time, global rating scales with qualitative input by the subject expert examiner have been preferred. They have been found to be better measures in terms of reliability and validity (Regehr et al, 1998). The choice of type of marking must depend on the task at the station, the competencies observed and the expertise of the observer. Soft skills are better marked on a global rating scale while procedural skills may be better marked on an itemized checklist or a combination. A less experienced examiner or a standardized patient may do better with an itemized checklist.

- **Blueprinting:** Blueprinting while planning the OSCE contributes to an improved validity of this tool. A well-planned rubric of competencies to be tested and the subject areas to be assessed can better align assessment with the expected outcomes. Additionally, it is suggested that resource availability, and feasibility must also be factored in while deciding the level of skill testing in the blueprint.
- **Emphasis on 'soft skills' assessment:** A deliberate effort is now made to include observation and assessment of 'soft skills' at OSCE stations, e.g., behavior during history taking or examination, counseling skills, body language, and professional behavior. Inclusion of these items in the marking sheet reflects their importance and conveys the same to students. The OSCEs provide a safe setting for assessing and learning these skills.
- **Emphasis on immediate or early feedback:** After the trainee has carried out the task and has been marked for it at a station, the last few minutes after completion of the examination are kept for provision of feedback by the observer. Providing immediate or early feedback augments the formative function of assessment. In fact, feedback by the observing examiner is now sometimes incorporated as a part of an OSCE station.

The *strength* of the OSCE lies not so much in being standardized or objectivized, but in that it presents a unique opportunity for wider content sampling, direct observation of the trainee, and a provision for immediate feedback (Sood & Singh, 2012). The major *limitations* of OSCE are that it is conducted in examination settings and not in authentic settings, and that it is inherently resource- and effort-intensive. It has been tried with success as a tool for in-training assessment in limited institutions in India but with time, more institutions are gradually adopting it (Gupta et al., 2010).

Mini-clinical Evaluation Exercise

Like the OSCE, the origin of the mini-Clinical Evaluation Exercise (mini-CEX) was developed to improve the traditional long case. The focus was on making it observable rather than objectivizing or standardizing it. In the 1970s, the American Board of Internal Medicine (ABIM) replaced the traditional long case viva voce examination with the CEX, wherein the examiner observed the trainee during the entire process of history taking and physical examination of a new real patient, and this was followed by case presentation and discussion (Norcini, 2005). The whole exercise took about 2 hours and the trainee was assessed only on 1–2 clinical conditions in the entire examination. The use of real patients contributed to the authenticity of the assessment; however, its duration posed a limitation since in real situations, the patient encounters are much shorter and there is much less time to assess, comprehend, and develop a plan of management. The number of examiners in this form of assessment was also limited.

The mini-CEX was introduced as a more focused and a shorter form of CEX, with multiple clinical encounters spread over a longer duration of training. Described by Norcini et al. in 1995, this tool has been widely used in the Western world during residency training (Norcini, 2005). While only a few institutions in India have utilized it on a regular basis, the reports of its use are encouraging (Singh & Sharma, 2010). The mini-CEX involves observation of the trainee by a supervising faculty or senior resident during an actual clinical encounter with a real patient in real clinical setting. The setting could be outpatient clinic, inpatient ward or even emergency care service. The entire exercise lasts about 10–20 minutes. The observation of the trainee's interaction with patient is followed by a discussion between the observing faculty and the trainee to assess clinical reasoning/ management approach, and to provide constructive feedback. This tool can be used to assess a wide range of core clinical skills such as history taking, examination, clinical judgment, communication skills, counseling skills, or even humanistic qualities such as empathy that are difficult to assess by traditional methods. However, all of these may not be assessed in a single encounter. About 6–8 encounters are recommended per trainee per year using a variety of clinical settings, clinical problems, examiners, and competencies in focus (Norcini 2005). The observer and the trainee mutually agree upon the focus area(s) for a particular encounter such as data gathering, diagnosis, therapy or counseling. An assessment of overall clinical competence can also be made.

Process: mini-CEX assesses trainees on the seven core skills: (1) medical interviewing, (2) physical examination, (3) professionalism, (4) clinical judgment, (5) counseling, (6) organization and efficiency, and (7) overall clinical competence. A global rating is given on a 9-point scale, where 1–3 is unsatisfactory, 4–6 is satisfactory, and 7–9 is superior performance. A faculty member observes the trainee-patient encounter and scores the performance using the rating form. The encounters are brief, generally lasting 10–15 minutes, and are followed by a feedback session which focuses on what was done well and what could be improved. A trainee is observed during several such encounters covering different aspects of patient care and is generally observed by different faculty members.

The faculty observer records her observations using a structured assessment form. One of the most popular formats is the one used by the ABIM for residency training programs available at their website: *https://www.abim.org/pdf/paper-tools/minicex.pdf* and is reproduced here in **Figure 9.1** (Norcini & Burch, 2007). The form provides spaces for recording names of the evaluator and the resident, the stage of training, and the focus area(s) of clinical competence for that encounter. The clinical setting in which the exercise is being carried out is noted, as is relevant clinical information about the patient

Mini-clinical evaluation exercise (mini-CEX)

Evaluator:_____
Date:_____

Resident:_____ OR-1   OR-2   OR-3

Patient Problem/Dx:_____

Setting: ☐ Ambulatory   ☐ Inpatient   ☐ ED   ☐ Other

Patient: Age:_____   Sex:_____   ☐ New   ☐ Follow-up

Complexity: ☐ Low   ☐ Moderate   ☐ High

Focus: ☐ Data Gathering   ☐ Diagnosis   ☐ Therapy   ☐ Counseling

1. Medical Interviewing Skills (☐ Not Observed)

| 1 | 2 | 3 | 4 | 5 | 6 | 7 | 8 | 9 |

Unsatisfactory   Satisfactory   Superior

2. Physical Examination Skills (☐ Not Observed)

| 1 | 2 | 3 | 4 | 5 | 6 | 7 | 8 | 9 |

Unsatisfactory   Satisfactory   Superior

3. Humanistic Qualities/Professionalism (☐ Not Observed)

| 1 | 2 | 3 | 4 | 5 | 6 | 7 | 8 | 9 |

Unsatisfactory   Satisfactory   Superior

4. Clinical Judgment (☐ Not Observed)

| 1 | 2 | 3 | 4 | 5 | 6 | 7 | 8 | 9 |

Unsatisfactory   Satisfactory   Superior

5. Counseling Skills (☐ Not Observed)

| 1 | 2 | 3 | 4 | 5 | 6 | 7 | 8 | 9 |

Unsatisfactory   Satisfactory   Superior

6. Organization/Efficiency (☐ Not Observed)

| 1 | 2 | 3 | 4 | 5 | 6 | 7 | 8 | 9 |

Unsatisfactory   Satisfactory   Superior

7. Overall Clinical Competence (☐ Not Observed)

| 1 | 2 | 3 | 4 | 5 | 6 | 7 | 8 | 9 |

Unsatisfactory   Satisfactory   Superior

Mini-CEX Time: Observing _____ Mins   Providing Feedback: _____ Mins

Evaluator Satisfaction with Mini-CEX

1   2   3   4   5   6   7   8   9
    Low   High

Resident Satisfaction with Mini-CEX

1   2   3   4   5   6   7   8   9
    Low   High

Comments:
_____
_____
_____

_____   _____
Resident signature   Evaluator signature

Medical interviewing skills: Facilitates patient's telling of story; effectively uses questions/directions to obtain accurate, adequate information needed; responds appropriately to affected, nonverbal cues.

Physical examination skills: Follows efficient, logical sequence; balances screening/diagnostic steps for problem; informs patient; sensitive to patient's comfort, modesty.

Humanistic qualities/professionalism: Shows respect, compassion, empathy, establishes trust; attends to patient's needs of comfort, modesty, confidentiality, information.

Clinical judgment: Selectively orders/performs appropriate diagnostic studies, considers risks, benefits.

Counseling skills: Explains rationale for test/treatment, obtains patient's consent, educates/counsels regarding management.

Organization/efficiency: Prioritizes; is timely; succinct.

Overall clinical competence: Demonstrates judgment, synthesis, caring, effectiveness, and efficiency.

Fig. 9.1: Format of mini-clinical evaluation exercise form.
From the American Board of Internal Medicine, www.abim.org

such as age, gender, new or follow-up patient, and complexity of the clinical condition. Below these details is space for recording the assessment of observed clinical skills. It allows the evaluator to mark 'not observed' for any skill that was not observed during the exercise. The rating scale is numerical and has corresponding qualifiers such as 'unsatisfactory', 'satisfactory' or 'superior'. It is a global-rating scale rather than a checklist-based scale, and hence places value on subject expert's overall judgment. There is a space for any additional comments, and time spent on observing and providing feedback, respectively. Another notable feature is a record of the overall level of satisfaction of the trainee and the assessor with the exercise.

For the mini-CEX, a global rating is given rather than the checklist-based recording typical of the OSCE. Whereas checklists usually capture a dichotomous division or nominal rating (right or wrong), global ratings capture ordinal information. Like other global ratings, some subjectivity may be involved. In fact, the assessor can use his/her discretion and calibrate the ratings according to the performance expected depending on the level of trainee, case setting (ambulatory, emergency, etc.), and complexity of the patient's problem(s).

The fact that it can be carried out during routine clinical work makes it feasible for use in resource poor settings with a heavy clinical workload. The authentic clinical setting, actual patient interaction and its potential to assess whole competencies rather than individual skills, contribute to its validity. This can be improved by varying the clinical settings and case selection. Increase in number of encounters and use of different examiners increase the reliability of assessment. It has been shown that with 6–8 encounters per trainee per year the reliability is about 0.8 (Pelgrim et al., 2011). Inbuilt immediate and contextual feedback makes it very valuable as a formative assessment tool especially for resident trainees. With some modifications, it has been used for undergraduate medical students as well (Norcini & Burch, 2007). The salient features and strengths of mini-CEX are summarized in **Table 9.2**.

Role of the assessor: Direct observation of the trainees is an important prerequisite for the teachers to provide educationally useful formative feedback. Even in situations where such training is largely based on simulated patients, the importance of direct observation on actual patients is being recognized (Holmboe & Hawkins, 1998; Vleuten & Swanson, 1990). Direct observation of performance helps in generating high-quality real-time feedback, which is more authentic (Norcini et al., 1995). From this perspective, the mini-CEX appears to be an authentic assessment of students' performance, useful not only for grading but, more importantly, for helping trainees to improve their clinical skills.

Although mini-CEX decisions are based on the subjective judgments of the faculty, there are important issues pertaining to this. The first relates to the use of a recording form, which provides a structure to the encounter. The second relates to the number of assessors. Since these clinical encounters are observed by different faculty members, the trainees have the advantage of receiving feedback based on varied strengths and experiences of faculty members. Thirdly, the variety of situations in which the encounters are observed samples a wider area of clinical competence. Putting all this together, the mini-CEX has strengths compared to a traditional case presentation or an

TABLE 9.2: Salient features and strengths of mini-Clinical Evaluation Exercise

Salient features	Strengths
❖ Observation of trainee by a faculty/superior during clinical encounter with a real patient in actual clinical settings. A single exercise usually takes 10–20 minutes. ❖ Discussion with trainee to explore clinical reasoning and approach. ❖ Recording of assessment of observed area of competency on a standard format that utilizes global rating based on expert judgment. Space for additional qualitative comments also provided. ❖ Immediate feedback to trainee. Feedback from trainee about her own experience of the exercise. ❖ Schedule 6–8 such encounters per trainee per year, set in different clinical areas with different faculty members and a varied spectrum of clinical conditions.	❖ Actual workplace settings make the discussion and feedback contextual, easy to implement and contribute to the authenticity and hence validity of assessment. ❖ Time, space, and effort of arranging an examination set-up is reduced. ❖ Feasible even in busy clinical areas such as the outpatient with minimal disruption of work. ❖ The assessment of ability to perform a whole task or competency (or subcompetency) is possible, hence directly relevant to actual future working. ❖ Feedback is immediate and contextual, and hence likely to be effective. ❖ Multiple encounters in multiple settings with multiple examiners and a wide case variation contribute to the reliability of assessment. ❖ Prior training of the faculty in using the method effectively and sensitization of trainees will contribute to its acceptability.

OSCE. Its validity and reliability derive from the fact that trainees are observed while engaged with a series of real patients in real clinical settings and are being observed by experienced educators who bring different strengths and perspectives to the process (Norcini, 2005). However, at no point, should the mini-CEX be taken as a replacement for other means of assessment—rather it should be used to complement the information available from case presentation or OSCE. Factor analysis has showed that mini-CEX appears to measure the single global dimension of clinical competence. The six mini-CEX domains correlate highly; so for measuring discrete clinical skills, it may need to be supplemented with other measures of competence. For this reason, use of mini-CEX in its present form is generally limited for high-stakes summative assessment (Cook et al., 2010).

The recording forms serve as useful records of the assessment. They can be used with other tools like portfolios to document the progress of the student over time; they can also be used to ensure that the competencies required for a given curriculum are being addressed. If, for example, taking care of healthy children is part of pediatric training, then one of the encounters should be in a well-baby clinic. This helps to build the content validity of the process. Certain modifications have been proposed in the recording form to make it useful for undergraduate students as well (Hill & Kendall, 2007).

Preparing to use: It stands to reason that trainees as well as faculty need to be prepared to adopt this method of learning and assessment. Especially in the Indian context, where students may not be used to direct observation of their performance, it may come as a culture shock. Similar feelings have been reported where students expressed anxiety on the introduction of the OSCE/objectivey structured practical examination (OSPE). Since it serves the dual purpose of assessment as well as education, trainees are likely to feel a conflict between the two roles (Malhotra et al., 2008). However, in many studies, mini-CEX has been shown to foster self-directed learning (de Lima et al., 2005; Ringsted et al., 2004). These differences might be attributable to sampling differences and to the prior exposure of postgraduates to such method of assessment. There is good evidence that formative feedback will improve learning (Burch et al., 2006). Students perceived it to be beneficial and up to 90% of planned encounters were completed (Kogan et al., 2003) in some of the reported studies.

Similarly, assessors need to reorient their role from an information provider to someone providing developmental feedback. The most significant aspect of using mini-CEX is the one-to-one observation of the students and the authentic feedback this observation generates. The pattern of feedback in the mini-CEX is based on what was done well, what could be better, and a plan for future action is agreed upon. This helps to take care of inhibitions associated with giving and taking feedback. The quality of feedback can be improved by faculty training (Fernando et al., 2008).

Psychometrics: Holmboe et al. (2003) reported strong construct validity of the mini-CEX. They also found that the difference in ratings between depicted levels of performance was *educationally* as well statistically significant (emphasis added). Durning et al. (2002) argued that the mini-CEX has concurrent validity by demonstrating correlations between the mini-CEX scores and monthly evaluation forms.

Unlike oral examinations, there is no significant difference related to examiner predisposition. Complexity of the case, setting of the mini-CEX, and background of the examiners do not seem to have a significant influence on the ratings (Norcini et al.,1997). In addition, by using several examiners to rate the trainees in a variety of settings, such differences, if any, tend to get neutralized. This makes it possible to compare the ratings based on a variety of clinical problems for formative purposes (but not summative). Although inter-rater reliability is not high, overall reliability with repeated measures has been shown to be consistently high. Inter-rater reliability has not been shown to improve significantly with training. However, it is not really a limitation because the strength of mini-CEX is also in its diversity of feedback (Cook et al., 2008). Its discriminating ability between different levels of performances has also been reported to be high (Norcini et al., 2003).

The mini-CEX has measurement properties like other methods of performance assessment (Norcini et al., 2003). The reproducibility coefficient of the mini-CEX was reported as 0.77 and it correlated very significantly with inpatient ratings, outpatient ratings, and final course grades (Kogan et al., 2003). The mini-CEX has also been shown to discriminate between unsatisfactory, satisfactory, and superior performance in the domain of interviewing, examination, and counseling (Holmboe et al., 2003).

Generalizability coefficient of mini-CEX for 10 encounters was reported as 0.92 (Sidhu et al., 2009). There was a progressive increase in the coefficient by increasing the number of encounters from 1 to 10. Another study on internal medicine residents also showed a good correlation with other measures of residents' performance (Durning et al., 2002).

How can we use it? What place can mini-CEX have in the assessment of clinical competence? Enough evidence has accumulated to show that mini-CEX provides valid, reliable, and acceptable ratings of clinical competence. It takes such assessment to a higher level in terms of Miller pyramid by assessing the trainee in real work situations. There is evidence to support its construct and concurrent validity and its ability to differentiate between various levels of performances. Its strength lies in the trainee being observed in a variety of clinical settings, receiving developmental feedback from experienced clinicians, and its ability to be administered onsite and become a seamless part of routine clinical activity. Experiences with mini-CEX in a variety of settings in several institutions around the globe also help us to realize that subjective judgment of experts can be as reliable as check-list based assessment.

Issues about the predictive validity of mini-CEX, i.e., its ability to predict future performance remain. It is yet to be demonstrated that the faculty can pick the appropriate use of a skill as it would have an important bearing on the feedback that is given. A solution to this might be faculty training, especially to pick unsatisfactory performance.

A limitation of the mini-CEX is that the trainee is aware of being observed and assessed, and this itself may alter her behavior. Lack of training and hesitation in incorporating new methods in the assessment plan are perhaps the major hindrances to its popular use in our country. Faculty development and training, experience sharing, recognition of its valuable formative role in molding the learning process, and student sensitization are likely to increase its utilization.

A systematic review of 'tools of assessment by direct observation' by Kogan et al. (2009) reported 55 tools, and many of these test similar and overlapping domains and skills. The mini-CEX is the most used and has the strongest validity evidence. Direct Observation of Procedural Skills (DOPS) and Multisource Feedback (MSF) are the other tools in common use. Some of the other tools of assessment by direct observation are described here.

Direct Observation of Procedural Skills

Learning and acquisition of procedural skills during undergraduate as well as postgraduate training is often not observed by the supervisors (Hauer et al., 2011). Even if observed, it is not a conscious and formal observation of the whole task as an assessor with the purpose of giving specific feedback for improvement. Usually, the supervising faculty notices a trainee's practical skills, while assisting a procedure and provides occasional suggestions for improvement that mostly pertain to the technical steps of the procedure. Conventionally, the numbers of procedures assisted and performed were considered enough to assess and draw conclusions about competence in procedural skills, and the logbooks maintained by the trainees served the purpose.

Recognizing this problem, the Direct Observation of Procedural Skills (DOPS) was first introduced in the United Kingdom by the Royal College of Physicians to assess competence of residents in practical procedures (Wragg et al., 2003). It is analogous to mini-CEX, but for observed assessment of procedural or practical skills. In DOPS, the supervising faculty member observes a trainee performing a procedure on a real patient in an actual clinical setting. Observation and feedback are the two key steps in this assessment as they are for mini-CEX.

The procedure is usually a short diagnostic or interventional one, lasting 10-20 minutes. The observation spans the entire duration of procedure—from patient counseling, taking of consent to the actual performance of the task. The feedback takes another 5 minutes. The list of procedures to be assessed by DOPS for a given specialty may be drawn by consensus amongst the faculty members. Such a list would consider the developmental stage of the trainees. Thus, year 1 and year 2 of residency will have their respective lists of procedures.

The observations are noted on a standard DOPS assessment form (Format available from *https://ww2.health.wa.gov.au/~/media/Files/Corporate/general%20documents/Workforce/PDF/DOPS_form.ashx*) adapted for the specialty for which it is used. The form is structured like the mini-CEX form with details of the trainee, the assessor, clinical setting, number of times the procedure was performed, number of DOPS observed by the assessor earlier, level of difficulty, etc. The grading is done using a 6-point scale where a score of 3 is borderline performance. The areas that can be graded in an encounter are (Norcini & Burch, 2007): understanding of indication, relevant anatomy and technique of procedure, obtaining informed consent, appropriate post-procedure preparation, appropriate analgesia or safe sedation, technical ability, aseptic technique, seeking of help where appropriate, pre-procedure management, communication skills, professionalism, and overall procedural efficiency. The assessor has the option of marking one or more areas as 'unable to comment'. There is space provided for making a note of strengths of trainee and for making suggestions for improvement.

Like mini-CEX, each trainee should have 6–8 DOPS encounters in a year; and the process is trainee-driven, i.e., the trainee takes the initiative and approaches the faculty for arranging a DOPS session. A departmental schedule may also be developed for the purpose. However, unlike mini-CEX, the same faculty member may observe more than one DOPS encounters for different procedures, e.g., the trainee may have many DOPS sessions observed by the faculty members of a division that he or she is posted in for a few months (Singh et al., 2014). It can be used for formative assessment of procedural skills, as well as for certification of competence before moving to the next stage of training. You can find more discussion on DOPS in Chapter 13.

Acute Care Assessment Tool

The Acute Care Assessment Tool (ACAT) was developed to assess trainees in acute or emergency care settings and is very similar to mini-CEX and DOPS. Typically, the clinical supervisor observes the trainees during clinical work in emergency care and then provides developmental feedback (Johnson et al., 2009). In emergency, patients often present at odd hours with undiagnosed conditions, and physicians have to exercise judgment for early and appropriate action, coordinate and communicate with interprofessional and multispecialty teams, communicate effectively with the patient and caregivers, manage time, be adept at emergency procedures, keep records, and also give an effective handover of multiple patients to the team in the next shift (e.g., in emergency room or intensive care unit). The ACAT forms allow for recording observations on these aspects of physician behavior. The observations on specific behaviors as well as on overall performance may be marked as scores or be commented upon in the provided space. There is provision for noting down what was done well, suggested areas for improvement and for drafting an action plan for future.

A sample form by the Joint Royal Colleges of Physicians Training Board (JRCPTB) may be accessed at *https://www.ficm.ac.uk/sites/default/files/ACAT%202010%20JRCPTB.pdf*. With this basic design, minor variations in the form may be developed depending on the place and purpose for which it is used.

Professionalism Mini-evaluation Exercise

It is now agreed that professionalism must be taught and assessed as an explicit part of undergraduate and postgraduate medical curriculum. Lapses in professional behavior in medical schools are predictive of unprofessional conduct in future medical practice (Papadakis et al., 2005). Given this background, an imminent need to develop tools for assessing professionalism was recognized. The Professionalism Mini-Evaluation Exercise (P-MEX), adapted from the mini-CEX, was proposed and piloted by Cruess et al. in 2006. The supervisor consciously observes the student trainee's behavior during an actual clinical encounter or during meetings and rounds. The observations are noted on a structured form followed by feedback.

Though the mini-CEX form can be used for recording observations on 'humanistic qualities/professionalism', it does not name the specific behaviors. In P-MEX, this form has been modified to include behaviors that conform to professionalism. Professionalism is a complex construct of several attributes many of which are not amenable to observation and measurement. A list of 142 appropriate professional behaviors was derived by consensus during a faculty development workshop, of which 24 were included in the original form (Cruess et al., 2006). By factor analysis, these behaviors conformed to four factors: (1) doctor-patient relationship skills, (2) reflective skills, (3) time management, (4) and interprofessional relationship skills. The scoring is done on a 4-point scale with the options: exceeded expectations, met expectations, below expectations and unacceptable, and a fifth option of marking as 'not observed' or 'not applicable'. An example of P-MEX form may be viewed at: *https://www.acgme.org/Portals/0/430_Professionalism_MiniCEX.pdf*. Reports of its use from India are also beginning to appear (Kaur et al., 2020).

A systematic review of instruments for assessing medical professionalism by Li et al. in 2017 reported a good structural validity but poor cross-cultural validity for P-MEX (Li et al., 2017). This is understandable since many behaviors are culturally determined. Other modalities for assessing professionalism have been discussed in detail in Chapter 12.

Multisource Feedback

As the name suggests, this method entails assessment by collecting information from multiple sources or people who have had the opportunity of directly observing the trainee doctor at work. These include peers, senior residents, consultants, secretaries, nurses, and other health care workers. It was first introduced in the United States of America and Canada as Peer Review Assessment and subsequently was adopted in the United Kingdom and other countries (Abdulla, 2008). The Multisource Feedback (MSF) is also termed 360° assessment because the trainee is assessed from multiple perspectives by many stakeholders for an all-round evaluation. Thus, in addition to clinical skills it makes skills such as communication skills, professionalism, team working, leadership skills, humane qualities, and behavior amenable to assessment at the level of performance in real life. This aspect assumed further importance when it was demonstrated that the peer ratings for clinical/technical domain correlated well with the knowledge assessment tests or examination scores, but the ratings for humanistic qualities and communication correlated poorly with examination scores. Self-rating for these attributes has been found to correlate poorly with peer rating thereby suggesting a possible lack of insight in the erring physicians (Salmon & Pugsley, 2017).

A rather unique strength of the method is that the trainee is observed almost unawares. In mini-CEX or DOPS or similar planned real clinical encounter-based tools, the trainee is aware of being observed, and may consciously or subconsciously alter her behavior during the exercise, and this behavior may not truly represent what she does during the actual course of routine working. In MSF, however, though the trainee and potential observers are aware that observation-based information will be collected, it is always not possible to display a put-on behavior. Conversely, the knowledge that one is always being observed for assessment purposes at work may encourage a person to adopt good clinical and professional practices, improve behavior and be more productive as a team member. This again is very desirable as learning and improvement are after all the two major goals of any assessment.

The logistics of collecting information from multiple sources in a systematic and structured manner involves designing appropriate feedback forms according to specialty and setting. The key aspect of designing or selecting the instrument for collecting information is the purpose for which it is being collected. It can be used for resident training programs, for contributing to promotion decisions, or for improving inter-disciplinary collaboration and teamwork even in non-teaching set-ups such as district hospitals.

There are several questionnaire instruments/tools in use for collecting information for Multisource Feedback (MSF). The mini-Peer Assessment Tool (mini-PAT) is a popular and well-tested tool in use especially in the United Kingdom. The prefix 'mini' denotes that it is a shorter version of the original Sheffield Peer review assessment tool (SPRAT). A quick study of this tool gives an idea of the kind of information an MSF feedback form should carry (Norcini & Burch, 2007). The trainee nominates the assessors. For reliable results, 8–12 review ratings per round are recommended, and one such round once in 6 months is desirable (Ramsey et al., 1993). The broad categories of observation on the form include 'Good clinical care'; 'Maintaining good clinical practice'; 'Teaching, training, appraising and assessing'; 'Relationship with patients'; and 'Working with colleagues' (Norcini

& Burch, 2007). There are specific items that are to be rated under each of these. The 6-point rating with '3' as borderline is like that on the DOPS form. The completed forms are collected and collated for preparing individual feedback. While the comments included are verbatim, anonymity is maintained. The supervisor provides the feedback to the trainee based on these, and they together work out an action plan for improvement.

Another instrument like the mini-PAT for collecting feedback from multiple sources is the 360° Team Assessment of Behavior (TAB). This is more focused on evaluating the team behavior of the trainee. In this rating form, the categories are 'Maintaining trust/professional relationships with patients', 'Verbal communication skills', 'Team-working/working with colleagues', and 'Accessibility'.

The MSF assessment irrespective of the instrument used, banks on mutual trust, genuine interest, and honest feedback. In absence of these, the assessment is reduced to a paper exercise and at times a means of getting back at people. More often used in business and industry, this method has proven useful in medical field as well in terms of validity, reliability, and feasibility (Archer et al., 2008). Many studies have reported an overall improvement in performance of physicians after introduction of MSF although some studies have contested it (Abdulla, 2008; Salmon & Pugsley, 2017). This suggests that the implementation of the method perhaps plays a key role in determining its effect on physician behavior. Further, a training of the trainees in making an appropriate selection of raters can reduce the rater bias, and training of supervisors in providing effective feedback can augment its utility (Abdulla, 2008).

Objective Structured Long Examination Record

The Objective Structured Long Examination Record (OSLER) was introduced to overcome some of limitations of the traditional long case (Gleeson, 1997). It is discussed in depth in Chapter 7, and therefore is only briefly described here.

The strength of a long case lies in its authenticity because of use of real patients, and also because it tests comprehensive clinical approach to the patient as a whole. The limitations of long case include compromised generalizability as usually only 1-2 cases can be assessed in given time, unobserved student-patient interaction, and lack of a mechanism for providing feedback to the student. The OSLER improves upon the traditional long case through its three key characteristics:

1. **Observation:** In OSLER, the student is observed during the process of history taking and examination for about 20-30 minutes. Then the examiner discusses the diagnostic and management approach with the student and examines the student for clinical reasoning skills for about 10-15 minutes.

2. **Standardized and structured 10-item record form:** The examiner records her observations on a 10-item form. The ten items designate the core areas that must be observed by the examiner during the exercise. Of these ten, four pertain to history taking (pace, clarity, systematic, establishment of facts), three pertain to clinical examination (systematic, technique, signs demonstrated), and the remaining three are 'investigations', 'management', and 'diagnostic acumen'. The grading is done as P+, P, and P– that correspond to 'very good/excellent', 'pass/borderline pass', and 'below pass', respectively. Corresponding marks are also mentioned on the same form along with a guide for examiners for allocating marks. The examiner marks the difficulty level of the case before starting the examination. An itemized form ensures that the critical processes during the course are noted and commented upon, and that this is the standard observed for all students.
3. **Feedback:** While feedback can also be provided to the examinee after a traditional long case, the absence of structured observations makes it difficult, as well as likely to be incomplete and less specific. Structured observations about key areas of clinical competence make it easy to give feedback about specific areas of improvement.

Though the OSLER looks like a good way for improving the long case, it has not gained significant popularity. There are a few reports of its use in Indian medical colleges, but more as an educational innovation rather than as continued use for routine assessments.

Utility and Implementation of Observation-based Methods

The assessment characteristics that contribute to the utility of direct observation-based methods have several commonalities and some variations. The OSCE and the mini-CEX are the results of an effort to improve the traditional long case, and they are best presented in the context of, and in comparison, to the long case (**Table 9.3**). The table summarizes the characteristics, implementation, and utility of each. The methods such as the ACAT and the P-MEX are essentially derivatives of mini-CEX, and similar arguments apply to them.

The mini-CEX, DOPS, and MSF are the three most well-studied direct observation assessment methods that are carried out in the actual workplace, and among these the mini-CEX has the best validity evidence (Kogan et al., 2009). While classically it is desirable to discuss each method separately, more usable information is obtained when these methods are evaluated in combination. While a reliability coefficient of 0.80 was obtained for 8 mini-CEX, 9 DOPS, and 9 MSF rounds, it was more meaningful that the same reliability was found for 7 mini-CEX, 8 DOPS, and 1 round of MSF when combined in a portfolio (van Loon et al., 2013). This also goes out to support the long suggested programmatic approach to assessment (Vleuten, 2016) in preference to the method-based approach. It is only natural that the psychometrics of these be evaluated in combination than alone.

TABLE 9.3: Comparison of Long Case, Objective Structured Clinical Examination (OSCE), and mini-Clinical Evaluation Exercise (mini-CEX)*

Characteristic	Long case (traditional)	OSCE	Mini-CEX
Timing	Designated time for assessment	Designated time for assessment	During routine working: Integrated into daily clinical activity
Setting	Examination setting: Inpatient	Examination setting: Designated examination area or hall	Workplace (variety of settings): Inpatient, outpatient, emergency room, operation theater, procedure room
Initiated by	Examiner	Examiner	Trainee or examiner
Authenticity of task	Real but with limitations of being a part of formal assessment process. Unobserved clinical encounter	Artificially designed task for examination purpose (with real or standardized patients)	Real. Observed clinical encounter
Time required	1–2 hours per student	3–4 hours (for many students) for adequate reliability	10–20 minutes per encounter; 6–8 such encounters per trainee per year
Purpose	Assessment, mostly for summative purpose. Infrequent feedback when used for in training assessment.	Assessment with occasional feedback (mostly as a group feedback); some task stations with immediate feedback; summative as well as formative use	Feedback built into the method and always provided (immediate, specific, individual, contextual); mostly formative use
Observation by examiner	No	Yes (at the designated stations)	Yes (during an actual clinical interaction)
Number of examiners	Generally, 1–2	Multiple examiners; flexible depending on the number of observed stations	Multiple examiners; any number can be used depending on the number of trainees and number of encounters
Clinical contexts tested (reflects generalizability)	1–2	10–15 stations (good blueprinting contributes to better generalizability)	6–8 in 1 year (case and clinical setting variation contributes to better generalizability)
Competencies, domains, and skills tested	Presentation skills, clinical reasoning and problem solving (whole clinical problem)	Potential to test all four domains (cognitive, psychomotor, affective, communication); tendency to test small component skills rather than whole tasks or competencies	Potential for testing all four domains; one or multiple competencies may be tested during clinical encounter, e.g., interviewing skills, professionalism, clinical judgment, counseling skills

Contd...

Contd...

Characteristic	Long case (traditional)	OSCE	Mini-CEX
Marking by examiners	Examiner judgment as marking or global grading.	Standardized form for marking on specific components or skills observed—may have global rating scale or itemized checklist.	Standardized form with global rating for the competencies observed; space for qualitative remarks by the examiner; student and examiner satisfaction with process also noted.
Validity[†] considerations	Real patient whole clinical problem (construct validity); limited clinical cases and lack of clarity about what to assess among examiners (low content validity)	Examination settings and small component skills testing compromise the construct validity; content validity can be improved by wide sampling and blueprinting; directly observed tasks improve the validity	Good construct, criterion and content validity when the clinical encounters vary in setting and clinical contexts; direct observation contributes to validity
Reliability[†] (Reproducibility or consistency under similar circumstances)	1 hour: 0.60 2 hours: 0.75 3 hours: 0.86 (Wass et al., 2001) Inter-case variation more a reason for low reliability than inter-rater variation	1 hour: 0.47 2 hours: 0.64 3 hours: 0.78 (Petrusa et al., 2002) Improved by increasing number and duration of station, examiner training, item analysis and removal of problematic stations	1 hour: 0.60 2 hours: 0.75 3 hours: 0.86 (Norcini et al., 1997) Improved by increasing the encounters, varying the examiner and clinical setting/context
Equivalence[†] (Consistency across different institutions and cycles of testing)	Lack of standardized criteria for grading or marking may compromise equivalence.	Will depend on the faculty training and designing of stations. Of limited importance if being used for formative purposes	Faculty training will improve the equivalence across institutions, though of limited importance if being used for formative purposes
Feasibility[†]	High; minimal preparations and training of examiners	Lowered by being resource intensive; student sensitization and examiner training are a must	High, since it can be carried out during routine clinical work
Acceptability[†]	High; been in use for many years	Lowered by virtue of being resource and effort intensive, and requiring examiner training	Once trained, the acceptability by student and examiners is good
Educational effect[†] (Educational benefit derived from the motivation of trainees, students)	Limited. The trainees tend to focus more on presentation skills. Soft skills development is compromised	Blueprinting of stations to include varied skills and clinical contexts is likely to improve the educational effect. Feedback adds to effort at improvement.	Learners try and improve upon their overall clinical skills including soft skills such as communication. Feedback, multiple assessors, and multiple opportunities for learning contribute to the motivation.

Contd...

Contd...

Characteristic	Long case (traditional)	OSCE	Mini-CEX
Catalyst effect[†] (Results and feedback that motivates the stakeholders for future learning and improvement)	Limited. Informal feedback may be provided by some assessors	Has the potential of increasing the catalytic effect by early and mandatory feedback, and assessors trained in giving feedback	High because of feedback being built into the assessment methods. Proper implementation and assessor training will enhance it.
Developmental assessment	No (assessment at one point of time)	No (assessment at one point of time)	Yes (spread over time; allows for developmental changes and for modulating the course of learning)
Summary: Major strengths	Real patient, authentic setting, clinical comprehensive approach to patient, low on resources and preparation; high acceptability.	Wide sampling of clinical contexts and skills in the same time; direct observation of some tasks; immediate feedback at some stations	Real patient, authentic setting, wide variation in clinical contexts, direct observation, competency assessment, standardized marking, mandatory feedback
Summary: Major limitations	Low generalizability, not observed; no feedback; varying standards applied by examiners	Examination setting; whole competencies usually not tested; resource intensive	Examiner training and student sensitization are a must for proper implementation; student aware of being observed and may alter behavior
Bottom-line	❖ Plan an assessment program for the entire course of training using a combination of assessment methods to draw the benefits from each, and to minimize (or counterbalance) the limitations of each and conforming to the developmental stage of the trainee. ❖ Consider the utility (and its determinants) of the entire assessment program with its combination of methods (composite) rather than of individual methods or tools.		

[†]As per the 2018 Consensus Framework for Good Assessment (Norcini et al., 2018).

The educational impact of observation-based methods has so far been a less studied area from among the attributes. However, a recent systematic review and meta-analysis by Lorwald et al., (2018) suggests that implementation characteristics, especially quality of implementation and participants' responsiveness are two key aspects that influence the educational impact of these methods. The effect size of DOPS was found to be ten times that of mini-CEX. This may be because the studies on DOPS have a specific area or procedure in focus, while the use of mini-CEX has been in more generic situations. An earlier systematic review by Miller & Archer (2010), reported a positive evidence for MSF as well. The fact remains that most of this evidence comes from studies that have evaluated level 1 (reaction) of Kirkpatrick's four-level model. Only four studies evaluated effect on trainee performance (Lorwald et al., 2018).

A qualitative analysis by Lorwald et al., (2018) identified the hindering and facilitating factors that affect implementation and hence also the educational impact of DOPS and mini-CEX. A perceived lack of time, poor understanding of the process by the supervisors, and a lack of training in giving effective feedback contributes to ineffective implementation. Trainees who had a prior exposure to any of these methods found them more useful. The learning culture in which mini-CEX and DOPS are embedded influenced their implementation, thereby emphasizing the role of educational environment. While this analysis considered only the studies with mini-CEX and DOPS, it is likely that the issues would be similar for other observation-based methods.

For effective observation-based assessment programs, it is crucial that besides the sensitization of learners and training of faculty supervisors, the organizational learning culture is made conducive (Kogan et al., 2017).

REFERENCES

Abdulla, A. (2008). A critical analysis of mini peer assessment tool (mini-PAT). *Journal of the Royal Society of Medicine, 101(1)*, 22–6.

Archer, J., Norcini, J., Southgate, L., Heard, S., & Davies, H. (2008). Mini PAT (Peer Assessment Tool): a valid component of a National Assessment Programme in the UK? *Advances in Health Sciences Education, 13(2)*, 181–92.

Burch, V.C., Seggie, J.L., & Gary, N.E. (2006). Formative assessment promotes learning in undergraduate clinical clerkships. *South African Medical Journal, 96(5)*, 430–3.

Cook, D.A., Beckman, T.J., Mandrekar, J.N., & Pankratz, V.S. (2010). Internal structure of mini-CEX scores for internal medicine residents: factor analysis and generalizability. *Advances in Health Sciences Education: Theory and Practice, 15(5)*:633–45.

Cook, D.A., Dupras, D.M., & Beckman, T.J. (2008). Effect of rater training on reliability and accuracy of mini-CEX. *Journal of General Internal Medicine, 24(1)*, 74–9.

Cruess, R., McIlroy, J.H., Cruess, S., Ginsburg, S., & Steinert, Y. (2006). The professionalism mini-evaluation exercise: a preliminary investigation. *Academic Medicine, 81(10 Suppl)*, S74–8.

De Lima, A.A., Henquin, R., Thierer, J., Paulin, J., Lamari, S., Belcastro, F., et al. (2005). A qualitative study of the impact on learning of the mini clinical evaluation exercise in postgraduate training. *Medical Teacher, 27(1)*, 46–52.

Durning, S.J., Cation, L.J., Markert, R.J., & Pangaro, L.N. (2002). Assessing the reliability and validity of the mini-clinical evaluation exercise for internal medicine residency training. *Academic Medicine, 77(9)*, 900–4.

Epstein, R.M. (2007). Assessment in medical education. *New England Journal of Medicine, 356(4)*, 387–96.

Fernando, N., Cleland, J., McKenzie, H., & Cassar, K. (2008). Identifying the factors that determine feedback given to undergraduate medical students following formative mini-CEX assessments. *Medical Education, 42(1)*, 89–95.

Gleeson, F. (1997). AMEE Medical Education guide no. 9: Assessment of clinical competence using the objective structured long examination record (OSLER). *Medical Teacher, 19(1)*, 7–14.

Gupta, P., Dewan, P., & Singh, T. (2010). Objective structured clinical examination (OSCE). *Indian Pediatrics, 47(11)*, 911–20.

Harden, R.M., Stevenson, M., Downie, W.W., & Wilson, G.M. (1975). Assessment of clinical competence using objective structured examination. *British Medical Journal, 1(5955)*, 447–51.

Hauer, K.E., Holmboe, E.S., & Kogan, J.R. (2011). Twelve tips for implementing tools for direct observation of medical trainees' clinical skills during patient encounters. *Medical Teacher, 33(1)*, 27–33.

Hill, F., & Kendall, K. (2007). Adopting and adapting the mini CEX as an undergraduate assessment and learning tool. *Clinical Teacher, 4(4)*, 244–8.

Holmboe, E.S., & Hawkins, R.E. (1998). Methods for evaluating the clinical competence of residents in Internal Medicine: A review. *Ann Intern Med, 129(1)*, 42-48.

Holmboe, E.S., Huot, S., Chung, J., Norcini, J.J., & Hawkins, R.E. (2003). Construct validity of the mini clinical evaluation exercise. *Academic Medicine, 78(8)*, 826–30.

Holmboe, E.S., Sherbino, J., Long, D.M., Swing, S.R., & Frank, J.R. (2010). The role of assessment in competency-based medical education. *Medical Teacher, 32(8)*, 676–82.

Johnson, G., Wade, W., Barrett, J., & Jones, M. (2009). The acute care assessment tool: a new assessment in acute medicine. *Clinical Teacher, 6*, 105–9.

Kogan, J., Bellini, L., & Shea, J. (2003). Feasibility, reliability, and validity of the mini-clinical evaluation exercise (mCEX) in a medicine core clerkship. *Academic Medicine, 78(10 Suppl)*, S33–5.

Kogan, J.R., Hatala, R., Hauer, K.E., & Holmboe, E. (2017). Guidelines: The do's, don'ts and don't knows of direct observation of clinical skills in medical education. *Perspectives on Medical Education, 6(5)*, 286–305.

Kogan, J.R., Holmboe, E.S., & Hauer, K.E. (2009). Tools for direct observation and assessment of clinical skills of medical trainees: a systematic review. *Journal of the American Medical Association*, 302(12), 1316–26.

Kaur, T., Jain, R., Thomas, A.M., & Singh T. (2020). Evaluation of Feasibility, Acceptability and Utility of Professionalism Mini Evaluation Exercise (P-MEX) Tool in Dental Students of India: A Preliminary Report. *J Res Med Educ Ethics, 10*, 147-151.

Li, H., Ding, N., Zhang, Y., Liu, Y., & Wen, D. (2017). Assessing medical professionalism: a systematic review of instruments and their measurement properties. *PLoS One, 12(5)*, e0177321.

Lorwald, A.C., Lahner, F.M., Greif, R., Berendonk, C., Norcini, J., & Huwendiek, S. (2018): Factors influencing the educational impact of mini-CEX and DOPS: a qualitative synthesis. *Medical Teacher, 40(4)*, 414–20.

Lorwald, A.C., Lahner, F.M., Nouns, Z.M., Berendonk, C., Norcini, J., Greif, R., et al. (2018). The educational impact of mini-clinical evaluation exercise (mini-CEX) and direct observation of procedural skills (DOPS) and its association with implementation: a systematic review and meta-analysis. *PLoS One, 13(6)*, e0198009.

Malhotra, S., Hatal, R., & Courneya, C. (2008). Internal medicine residents' perceptions of the mini-clinical evaluation exercise. *Medical Teacher, 30(4)*, 414–9.

Miller, A., & Arthur, J. (2010). Impact of workplace based assessment in doctors' education and performance: a systematic review. *BMJ*, 341, c5064 (DOI:10.1136/bmj.c5064)

Miller, G.E. (1990). The assessment of clinical skills/competence/performance. *Academic Medicine, 65(9 Suppl)*, S63–7.

Modi, J.N., Gupta, P., & Singh, T. (2015). Competency-based medical education, entrustment and assessment. *Indian Pediatrics, 52(5)*,413–20.

Norcini, J., Anderson, M.B., Bollela, V., Burch, V., Costa, M.J., Duvivier, R., et al. (2018). 2018 consensus framework for good assessment. *Medical Teacher, 40(11)*, 1102–9.

Norcini, J.J. (2005). The mini clinical evaluation exercise (mini-CEX). *Clinical Teacher, 2(1)*, 25–30.

Norcini, J., Blank, R., Arnold, G., & Kimball, H. (1995). The mini-CEX: A preliminary investigation. *Ann Intern Med, 123*, 795–799.

Norcini, J.J., Blank, L., Arnold, G.K., & Kimball, H.R. (1997). Examiner differences in the mini CEX. *Advances in Health Sciences Education, 2(1)*, 27–33.

Norcini, J.J., Blank, L.L., Duffy, D., & Fortna, G.S. (2003). The mini-CEX: a method for assessing clinical skills. *Annals of Internal Medicine, 138(6)*, 476–81.

Norcini, J.J., & Burch, V. (2007). Workplace-based assessment as an educational tool: AMEE guide no. 31. *Medical Teacher, 29(9)*, 855–71.

Papadakis, M.A., Teharani, A., Banach, M.A., Knettler, T.R., Rattner, S.L., Stern, D.T., et al. (2005). Disciplinary action by medical boards and prior behavior in medical school. *New England Journal of Medicine, 353(25)*, 2673–82.

Pelgrim, E.A., Kramer, A.W., Mokkink, H.G., van den Elsen, L., Grol, R.P., & van der Vleuten, C. (2011). In-training assessment using direct observation of single-patient encounters: a literature review. *Advances in Health Sciences Education, 16(1)*, 131–42.

Petrusa, E.R. (2002). Clinical performance assessment. In C.P.M. van der Vleuten, G.R. Norman, I. Newbie (Ed.), *International handbook for research in medical education* (pp 673-709). Dordrecht: Kluwer Academic Publisher,

Ramsey, P., Wenrich, M.D., Carline, J.D., Inui, T.S., Larson, E.B., & LoGerfo, J.P. (1993). Use of peer ratings to evaluate physician performance. *Journal of the American Medical Association, 269(13)*, 1655–60.

Regehr, G., MacRae, H., Reznick, R.K., & Szalay, D. (1998). Comparing the psychometric properties of checklists and global rating scales for assessing performance on an OSCE-format examination. *Academic Medicine, 73(9)*, 993–7.

Ringsted, C., Pallisgaard, J., Østergaard, D., & Scherpbier, A. (2004). The effect of in-training assessment on clinical confidence in postgraduate education. *Medical Education, 38*, 1261–9.

Salmon, G., & Pugsley, L. (2017). The mini-PAT as a multi-source feedback tool for trainees in child and adolescent psychiatry: assessing whether it is fit for purpose. *BJ Psych Bulletin, 41(2)*, 115–9.

Sidhu, R.S., Hatala, R., Baron, S., Broudo, M., Pachev, G., & Page, G. (2009). Reliability and acceptance of the mini-clinical evaluation exercise as a performance assessment of practicing physicians. *Academic Medicine*, 84(10 Suppl), S113–5.

Singh, T., Kundra, S., & Gupta, P. (2014). Direct observation and focused feedback for clinical skills training. *Indian Pediatrics, 51(9)*, 713–7.

Singh, T., & Sharma, M. (2010). Mini-clinical examination (CEX) as a tool for formative assessment. *National Medical Journal of India, 23(2)*, 100–2.

Sood, R., & Singh, T. (2012). Assessment in medical education: evolving perspectives and contemporary trends. *National Medical Journal of India, 25(6)*, 357–64.

van der Vleuten, C.P.M. (2016). Revisiting 'assessing professional competence: from methods to programmes'. *Medical Education, 50(9)*, 885–8.

van der Vleuten, C.P.M., & Schuwirth, L.W. (2005). Assessing professional competence: from methods to programmes. *Medical Education, 39(3)*, 309–17.

van der Vleuten, C.P.M., & Swanson, D.B. (1990). Assessment of clinical skills with standardized patients: state of the art. *Teaching and Learning in Medicine, 2(2)*, 58–76.

van Loon, M., Overeem, K., Donkers, H., van der Vleuten, C.P.M., & Driessen, E.W. (2013). Composite reliability of a workplace-based assessment toolbox for postgraduate medical education. *Advances in Health Sciences Education, 18(5)*, 1087–102.

Wass, V., Jones, R., & van der Vleuten, C.P.M. (2001). Standardized or real patients to test clinical competence? The long case revisited. *Med Educ, 35*, 321–5.

Wragg, A., Wade, A., Fuller, G., Cowan, G., & Mills, P. (2003). Assessing the performance of specialist registrars. *Clinical Medicine, 3(2)*, 131–4.

Chapter 10

Oral Examinations

Anshu

KEY POINTS

- Oral examination allows assessors to probe the breadth and depth of students' knowledge.
- It can test clinical reasoning, decision-making, and problem-solving abilities.
- Structured oral examination can improve the inter-rater reliability of oral examination.
- Multiple mini-interviews have been used for selection during high-stakes examinations and have high predictive validity.

The oral examination or the *viva voce* refers to a format of assessment that calls on students to use the spoken word to express their knowledge and understanding. Most people are familiar with the viva which accompanies doctoral dissertations. Oral assessments may also accompany a clinical case, where a student is asked questions by examiners to explore his/her knowledge, understanding, problem-solving, and other abilities.

Although this mode of assessment has largely been abandoned in undergraduate education in North America, large parts of the United Kingdom and almost all medical schools in India continue to use this form of assessment. In some universities in India, the oral examination is only used to determine pass-fail decisions in borderline candidates, or to decide whether to award a distinction to very good performers.

The oral examination is an assessment method which allows the examiner to probe into the breadth and depth of a student's knowledge and decision-making abilities. However, this method has been criticized for being too subjective and for its inability to produce standardized results. In this chapter, we will look at some strategies by which the reliability and validity of the oral examination can be improved.

Abilities that can be Tested by Oral Examination

The oral examination allows examiners to probe students' depth of knowledge and their higher levels of understanding. One of the most important characteristics of the oral examination is that follow-up questions can be used to determine the limits of what a student knows. Students prepare themselves more thoroughly by understanding (rather than mere memorization) to handle questions they cannot predict, and this promotes learning (Joughin, 2010). Learning is often more effective when students see the need to argue a case rather than simply reiterate what is known (Ong, 2002).

A good educational principle is that assessment should simulate the actual behavior expected of a student in practice (Tyler, 1950). In practice, a doctor will come across several complex scenarios. The oral examination is useful to explore the students' cognitive processes during problem-solving or decision-making. Medicine is also a profession where communication skills are central to practice and the ability of candidates to listen to their patients, respond appropriately, explain treatment or prognosis or teach students need to be developed. Their ability to express their thoughts and articulate their ideas incorporating their knowledge, beliefs, and feelings need to be assessed. One can also test a student's ability to discuss and defend professional decisions and rationale for interventions. The oral examination can also be used to assess confidence, self-awareness, and other aspects of professionalism which may not be assessed by other modes of assessment **(Table 10.1)**.

TABLE 10.1: What can be assessed by the oral examination?

- Concepts and theories
- Breadth and depth of a given topic
- Applied problem solving
- Interpersonal competence
- Interpersonal qualities
- Integrated practice
- Verbal and non-verbal communication skills
- Interviewing skills
- Attitudes, professionalism, ethics
- Personal abilities

Flaws of the Traditional Oral Examination

Some of the challenges of the traditional oral examination are as follows:

Objectivity Issues

The oral examination has often been criticized for being very subjective and being influenced by the learning and bias of the examiner. Since the student's identity is not anonymous, results are frequently affected by extraneous factors like outward appearance, gender, accent, and confidence. Students from vernacular medium who have difficulty in speaking English are often judged on language and vocabulary rather than knowledge. Student's level of confidence has been stated to be a key factor influencing the scores (Thomas et al., 1993). Goldney & McFarlane (1986) suggested that students who were successful in oral examinations were more able to pick up cues and respond appropriately to examiners. All these seem to bring in an element of construct irrelevance variance in the process.

The viva suffers from several errors including the *halo effect*, where judgment of one attribute may influence other attributes. For example, a student who speaks fluently may score more though his content knowledge may be poor. Studies have shown that scores are directly proportional to the number of words and speaking time used by the examinee, and inversely proportional to the number of words and speaking time used by the examiner (Evans et al., 1966). Scoring patterns in the oral examination tend to bend toward leniency and tend to cluster around the middle (*error of central tendency*) and scores are affected by impressions left by preceding candidates (*error of contrast*) (Miller, 1962). Examiners do not seem to be using the extremes of scores, in effect shrinking the scale on which students are being measured.

Reliability Issues

The reproducibility of scores is affected by differences in examiner judgments, difficulty level of questions asked, candidate anxiety, and test conditions. Since these examinations are difficult to grade in a standardized manner, content specificity would also include a certain degree of unreliability.

Candidate performance across cases or questions (intercase reliability) is variable in oral examinations. The main reason for loss of reliability arises from limited sampling of content. One candidate may be questioned on matters with which they are most familiar, while another candidate can face quite the opposite (Memon et al., 2010).

The main criticism against the oral examination stems from inter-rater reliability. Some examiners tend to be stringent in assigning marks, while others are lenient. Agreement between examiners is usually poor. However, failure rates in viva are usually less, as poor agreement between examiners makes it unlikely that any two will agree to fail a student, unless one convinces the other (Thomas et al., 1993).

The oral examination is one mode of assessment which gives immediate feedback to students, teachers, as well as the educational process itself. Vu et al. (1981) reported that students felt that the oral examination was a fairer evaluation of the students' knowledge database and provided an opportunity for immediate feedback which supported learning. However, the amount of feedback given to students varies widely. Evans et al. (1966) found that there was approximately twice as much feedback from examiners who asked the least number of questions. Further, examiners giving more feedback tend to grade more leniently. Student performance in the viva gives additional information upon which a grading decision for a student who is marginal may be based. It also helps identify students who have poor clinical reasoning abilities.

The environment in which the examination is conducted also has a bearing on the performance of the candidate. The examiner-student encounter is often confrontational, rather than comfortable. Anxiety and mental fatigue on the part of the student that interfere with student performance may not give a true indication of the student's ability. Similarly, emotions and fatigue on the part of the examiner do affect the outcome of the assessment. Gibbs et al. (1988) list problems for examiners as: balancing the need to ask challenging questions with the need to help the examinee relax; encouraging the examinee to talk while keeping him or her on track; discriminating between what the examinee says and how he or she says it; making a sound judgment on the basis of a small amount of evidence; and justifying a mark in the absence of written evidence, especially in the case of student appeals. They also note three problems for examinees: (1) a lack of skill in what is an infrequently experienced type of assessment; (2) the unpredictability of questions which makes preparation more difficult; and (3) the potential for stress. There is also variability in the time spent by examiners in assessing each candidate.

Validity Issues

Assessment is valid when it allows students to fully demonstrate what they know about the subject they have been studying. When the oral examination is used to test only lower cognitive levels, it fails to serve its purpose. One study (Evans et al., 1966) showed that as many as 76% of questions asked are based on recall rather than on higher levels of understanding. Some authors feel (Jayawickramarajah, 1985) that examiners merely act as 'quiz masters' and abilities routinely being tested in oral examinations could easily be tested in a written examination. Generally, examiners tend to focus on what students do not know rather than trying to gauge what they know. And it is a tendency of most examiners to ask questions related to their special areas of interest (Mitchell, 1959).

Cost-effectiveness

The well-planned oral examination can be pretty time consuming, especially if large numbers of students are examined. McGuire (1966) questioned the cost-effectiveness of oral examinations. While the logistics of setting up an oral examination is simple, in terms of professional time and energy expended by examiners weighed against its reliability in measuring professional competence, the effort may not seem 'educationally profitable'.

Strategies to Improve the Oral Examination

Doubts about the reliability of oral examinations can be tempered by attention to structure, careful selection, training, standardization and monitoring of examiners, and purposive sampling of content (Spike & Jolly, 2003).

Structured oral examinations have been introduced in several universities to offset the poor reliability of oral examination as explained earlier.

In this format, all candidates are exposed to either the same or equivalent tasks which are administered under the same conditions. Quite often, structured oral examinations can be based on a clinical case. Here the objectives of using the case must be defined clearly. Questions which can give an insight into the candidate's clinical knowledge, problem-solving ability, attitudes, and decision-making skills should be preferred (Kearney et al., 2002).

This requires proper training of examiners and is very resource-intensive. Before conduct of an examination, the panel of examiners must decide detailed content to be assessed. It must be remembered that students might not perform consistently in all areas. So, it is essential to sample broad areas across the subject and include as many different cases in different content and contexts as possible in the available time, ensuring against repetition and overlap. All areas of competence specified for the examination (e.g., diagnosis, problem solving, management, communication skills, ethics, etc.) must be explored. **Table 10.2** shows a sample blueprint which plans how many different content areas can be sampled. All examiners agree to what the correct answers are. In order to make the scoring more objective, a rubric is also created.

TABLE 10.2: Sample oral examination plan

Competency to be tested	Communication skills	Professionalism	Personal and professional development
Patient care	Breaking bad news	Informing about procedural risks	
Managerial skills		Documentation/ Record keeping	
Interpersonal skills		Working in a health care team	
Lifelong learner			Ability to see gaps in learning/action plan for improvement

The structured format tests the ability of the students to create a reasonable list of the patient problems, their clinical reasoning skills, and their ability to correlate symptoms and signs to diseases. **Table 10.3** shows an example of how to prepare a structured oral examination based on a clinical case of pulmonary consolidation.

Several authors have showed that the inter-rater reliability of structured examinations is much better than the traditional oral examination (Anastakis et al., 1991; Swing & Bashook 2000).

While concepts and procedures lend themselves to assessment by other formats, this mode can be used to probe deeper into students' understanding and assessing it in the context of application. They can be called upon to apply their knowledge to real and hypothetical complex situations.

It is important to look for evidences for validity. Do the questions comprehensively cover course content? Are student performances in oral examination markedly different from their performances in the theory examinations? Is the examination pattern promoting deep student learning and not encouraging rote learning? It is important to continuously evaluate the manner in which the examination is conducted and examiners are assessing candidates, so that the obvious flaws can be rectified at each step.

Structure is concerned with how far the assessment follows a more or less predictable plan. However, overt structuring can lead to loss of flexibility, which is the strength of the oral examination. The capacity to ask probing follow-up questions must not be lost.

Students must be familiar with the pattern of the examination and all attempts must be made to alleviate their anxiety levels. The examination must be conducted in a fair and transparent manner. Students must be confident that the judgments based on this examination are sound, reliable, and fair. All students must be given equal time and opportunity to display their learning. It is a good idea to videotape the examination for future use in case of appeal against the examination process. The presence of more than one examiner usually ensures 'fair play' (Thomas et al., 1993); however, this may limit the content that is being tested. Putting one examiner at each place and testing more content may give more generalizable results.

Oral Examinations for High-stakes Selection Process: Multiple Mini-Interviews

Selection of trainees for health professions courses require evaluation of academic and non-academic factors. While most schools use scholastic grades or tests to determine candidates' potential, these are not the only determinants of future performance in the field. One of the problems with unstructured interviews is their unacceptably low predictive validity.

TABLE 10.3: Example of a case in a structured oral examination for final year medical students

Name of Student:_____
Roll No. :_____
Case: Presenting complaints
A 55-year-old male smoker presented with complaints of breathlessness, fever, and cough of 5 days duration.
I. History: 5 minutes   20 marks
What further information would you like to obtain?

	Answered correctly	Answered on prompting	Wrong answer	Blunder/ irrelevant answer	Remarks
Analysis of presenting complaints					
❖ Breathlessness—mild shortness of breath, no orthopnea, no paroxysmal nocturnal dyspnea (PND), no diurnal variation	☐	☐	☐	☐	
❖ Fever—gradual onset, continuous, associated with chills	☐	☐	☐	☐	
❖ Cough—productive, rusty sputum, not foul smelling	☐	☐	☐	☐	
❖ History of weakness. No history of chest pain, loss of appetite, loss of weight	☐	☐	☐	☐	
❖ History—no history of diabetes or hypertension or asthma	☐	☐	☐	☐	
❖ Social history—smoker since 25 years, no history of contact with tuberculosis (TB) patients	☐	☐	☐	☐	
❖ Socioeconomic history—works as farmer	☐	☐	☐	☐	

Final marks   /20

II. Physical examination: 3 minutes   10 marks
Based on this information, what relevant physical signs do you want to examine in this patient?

	Answered correctly	Answered on prompting	Wrong answer	Blunder/ irrelevant answer	Remarks
❖ General look: ill, fatigued	☐	☐	☐	☐	
❖ Vital signs—temp = 101°F, pulse = 106, BP = 110/70, RR = 32/min, O_2 saturation = 90%	☐	☐	☐	☐	
❖ Chest examination—signs of consolidation and pleural effusion	☐	☐	☐	☐	
❖ Inspection—no deformity, reduced chest movement on left side	☐	☐	☐	☐	
❖ Palpation—trachea + apex beat not displaced, reduced chest expansion on left side, tactile vocal fremitus (TVF) reduced over left inframammary and infra-axillary area	☐	☐	☐	☐	
❖ Percussion—dullness in midclavicular line over left 6th intercostal space (ICS). dull note along the midaxillary line on left 6th–8th ICS	☐	☐	☐	☐	

Contd...

Contd...

	Answered correctly	Answered on prompting	Wrong answer	Blunder/ irrelevant answer	Remarks
❖ Auscultation—bronchial breath sound over left inframammary and infra-axillary area; increased vocal resonance over left inframammary and infra-axillary regions	☐	☐	☐	☐	
❖ Examination of abdomen, CVS-WNL	☐	☐	☐	☐	
❖ Systemic examination—cervical lymph nodes enlarged on left side	☐	☐	☐	☐	

Final marks /10

III: Differential diagnosis: 5 minutes   10 marks

List the problems that the patient has:
1. Fever, cough, breathlessness
2. Consolidation in left lower lobe of lung
3. Enlarged cervical lymph nodes

What is your differential diagnosis? Can you rationalize your answer?
1. Pulmonary consolidation in left lower lobe
2. Collapse of lung
3. Fibrosis of lung
4. Pulmonary tuberculosis
5. Bronchogenic carcinoma

Final marks /10

IV. Investigations: 8 minutes   20 marks
A. What investigations would you like to order? (5 marks)

	Answered correctly	Answered on prompting	Wrong answer	Blunder/ irrelevant answer	Remarks
❖ Chest X-ray (CXR), complete blood count (CBC), peripheral smear (PS), sputum, electrocardiography (ECG)	☐	☐	☐	☐	
❖ Chemistry, urinalysis, arterial blood gas (ABG)	☐	☐	☐	☐	
❖ Fine needle aspiration cytology (FNAC) of cervical lymph node	☐	☐	☐	☐	
❖ Septic workup (including blood culture)	☐	☐	☐	☐	

Final marks /5

B. Interpretation of investigation reports (15 marks) (Investigation reports provided)

	Answered correctly	Answered on prompting	Wrong answer	Blunder/ irrelevant answer	Remarks
❖ CBC, PS	☐	☐	☐	☐	
❖ Liver function test (LFT), kidney function test (KFT), urinalysis	☐	☐	☐	☐	
❖ CXR	☐	☐	☐	☐	
❖ ECG (normal)	☐	☐	☐	☐	
❖ FNAC	☐	☐	☐	☐	
❖ ABG	☐	☐	☐	☐	

Final marks /15

Contd...

Contd...

	Answered correctly	Answered on prompting	Wrong answer	Blunder/ irrelevant answer	Remarks
V. What is your final diagnosis now? Or do you want to revise your diagnosis: 3 minutes					**5 marks**
Final Diagnosis: Pulmonary consolidation in left lower lobe					
				Final marks	/5
VI. How would you manage this case? 6 minutes					**20 marks**
A. Nonpharmacological measures					
Admission to the hospital	☐	☐	☐	☐	
Nutrition and fluids	☐	☐	☐	☐	
				Final marks	/8
B. Pharmacological measures					
❖ Oxygen	☐	☐	☐	☐	
❖ Antibiotics coverage: ❖ What organisms:	☐	☐	☐	☐	
❖ Chest tube drainage	☐	☐	☐	☐	
❖ IV fluid, check electrolytes	☐	☐	☐	☐	
				Final marks	/12

VII. Professionalism + Overall performance + interaction (15 marks)

Marks	I. History	II. Physical examination	III. Differential diagnosis	IV. Investigation	V. Final diagnosis	VI. Management	VII. Overall	Total
	/20	/10	/10	/20	/5	/20	/15	/100

Examiner's name and signature: Date:

Around two decades ago, McMaster University developed and tested an OSCE-style interview process. These were subsequently called Multiple Mini Interviews (MMI) and adopted by several other schools. In this process, applicants go through a series of structured stations where they have to interact with interviewers on a one-on-one basis (Eva et al., 2004). MMIs allow examiners to interact with many candidates in a short period of time. To acquire adequate reliability, it is important that the interviewers are drawn from diverse fields with differing expertise and widespread experience. This will enable to look at candidate's background and potential from different perspectives. Examiners must know exactly what the MMI is trying to accomplish.

Typically, 10–12 stations are used. These are structured based on the requirements, philosophy, and priorities of the educational institution. A structured station includes instructions for candidates, a statement informing everyone what qualities are being addressed by that station, some background information for the examiner about the basic principles around which the station is built, and some questions which examiners could use to initiate the discussion (Rosenfeld et al., 2008). Some stations are provided with rating scales where the examiners can evaluate the candidate. Examiners are trained so that they do not end up being too stringent or lenient (Eva et al., 2019).

Besides academic interest, the MMI seeks to look at other aspects such as sociodemographic and cultural backgrounds, ability to adapt to different circumstances, drive to excel, communication skills, professional demeanor, etc. Some applicants might be asked to reflect on past experiences. MMI allows the interviewers some flexibility and a chance to explore candidates' unique dimensions (Eva & Hodges, 2012).

Multiple mini-interviews have been reported to have a more acceptable reliability and validity. They are also reasonably cost-effective (Eva et al, 2004). In 2010, MMI was said to be an important contributor to competency-based health professional education, being the only measure of non-academic qualities with evidence of predictive validity and test-retest reliability (Prideaux et al., 2011).

Faculty Development

The ability to conduct oral examinations effectively requires the following attributes of examiners: knowledge and skills of the subject, knowledge of approach to practice of medicine and delivery of health care within acceptable limits, effective interpersonal skills and ability to work in a team toward the design and conduct of examination (Wakeford et al., 1995). Effective conduct of oral examinations requires commitment and effort. Careful selection and monitoring of a panel of examiners which is willing to expend this time and energy is mandatory.

Contrasting examiner behavior (hawk versus dove; theatrical versus restrained) and stringency or leniency in marking can be contained by training (Raymond et al., 1991). Intra-rater and inter-rater variability of marking must be reduced by training and agreement in the examiner panel. A rubric can be worked out by consensus. The reliability of global judgment is considered better than the reliability of averaged item scores (Daelmans et al., 2001).

Increasing the number of questions and teams of examiners appears to increase inter-rater reliability. However, many orals are needed to achieve a reliable score, requiring at least 9-10 occasions or 5 hours of testing time (Daelmans et al., 2001). However, Wass et al. (2003) found that structured oral examinations can achieve reliabilities appropriate to high-stakes examinations.

Examiners selected for the membership examination of the Royal College of General Practitioners (MRCGP) (Wakeford et al., 1995) are required to undertake a written examination of recent questions, and in turn act as candidate, examiner, and observer in simulated oral examinations. Experts judge their approach and interpersonal and communication skills and review their performance independently. When there is serious concern about a potential examiner's performance, they are not invited to be part of the panel. It needs to be mentioned that examiner skills are not analogous to clinical skills and rejection as an examiner is no criticism of a doctor's clinical acumen.

Questioning is an art and examiners need to learn how to move in a structured manner to higher levels of questions which test understanding. Examiners need to be trained how to move from asking factual information to questions which gauge problem-solving and decision-making ability (DesMarchais, et al., 1989). It may be necessary to plan tactics for difficult candidates. A slow spoken candidate may need nonverbal encouraging gestures or remarks. Overbearing garrulous ones may need to be slowed down by interrupting and asking for clarifications.

Oral examinations have been described as a 'rite of passage' and a tradition, which is hard to give up (Davis & Karunathilake, 2005). Marshal & Ludbrook (1972) pointed out that 'we are not measuring anything, but merely judging that the student is or is not fit to join the club'. However, a face-to-face encounter with a student adds a unique dimension to the assessment procedure. The strength of the oral examination is the flexibility it offers in assessing various aspects of competence. Variability in scoring can be reduced by careful examiner selection, training, and monitoring, increasing the number of raters, number of encounters, and randomly assigning examiners to candidates.

It must be remembered that no single assessment tool can provide judgment of anything as complex as clinical competence. And the viva voce is best used to supplement other tools in the assessment armamentarium to judge the quality of physicians we are producing for society.

REFERENCES

Anastakis, D.J., Cohen, R., & Reznick, R.K. (1991). The structured oral examination as a method for assessing surgical residents. *American Journal of Surgery, 162(1)*, 67–70.

Daelmans, H.E., Scherpbier, A.J., van der Vleuten, C.P.M., & Donker, A.J. (2001). Reliability of clinical oral examinations re-examined. *Medical Teacher, 23(4)*, 422–4.

Davis, M., & Karunathilake, I. (2005). The place of the oral examination in today's assessment systems. *Medical Teacher, 27(4)*, 294–7.

DesMarchais, J.E., Jean, P., & Delorme, P. (1989). Training in the art of asking questions at oral examinations. *Annals of the Royal College of Physicians and Surgeons of Canada, 22*, 213–6.

Eva, K.W., & Hodges, B.D. (2012). Scylla or Charybdis? Can we navigate between objectification and judgement in assessment? *Medical Education, 46(9)*, 914–9.

Eva, K.W., Macala, C., & Fleming, B. (2019). Twelve tips for constructing a multiple mini-interview. *Medical Teacher, 41(5)*, 510–6.

Eva, K.W., Rosenfeld, J., Reiter, H.I., & Norman, G.R. (2004). An admissions OSCE: the multiple mini-interview. *Medical Education, 38(3)*, 314–26.

Eva, K., Rosenfeld, J., Reiter, H., & Norman, G. (2004). The ability of the multiple mini-interview to predict preclerkship performance in medical school. *Academic Medicine, 79(10 Suppl)*, S40–2.

Evans, L.R., Ingersoll, R.W., & Smith, E.J. (1966). The reliability, validity, and taxonomic structure of the oral examination. *Journal of Medical Education, 41(7)*, 651–7.

Goldney, R.D., & McFarlane, A.C. (1986). Assessment in undergraduate psychiatric education. *Medical Education, 20(2)*, 117–22.

Gibbs, G., Habeshaw, S., & Habeshaw, T. (1988). *53 Interesting ways to assess your students*. Bristol: Technical and Educational Services Ltd.

Jayawickramarajah, P.T. (1985). Oral examinations in medical education. *Medical Education, 19(4)*, 290–3.

Joughin, G. (2010). *A short guide to oral assessment*. Leeds Metropolitan University. [online] Available from https://www.qub.ac.uk/directorates/AcademicStudentAffairs/CentreforEducationalDevelopment/FilestoreDONOTDELETE/Fileotupload,213702,en.pdf [Last accessed August, 2020].

Kearney, R.A., Puchalski, S.A., Yang, H.Y., & Skakun, E.N. (2002). The inter-rater and intra-rater reliability of a new Canadian oral examination format in anesthesia is fair to good. *Canadian Journal of Anesthesia, 49(3)*, 232–6.

Marshal, V.R., & Ludbrook, J. (1972). The relative importance of patient and examiner variability in a test of clinical skills. *British Journal of Medical Education, 6*, 212–7.

McGuire, C.H. (1966). The oral examination as a measure of professional competence. *Journal of Medical Education, 41*, 267–74.

Memon, M.A., Joughin, G.R., & Memon, B. (2010). Oral assessment and postgraduate medical examinations: establishing conditions for validity, reliability, and fairness. *Advances in Health Sciences Education: Theory and Practice, 15(2)*, 277–89.

Miller, G.E. (1962). *Teaching and learning in medical school*. Cambridge, Massachusetts: Harvard University Press. pp.212–3.

Mitchell, J.M. (1959). Medical education and specialty boards. *Journal of Medical Education, 34(6)*, 555–60.

Ong, W. (2002). *Orality and literacy: the technologizing of the word*, (2nd ed). New York: Routledge.

Prideaux, D., Roberts, C., Eva, K., Centeno, A., McCrorie, P., McManus, C., et al. (2011). Assessment for selection for the health care professions and specialty training: consensus statement and recommendations from the Ottawa 2010 Conference. *Medical Teacher, 33(3)*, 215–23.

Raymond, M.R., Webb, L.C., & Houston, W.M. (1991). Correcting performance-rating errors in oral examinations. *Evaluation and the Health Professions, 14*, 100–22.

Rosenfeld, J.M., Reiter, H.I., Trinh, K., & Eva, K.W. (2008). A cost efficiency comparison between the multiple mini-interview and traditional admissions interviews. *Advances in Health Sciences Education: Theory and Practice, 13(1)*, 43–58.

Spike, N., & Jolly, B. (2003). Are orals worth talking about? *Medical Education, 37(2)*, 92–3.

Swing, S., & Bashook, P.G. (2000). *Toolbox of assessment methods.* Evanston, IL: Accreditation Council for Graduate Medical Education and American Board of Medical Specialties.

Thomas, C.S., Mellsop, G., Callendar, J., Crawshaw, J., Ellis, P.M., Hall, A., et al. (1993). The oral examination: a study of academic and non-academic factors. *Medical Education, 27(5),* 433–9.

Tyler, R.W. (1950). *Basic principles of curriculum and integration.* Chicago: University of Chicago Press. pp.71-2.

Vu, N.V., Johnson, R., & Mertz, S.A. (1981). Oral examination: a model for its use within a clinical clerkship. *Journal of Medical Education, 56(8),* 665–7.

Wakeford, R., Southgate, L., & Wass, V. (1995). Improving oral examinations: selecting, training, and monitoring examiners for the MRCGP. Royal College of General Practitioners. *British Medical Journal, 311(7010),* 931–5.

Wass, V., Wakeford, R., Neighbour, R., & van der Vleuten, C.P.M. (2003). Achieving acceptable reliability in oral examinations: an analysis of the Royal College of General Practitioners membership examination's oral component. *Medical Education, 37(2),* 126–31.

Chapter 11

Portfolios for Assessment

Medha A Joshi

KEY POINTS

- ☞ Portfolio is an excellent tool to assess the students' learning over time.
- ☞ The purpose of portfolio should be defined and communicated to the students.
- ☞ Mentors play a major role in guiding and supporting portfolio learning.
- ☞ Portfolio encourages reflective practice.
- ☞ An assessment based on qualitative principles will make portfolio credible and valid, especially with multiple raters.
- ☞ Implementation and sustainability of portfolio depends on a well-thought-out plan and a strong organizational support.

The move towards competency-based medical education has created the need for newer instruments to support and assess development of competence. There are competencies that can be assessed using conventional assessment methods, and then there are those which cannot be assessed similarly. For assessment of competencies which are 'difficult to measure', we have assessment tools such as the portfolio.

▌What is a Portfolio?

The concept of a portfolio has been drawn from the study of art where the term signifies a *purposeful* collection of work. Portfolios have been used to assess the work of the artists and architects since a long time. Although they have been introduced in medical education relatively recently, they have been accepted as one of the valid tools for assessment at the undergraduate and postgraduate level, and for continuing medical education (Challis, 1999).

Davis and Ponnamperuma (2005) define a modern-day portfolio as 'a collection of papers and other forms of evidence to show that learning has taken place, annotated with the student's reflections on what has been learnt in terms of learning outcomes, over a period of time'. The important features of the contemporary portfolio are the evidence of learning through the learner's reflections over a period of training.

A portfolio can be considered as an educational tool that compiles learning over many learning opportunities to optimize learning. A learning opportunity is any event which triggers learning. This could be in the form of an interaction with a patient in an outpatient department, or a visit to a primary health center, or an assignment submitted and graded by the instructor. It is a collection of a student's work that demonstrates the efforts put in by students, their progress, their breadth of learning and achievements over a specified time-period (Martin-Kneip, 2000).

Portfolios are used in various forms and for diverse purposes in medical education in many parts of the world. Their uses are widely accepted as complementary to other conventional methods of learning and assessment (David et al., 2001).

Portfolios for Learning

Portfolio-based learning has been shown to be consistent with the principles of adult learning theory (Dennick, 2014). Introducing portfolios early in the curriculum can achieve several objectives. They help students connect theory to practice and teach them to reflect on their learning (Gall et al., 1996). They can help in creation of a robust mentoring system, and make students more responsible for their learning. In some health professions such as nursing, portfolios have been used to record career and professional development through formal and experiential learning. They also stimulate critical thinking and self-directed learning. Portfolios can cater to different learning styles.

Contents of a Portfolio

The purpose of the portfolio will determine the content included in it. One common feature is the cumulative nature of the content showing progression of the students' learning over a longitudinal period of time. There are two main ingredients to a portfolio: (1) portfolio content and (2) learning outcomes.

Usually, it is the learning outcomes stipulated in the course curriculum that mandate the development of a portfolio. Each discipline should identify learning outcomes that best suit their discipline. Common learning outcomes that can be used to develop a portfolio are in areas such as—clinical skills, investigations, procedural skills, patient management, health promotion and disease prevention, communication skills, information handling, basic social and clinical sciences knowledge, ethics, attitudes and legal responsibilities, problem solving, ethical/clinical reasoning and higher-order thinking, role of the doctor in a health care team (e.g., teamwork, leadership, educating others), and professionalism, and lifelong learning (Davis et al., 2001).

The portfolio builder should select portfolio content to illustrate achievement of learning outcomes. Portfolios should contain students' ongoing work over time, which may provide evidence for learning and progress toward educational and professional outcomes or learning objectives. Portfolios should contain students' reflections on the submitted evidence. Some examples of evidence of learning that can be included in the portfolio are (David et al., 2001):

- Written reports or research projects
- Samples of assessment of performance, e.g., teacher reports from clinical attachments
- Records of practical procedures undertaken (logbooks)
- Annotated patient records
- Letters of recommendation
- Curriculum vitae
- Peer assessments
- Patient surveys
- Videotapes of interactions with patients or peers (should be done with patient's content and by maintaining anonymity)
- Literature searches
- Quality-improvement projects
- Any other type of learning material
- Written reflection on the evidence and on professional growth (Martin-Kneip, 2000).

As portfolio content is very personalized, it is left to the creativity of the individual to make it as exclusive as possible. If the portfolio is too structured, it leaves no room for student reflection and creativity, it might end up in showing a forced study behavior and restricting to ticking checklists to show that they have met the expected objectives. It is necessary that students take ownership to stimulate reflection. On the other hand, if no structure is provided, students have no idea as to how to compile a portfolio especially if they are doing it for the first time.

A midway solution would be to provide probing questions related to the each of expected professional competencies. Posing probing questions (Sandars, 2009) will encourage students to reflect on their learning and will guide them in their thought processes. To support this, a manual can be provided to students in which each competency can be explained. Possible questions that students may ask themselves and potential sources of information that may be used to document their advancement in the areas of competence in question may also be included in the manual.

Table 11.1 gives examples of competencies and some of the documents that can be included in the portfolio to demonstrate progression toward these competencies. Reflective writing should be included as a part of evidence too (Roh et al., 2015).

TABLE 11.1: Examples of competencies and some of the evidences

Competency	Evidence
Patient care	Preliminary patient encounter in the outpatient department Case presentation in the ward Direct observation of procedural skills (DOPS) Mini-clinical evaluation exercises (mini-CEX) Discharge summary
Problem solving and critical thinking	Case discussion Framing of research question
Effective communication	Multisource feedback
Leadership	Multisource feedback
Professionalism	Medical ethical dilemma discussion Multisource feedback
Lifelong learning and reflection	Reflective writing Learning plan
Using basic science in the practice of medicine	Case discussion Journal article discussion
Understanding and application of scientific methods	Research projects

How do Portfolios Promote Reflection?

It is reflection on the learning experience that differentiates the portfolio from the logbook. Many definitions can be found of reflection. Pee et al., (2002) define reflection as a "deliberate, purposive exploration of experience, undertaken in order to promote learning, personal and professional development, and improvement of practice". Boud et al., (2013) define reflection as "a generic term for those intellectual and affective activities in which individuals engage to explore their experiences in order to lead to a new understanding and appreciation".

As very aptly discussed by Challis (1999), "a portfolio's purpose is to demonstrate learning, not to chronicle a series of experiences. Learning from experience will only happen once reflection and application of resulting modifications in practice have taken place. It is evidence of how the learning has been, or will be applied that will form the basis of the review or assessment". Therefore, reflection is the principal activity that exemplifies improvement of practice, as opposed to the mere documentation of learning, as typically done through a logbook.

Improvement of practice can only be achieved through the process of reflection. Portfolio assessment promotes learner reflection which makes an important contribution to the triangulation of information in the assessment process (Sandars, 2009). It should be noted that the use of portfolio does not necessarily lead to reflection. To stimulate reflective abilities in students, a portfolio should include (Driessen et al., 2005) an introduction, its intended use, clear guidelines and a structure, a mentoring system that will help in formative assessment and finally the student ownership of the content.

The reflective component of portfolios stimulates students to develop new understanding and appreciation of their experiences, recognize the link between different aspects of these experiences, and formulate insights to be tested in future similar situations.

The process of reflecting on experiences, and identifying and recording evidence of learning involves a process of self-assessment, which is an essential component of autonomous learning. Reflection also forms the basis for identifying further learning needs and setting goals for the future.

A number of models have been described in literature for reflection. The most widely used model is the one proposed by Kolb & Kolb (2012) **(Fig. 11.1)**.

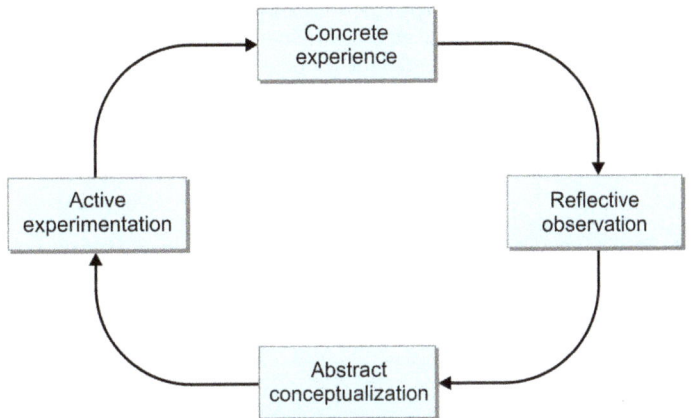

Fig. 11.1: Kolb's cycle.

Kolb proposed reflection as a four-stage process and this has been further simplied into the following five questions:
1. What was the learning experience?
2. What did I learn?
3. What more do I have to learn?
4. How can I learn it?
5. What is the evidence for learning?

A brief clarification on each question (Ponnamperuma, 2014) and an example of reflection is given in **Table 11.2**. Competency addressed here is *patient care*.

TABLE 11.2: A brief clarification on each question and an example of reflection

Question	Clarification	Example
What was the incident/event that triggered reflection?	An incident or an event that either ended well or otherwise, and has sufficient material to plan further learning, with an intention that if a similar situation arises it could be handled more efficiently.	I auscultated the chest of the patient in the intensive care unit (ICU) and then planned the treatment. Nursing staff helped with suctioning from the tube. I was able to identify the block in the tube while suctioning, but was not very confident of my findings. Soon the patient began to gasp, the vitals started falling and I panicked. Nurse called the emergency team and patient was revived.
What was the learning from this event?	Any event whether successfully carried out or not offers a lot of potential 'lessons' to modify future practice. These lessons should be stored to be applied in a similar situation in future without further refinement.	If my decision making was effective and I was confident of my findings, this emergency would have been avoided. During the chest auscultation, I restricted myself to the findings of crepitations and planned the treatment accordingly. If only I had taken into consideration the reduced breath sounds, I could have confirmed the blockage of the tube and acted upon it immediately. I was not confident of my auscultation skills and depended on the nurse to confirm my finding of tube block.
What is the gap in my knowledge that needs additional learning?	This is the gap in the knowledge or skill identified from the above experience and is the 'learning need'. Such need must be acted upon through further learning in order to deal with a similar event successfully in the future.	1. Need to learn more about how to identify tube blockage on auscultation and take immediate action. 2. Improve my clinical reasoning and decision making skills. 3. Should learn about the roles and responsibilities of each team member in a multidisciplinary team.
How can I learn it?	These are the methods applied to achieve the learning need/s identified in the previous question.	1. Will make use of the skills lab to gain proficiency in identifying different auscultatory findings. 2. Read about how to improve clinical decision making. 3. Read about multi-disciplinary teams in health care.
What is the evidence for the new learning?	The next step would be to apply the new learning in a similar or the same situation and provide an evidence. The evidence could be gathered on two counts. Firstly evidence for change of practice in form of direct observation by a senior person or a video recording, and secondly, evidence of the resources used to achieve the new learning such as journal articles, books, and other resources used for learning. A summary of the new learning can be added as an evidence.	I had a similar case during my next postings in ICU and was able to identify the block and act upon it immediately and confidently. My interaction with the nursing and other support staff has improved as observed by my senior faculty member. I have written a protocol to be followed in case of tube blockage and presented it in my department.

Reflective writings usually belong to one of the three levels: (1) descriptive, (2) analytical, or (3) evaluative (Epstein, 1999). Reflective writing falls into the 'descriptive' level when each of the five questions within the reflective cycle have been addressed as mere descriptions. The same entry can be upgraded to the 'analytical' level, if the candidate answers the question 'why' within each of the five questions. Once the portfolio developer identifies the reasons for each stage of the cycle, the same reflective process can be upgraded to the 'evaluative' level by selecting the best possible reason(s). Such selection of the best reason(s) should be accompanied by a justification as to why the chosen reason(s) could be considered as the best.

Role of Mentors

Teachers' perceptions of use and usefulness of portfolio, their ability to demonstrate reflective practice and motivation determines how easily students learn to reflect (van Schaik et al., 2013). Students may not be able to reflect if they belong to one of the three categories identified as poor portfolio compilers: (1) students who lack analytical ability, (2) those who think assembling a portfolio is pointless, and (3) students who are not motivated. The first two groups of students are incompatible with preparing a reflective portfolio. It is important to identify the first group as the quality of reflection is considered to be a vital skill for medical practitioners. Such students can be identified by discussing the portfolio with them. A teacher/mentor plays a vital role in motivating the third group of students.

Mentors have a very special role to play in assisting students in creating the portfolio (Bashook et al., 2008). First, they can aid students in recognizing their learning needs and help them develop a learning schedule. Secondly, mentors can ensure that students learn not just the practical, but also the emotional aspects of interacting with patients. This is often neglected. The personal relationship between the mentor and student facilitates the documentation of the progress, as the mentor is able to validate the portfolio materials and appreciate the evidence compiled by the student (van Tartwijk & Driessen, 2009).

Portfolios for Assessment

Portfolios can be used both for formative and summative assessment. They can be used to assess a wide range of outcomes that are difficult to assess with traditional methods, such as, professionalism and attitudes. While portfolios are considered to be excellent tools for formative assessment, they also enable assessment within a framework of transparent and defined criteria and learning objectives making them equally suitable for summative assessment.

Broadly, the aim of portfolio assessment may be any or all of the following:
- ❖ To provide feedback to learners so that they can learn from mistakes and build on achievements
- ❖ To motivate learners and focus on their sense of achievement
- ❖ To enable learners to correct errors and remedy deficiencies
- ❖ To consolidate learning
- ❖ To help learners apply abstract principles to practical contexts
- ❖ To classify or grade learner achievement
- ❖ To give teachers feedback on how effective they are at promoting learning (Brown & Knight, 2012).

Features of Assessment Portfolios

The main features of assessment portfolios are as follows:
1. Portfolios focus on the formative and summative aspects where students gather evidence of their own performance for feedback, for diagnostic purposes, interventions and pass/fail decisions. The formative value of the portfolio, when linked to summative decisions, makes it a very powerful assessment tool.
2. An important feature of assessment portfolios is the combined qualitative and quantitative approach. This is unlike many other performance assessment methods that rely entirely on the quantitative aspect of performance. Portfolios contain descriptive written material as well as reflections which can be graded by an assessor. This approach to assessment allows a more comprehensive interpretation of student achievement.
3. Student is actively involved in creating the portfolio. The role of teacher is to monitor and guide this student-centered activity.
4. Unlike other forms of assessment such as the Objective Structured Clinical Examination (OSCE) which focus on standardization of the process, portfolios are highly personalized endeavors. Here students select evidence to demonstrate their learning, reflect on it and are able to defend their work.
5. Though portfolios seek to balance the personalized approach to assessment and the standardization of the process and content to increase their reliability, this is not very easy to achieve. Nevertheless, the standardization process is critical to the reliability and validity of portfolios.

Some suggestions for bringing in standardization (David et al., 2001) are summarized below:
- ❖ The portfolio should be complied in such a way that its content will illustrate achievement of learning outcomes. When this aspect is taken care of, a great degree of standardization is brought in, because learning outcomes are specified in the course curriculum. Thus, all students will work toward achieving these outcomes.

- Tasks and criteria for assessment should be well defined and clearly outlined.
- Explicit guidelines should be provided to students for creating the portfolio.
- Grading of the portfolio content should follow standardized guidelines. This can be achieved by providing written instructions and training workshops for assessors.
- An oral questioning/discussion of the portfolio with the student can follow using standard guidelines.

Portfolio assessment is best carried out within a set of principles that will guide the assessor to decide whether the evidence presented in the portfolio is valid and sufficient to infer that appropriate learning has indeed taken place. Portfolios are therefore, almost by definition, assessed on the basis of previously decided criteria, and comparison between learners becomes inappropriate.

The following guidelines could be taken into consideration while developing an assessment framework for portfolios:

1. Assessment is carried out within a criterion-referenced rather than a norm-referenced framework.
2. 'Grading' portfolios, while not impossible, are counterproductive to the learner-centered philosophy underpinning the use of portfolios.
3. The criteria for assessment, that is the standards against which the evidence of learning will be measured should be explicit, and known both to the learner and the assessor
4. Criteria should link to specific learning outcomes, which should be written in such a way that the evidence of their attainment can be assessed. Example: Instead of stating 'demonstrates the understanding of', use active, measurable verbs such as 'explain', 'evaluate', 'analyze', 'illustrate' which will enable both the learner and assessor to approach the evidence of learning from a common perspective.
5. The evidence of learning should be accompanied by a reflective explanation of why each piece of evidence has been included, the learning that has happened and the part it has played in the progression of the learner's thought process and practice.
6. Evidence must be attributable as either by or about the learner (authentic), be appropriate to demonstrate the learning claimed (valid), and of sufficiently recent origin for the assessor to infer that the learning is current (van Tartwijk & Driessen, 2009).

Advantages and Limitations of Portfolios

Advantages

Portfolio learning and assessment offer certain advantages over conventional teaching-learning and assessment activities. Some of these are enumerated here:

- It encourages and fosters self-directed learning which is triggered by an incident experienced by the learner.

- Since it is based on the real experience of the learner, it enables the consolidation of the connection between theory and practice.
- It is suitable for diverse learning styles.
- It provides a model for lifelong learning and continuing professional development.
- It is a compilation of evidences of learning from a range of different contexts.
- It enables assessment within a framework of transparent and defined criteria and learning objectives.
- It is amenable to continuous and longitudinal assessment.
- In addition to assessing knowledge and skills, portfolios are useful to assess attitudes, professionalism, teamwork, and leadership.
- Portfolios provide a basis for both formative and summative assessment, based on either personally derived or externally governed learning objectives.
- It is a 'framework' for assessment and not a just a 'method' of assessment, meaning that portfolios can be used as the framework to include the results of many assessments from all four levels of the Miller pyramid (Davis et al., 2001). This could include written and clinical assessments conducted under a variety of examination conditions, and workplace-based assessment along with the reflective write-up. Portfolios can build a realistic, inclusive picture of the learner that cannot be achieved by any other form of assessment.

Limitations

Students and faculty members may find it time-consuming, less important or distractive from other types of learning and assessment. These limitations can be overcome with a carefully planning for development and implementation of the process (Fida & Shamim, 2016). Reliability of the assessment is one of the weaker aspects of portfolio use. Inter-rater reliability may be improved by three strategies: (1) by portfolio standardization, (2) by using analytical criteria for assessment, and (3) by increasing the number of assessors. Portfolio standardization and the use of analytical criteria with the aim of improving reliability will threaten validity, as this restricts the scope for describing students' personal learning experiences in different authentic situations. This may also limit the type of reflection prompted by the process itself. Aspects of great personal worth may be omitted or reduced in order to meet the criteria against which assessment is likely to be carried out. Yet these may be the very areas in which the student has the greatest learning needs or highest achievements. The third strategy for enhancing inter-rater reliability, i.e., increasing the number of assessors, is an effective strategy in theory, because for most educational institutions this strategy is too expensive to be applied, especially when large numbers of students need to be assessed (Driessen et al., 2006).

Portfolios are not the appropriate method of assessment if the purpose is to see whether the learner can recall information and apply it in a specific, time-limited context. Also, they cannot be used if it is important to be able to rank learners or grade their learning. On the other hand, portfolio may offer the breadth of information about the learner's progress and achievement that could be considered an appropriate addition to traditional modes of assessment. There will be a great degree of subjectivity associated with portfolio assessment that should be borne in mind when including it as an assessment tool (Challis, 1999).

Steps in Implementing the Portfolios

Following the steps for implementation is likely to meet the process with greater acceptance and success (Donato & George, 2012; Fida & Shamim, 2016; van Tartwijk & Driessen, 2009).

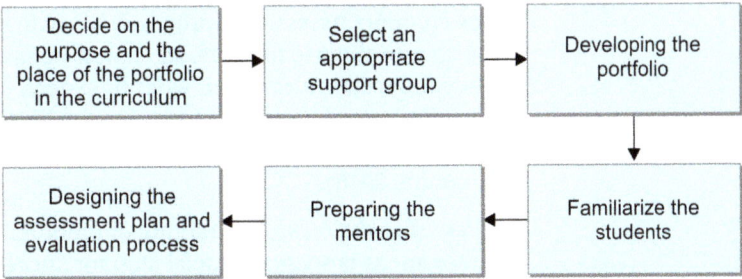

Decide on the purpose and the place of the portfolio in the curriculum: The goal of introducing portfolio should be made known to all stakeholders in advance. The goal may vary from collection of material for formative feedback and improvement to its use in summative assessment for pass/fail decision. Acceptance by students and faculty members may be facilitated by developing and sharing the goals in advance. Introducing portfolios for learning from early undergraduate courses will prepare the students to reflect when they come to clinical years. The competencies and learning outcomes to be achieved through portfolios should be clearly defined. Starting early might help improve the reflective and communicative skills.

Select an appropriate faculty support group: Faculty buy-in is essential as they will have to be fully convinced of the benefits of putting in extra efforts in terms of time for giving feedback and guiding the students plan their learning (Donato & George, 2012). Selecting the initial support group to start the process is most difficult; however, once the plan gets implemented many faculty members get motivated to join the group. The faculty support can be enhanced by conducting workshops and faculty development programs. Unless they perceive the educational advantages of portfolio especially in competency based education, the portfolio may not take off (Driessen et al., 2005). Faculty participation can be improved by rewarding innovative curricular activities.

Developing the portfolio: Once the appropriate competencies and other objectives are set, the structure and the content can be decided by the team. A plan for how the collected material will be used for students' assessment should also be developed at this point. Starting with a long-term vision that is accepted by both administrators and faculty members, and then planning a step-wise approach is likely to meet with a greater success than trying to implement a full-fledged portfolio covering all competencies. Including contents which are less time-intensive and are learner-relevant will make it suitable in the initial stages, for example, a curriculum vitae, reflections on their first day in the anatomy dissection hall or their first clinical posting.

Familiarize students: Students must get convinced of the value added by compiling a meaningful portfolio. Developing clear instructions that describe the goals clearly without being too prescriptive regarding the contents, assessment processes, marking system, and benefits that pertain to the use of portfolio should be made known to students. If they are well informed on what to expect, students are less likely to feel threatened; thereby, increasing the likelihood of a successful and meaningful learning experience (Dannefer & Henson, 2007; Fida & Shamim, 2016).

Preparing the mentors: Training of mentors in portfolio learning and assessment is seen as crucial step for success (Driessen et al., 2007) and lack of it instrumental for failure of the project (Ryland et al., 2006). Arranging regular meetings among the mentors helps to resolve common issues faced by students.

Designing the assessment plan and evaluation process: This process must cover decisions regarding the type of assessment (formative or summative), frequency of assessment for students at different levels as well as regarding marking criteria for the content of portfolios, training for examiners, and the time, place and methods to be used for assessment. The evaluation process for improvement and quality assurance should be in place from the start of implementation of the project.

Challenges and Issues

Despite their proven utility, portfolios may face issues, especially from faculty (and students). Often, no value is seen in the effort. Assessment of portfolios requires time and effort, which does not match the perceived benefits. Absence of feedback and mentoring support may further confound the issues. There may be logistic and administrative issues as well, especially non-availability of technology, faculty shortage, and lack of enough weight to the entire exercise. Similarly, lack of training in reflecting and assessing reflections may limit the utility. Enough thought and attention should be given to these issues to make optimum use of portfolios as learning and/or assessment tools (Springfield, 2011).

Place of Portfolio in Medical Education

Though the use of portfolios as a learning and assessment tool is comparatively new to the medical field, they have been used successfully in other health care professions like nursing, pharmacy, and physiotherapy. In medical education, introduction of portfolio early during undergraduate training helps students develop reflective ability. For postgraduates, this is an excellent tool to document not only their ability in the technical domain, but also to capture and document attitudes, ethics, professionalism, teamwork, and leadership. Since the initiative for learning in this method of learning is entirely decided by the learners themselves, with little or no external stipulations, such as those imposed by a formal curriculum, portfolios are considered ideal for continuing professional development (du Boulay, 2000). When the portfolios are developed for continuing professional development, they can be created using the learning opportunities offered within the workplace. This makes portfolio a desirable tool for learning and assessment for all levels of practice—from undergraduate training to postgraduate training and to continuing professional development.

REFERENCES

Bashook, P.G., Gelula, M.H., Joshi, M., & Sandlow, L.J. (2008). Impact of student reflective e-portfolio on medical student advisors. *Teaching and Learning in Medicine, 20(1),* 26–30.

Boud, D., Keogh, R. & Walker, D. (2013). *Reflection: turning experience into learning.* London: Routledge.

Brown, S. & Knight, P. (2012). *Assessing learners in higher education.* London: Routledge.

Challis, M. (1999). AMEE Medical Education Guide No. 11 (revised): Portfolio-based learning and assessment in medical education. *Medical Teacher, 21(4),* 370–86.

Dannefer, E.F., & Henson, L.C. (2007). The portfolio approach to competency-based assessment at the Cleveland Clinic Lerner College of Medicine. *Academic Medicine, 82(5),* 493–502.

David, M.F., Davis, M.H., Harden, R.M., Howie, P.W., Ker, J., & Pippard, M.J. (2001). AMEE Medical Education Guide No. 24: Portfolios as a method of student assessment. *Medical Teacher, 23(6),* 535–51.

Davis, M.H., & Ben-David, M.F., Harden, R.M., Howie, P., Ker, J., McGhee, C., et al. (2001). Portfolio assessment in medical students' final examinations. *Medical Teacher, 23(4),* 357–66.

Davis, M.H., & Ponnamperuma, G.G. (2005). Portfolio assessment. *Journal of Veterinary Medical Education, 32(3),* 279–84.

Dennick, R. (2014). Theories of learning: constructive experience. In: Matheson, D. (Ed). *An introduction to the study of education.* London: Routledge. pp.49–81.

Donato, A.A., & George, D.L. (2012). A blueprint for implementation of a structured portfolio in an internal medicine residency. *Academic Medicine, 87(2)*, 185–91.

Driessen, E., van Tartwijk, J., van der Vleuten, C.P.M., & Wass, V. (2007). Portfolios in medical education: why do they meet with mixed success? A systematic review. *Medical Education, 41(12)*, 1224–33.

Driessen, E.W., Overeem, K., van Tartwijk, J., van der Vleuten, C.P.M., & Muijtjens, A.M. (2006). Validity of portfolio assessment: which qualities determine ratings? *Medical Education, 40(9)*, 862–6.

Driessen, E.W., van Tartwijk, J., Overeem, K., Vermunt, J.D., & van der Vleuten, C.P.M. (2005). Conditions for successful reflective use of portfolios in undergraduate medical education. *Medical Education, 39(12)*, 1230–5.

du Boulay, C. (2000). From CME to CPD: getting better at getting better? Individual learning portfolios may bridge gap between learning and accountability. *British Medical Journal, 320(7232)*, 393-4.

Epstein, R.M. (1999). Mindful practice. *Journal of the American Medical Association, 282(9)*, 833–9.

Fida, N.M., & Shamim, M.S. (2016). Portfolios in Saudi medical colleges: why and how? *Saudi Medical Journal, 37(3)*, 245–8.

Gall, M.D., Borg, W.R. & Gall, J.P. (1996). *Educational research: an introduction*. New York: Longman Publishing.

Kolb, A.Y., & Kolb, D.A. (2012). Experiential learning theory. In: Seel, N.M. (Ed). *Encyclopedia of the Sciences of Learning*. Boston, MA: Springer. pp.1215–9.

Martin-Kneip, G.O. (2000). *Becoming a better teacher: eight innovations that work*. Alexandria, VA: ASCD.

Pee, B., Woodman, T., Fry, H., & Davenport, E.S. (2002). Appraising and assessing reflection in students' writing on a structured worksheet. *Medical Education, 36(6)*, 575–85.

Ponnamperuma, G.G. (2014). Portfolio assessment. *Journal of the Postgraduate Institute of Medicine, 1*, E4:1–8.

Roh, H., Lee, J.T., Yoon, Y.S., & Rhee, B.D. (2015). Development of a portfolio for competency-based assessment in a clinical clerkship curriculum. *Korean Journal of Medical Education, 27(4)*, 321–7.

Ryland, I., Brown, J., O'brien, M., Graham, D., Gillies, R., Chapman, T., et al. (2006). The portfolio: how was it for you? Views of F2 doctors from the Mersey Deanery Foundation Pilot. *Clinical Medicine, 6(4)*, 378–80.

Sandars, J. (2009). The use of reflection in medical education: AMEE Guide No. 44. *Medical Teacher, 31(8)*, 685–95.

Springfield, E. *Starting a student portfolio program—a guide for faculty*. [online] Available from http://www.nursing.umich.edu/facultyresources/ePort/askYourself.html [Last accessed August, 2020].

Van Schaik, S., Plant, J., & O'Sullivan, P. (2013). Promoting self-directed learning through portfolios in undergraduate medical education: the mentors' perspective. *Medical Teacher, 35(2)*, 139–44.

Van Tartwijk, J., & Driessen, E.W. (2009). Portfolios for assessment and learning: AMEE Guide No. 45. *Medical Teacher, 31(9)*, 790–801.

Chapter 12

Assessment of Professionalism and Ethics

BV Adkoli

KEY POINTS

☞ Professionalism and ethics need to be assessed to ensure that students learn them.
☞ Observational methods such as supervisors' ratings, peer ratings, patient ratings, and multisource feedback provide useful inputs to assess these attributes.
☞ Feedback and reflection are important to promote learning.

Professionalism is a the current buzzword which has emerged, in response to the scathing attack against the credibility and sanctity of medical profession during the last two decades (Hafferty, 2006). While 'medical ethics' has existed for a long time, the term medical professionalism emerged in the late 1980s. If 'commercialization of medical profession' can be described as the greatest malady, professionalism is the only antidote which has the potential to cleanse its image. Whether it is a question of providing cost-effective, quality care to a large section of the Indian population or fighting against the evils of commercialization and corruption, the answer lies in strenghtehning professionalism.

In health professions education, the biggest challenge has been to ensure that new graduates develop values and attitudes indispensable to the health profession. The challenge, therefore, lies in how to teach and assess professionalism.

In this chapter, an attempt has been made to outline the meaning of professionalism, the challenges involved in the assessment of professionalism, and describe some methods which can be used in the context of undergraduate medical education.

What is Professionalism?

Professionalism is an integral part of competence. In the United States, the assessment of residents, and increasingly of medical students, is largely based on a model that was developed by the Accreditation Council for Graduate Medical Education (ACGME). This model uses six interrelated domains of competence: (1) medical knowledge, (2) patient care, (3) professionalism, (4) communication and interpersonal skills, (5) practice-based learning and improvement, and (5) systems-based practice (Epstein, 2007).

Epstein and Hundert (2002) define professional competence as the "habitual and judicious use of communication, knowledge, technical skills, clinical reasoning, emotions, values, and reflection in daily practice for the benefit of the individual and community being served". While knowledge, technical skills, and clinical reasoning constitute the biomedical aspects of the professional competence, emotions, values, and reflections belong to the humanistic aspects. The march toward professionalism marks a shift in emphasis, from the biomedical aspects to the humanistic aspects.

Ethics and professionalism are interwoven to such an extent that at times, it becomes difficult to differentiate between these concepts. Professionalism is derived from the word 'profession'. It denotes commitment to carry out professional responsibilities, adherence to ethical principles, and sensitivity to a diverse patient population. The word 'ethics' is derived from the Greek word 'ethos' meaning character. Ethics can be regarded as a set of values or principles, duties and obligations based upon standards of right and wrong that govern members of a professional group. Ethics tells us what we *should not do*, while professionalism deals with what *we should do* **(Table 12.1)**.

TABLE 12.1: Ethics and professionalism

Principles of Ethics	Attributes of Professionalism
❖ Beneficence: a practitioner should act in the best interest of the patient *(salus aegroti suprema lex)*	Altruism (absence of self-interest)
❖ Non-maleficence: 'first, do no harm' *(primum non nocere)*	Respect for others
❖ Autonomy: the patient has the right to refuse or choose the treatment *(voluntas aegroti suprema lex)*	Humanistic qualities (e.g., empathy)
❖ Justice: pertains to the distribution of scarce health resource, and the decision of who gets what treatment	Honesty, integrity, ethical and moral standards
❖ Dignity: the patient has the right to dignity	Accountability (accountability to the patient, profession, society)
❖ Truthfulness and honesty: this relates to the concept of informed consent	Excellence (commitment to lifelong learning)
	Duty/Advocacy (commitment to service)

Some universities also include teamwork, interpersonal skills, and communication skills in the list of professional qualities. The weightage given to these components varies from one university to the other. There is no universal agreement as to which of these components are more importantth an others.

Some interesting facts about Professionalism

Professionalism deals with values and attitudes. Naturally, they are influenced by biological inheritance and society. The type of personality, parental background, the type of upbringing *(sanskar)*, and early childhood experience—are all factors that definitely play an important role in molding professionalism. This leads us to question the way a medical student is selected and admitted (Albanese et al., 2003). Are we justified in selecting candidates based on their performance on multiple choice questions (MCQs), which are perhaps least capable of measuring professional qualities? Our assumption that we recruit the 'best material' for the medical course is therefore not correct.

Studies have shown that professionalism is acquired over several years as a product of two simultaneous, but diagonally opposite processes: (1) attainment and (2) attrition (Hilton, 2004). When medical students enter the profession, they are full of idealism but lack clinical competence. During the course of studies, they gain clinical competence but tend to lose idealism and develop cynicism. Why? This is mainly because professionalism is *caught* rather than *taught*. Students learn professional qualities by emulating their seniors and teachers as 'role models' through what is termed as 'hidden curriculum' (Kirk, 2007; Brainard & Brislen, 2007)). Both students and teachers are influenced by the 'external environment' that often works against altruism and promotes self-interest (Arnold, 2002).

Many medical schools in the West introduced modules on ethics and professionalism formally or informally in their curricula (Christianson et al., 2007). They also started 'white coat ceremonies', and administered Hippocratic Oath to the fresh graduates, only to realize that the inculcation of professional behavior is not an easy task.

General Principles and Specific Challenges in the Assessment of Professionalism

Assessment not only drives learning, but also directs and promotes learning. When we think of assessing professionalism, what comes to our mind is the Miller pyramid. The assessment of professional qualities should ideally fall under the topmost 'Does' category. It is, however, not easy to assess at this level because of the complexities involved.

Stern & Papadakis (2006) have emphasized the role of a three-pronged approach to the development of professionalism, viz., setting expectations, providing learning experience in an environment

that is conducive to professionalism, and evaluating outcomes in a comprehensive manner.
- ❖ Setting expectations or defining the rules of the game in a transparent manner is a challenging issue. Unless the professional standards are clearly defined, we cannot expect students to attain the same. If students are not told to follow a code of conduct, they are unlikely to do so. This lapse is often found in clinical rotations where the set of instructions (often unwritten) are likely to contradict each other.
- ❖ The approach to the assessment of professionalism must be both developmental and supportive. Providing an effective learning experience and a congenial environment are perhaps more challenging issues. You need teachers who can be role models who nurture students' professional qualities. They should not only assess professional qualities, but also give regular feedback and take remedial action. The observed behavior should be a true representation of a candidate's professionalism, not just random behavior on that occasion.
- ❖ A judicious reward and punishment system needs to be set in place, so that professional behavior can be rewarded and unprofessional behavior can be punished and modified. This implies an organizational culture rather than piecemeal efforts by individual teachers and trainees.
- ❖ Whether assessment of professionalism should be conducted as a part of assessment of clinical performance, or as a comprehensive entity is yet another unresolved issue. Combined with clinical teaching and assessment, it has the advantage of providing a great opportunity for building professional values in a holistic manner, rather than considering them as separate entities. But it has logistic problems which should be sorted out.
- ❖ A closely related issue is who should assess personal qualities? Physicians, peers, or others who come into contact with students? Which group is more suitable to assess a particular element of professionalism?
- ❖ Finally, are the tools and techniques can be effectively utilized to assess various professional qualities? No single tool can capture all the qualities, and none of the qualities can be ignored or omitted from assessment (Swing & Bashook, 2000).

Strategies for Overcoming the Challenges

In view of the challenges cited above, a medical school should develop an appropriate strategy for carrying out the assessment of professionalism. The key elements are:
- ❖ Every medical school should *define expected behavior*, which should be communicated to the students and the staff in the beginning of

the course. The consequences of flouting professional values should be announced clearly.
- Assessment of professional qualities requires *multiple methods (qualitative and quantitative)* as no single method can capture the assessment of all qualities.
- Assessment should be conducted by *a number of assessors* to minimize subjectivity involved in assessment, as well as to measure the behavior under different conditions. The assessment ratings made by the *faculty, residents, peers and other health professionals* must be triangulated to give a complete picture.
- Assessment should be carried out continuously over a *period of time. Continuous feedback* must be given to students to improve their behavior.
- Assessment should be based on *observations and reflections* made in a *real-life, authentic setting* and not artificial context.
- Professionalism training should be designed to involve *conflict situations*. A person is likely to express true behavior only in challenging circumstances.
- Assessment should be *fair and transparent*, such that everyone is evaluated similarly.
- Professionalism should be considered for *formative, as well as summative* assessment, for each one has a role.

Methods, Tools and Techniques

The methods used for the assessment of professionalism fall under the category of supervisor's assessment, peer assessment, self-assessment, and assessment by the patients **(Table 12.2)**. When we combine, we will get multisource feedback or 360-degree assessment which gives a comprehensive picture of professionalism. The main consideration for using a particular tool should be the domain that needs to be tested and the purpose for which it is used, viz., for providing feedback to the learner (formative use) or judging the overall performance at the end of the course (summative use).

Self-assessment

Self-assessment is highly appropriate for measuring qualities of self-regulation and self-reflection. One can imagine that self-assessment suffers from the bias of social desirability, hence its usefulness for formative assessment is doubtful. Studies have shown that good students' self-rating is closer to instructors' rating compared to that of weak students. Self-assessment plays more of a formative role, as it gives the opportunity for continuous improvement. If combined with peer assessment and supervisors' assessment, this can also be used for summative purposes.

TABLE 12.2: A framework for the assessment of professionalism.

Method	Domain	Use	Strength	Limitation
Supervisor ratings	Teamwork Excellence in work Ethical behavior	Summative and formative	Feedback value is high Valid Feasible Cost-effective	Subjective and less authentic; Based on second-hand reports
Self-assessment	Attitude, values, beliefs	Formative	Promotes reflection Encourages self-directed learning	Leads to over-rating Limited feedback
Peer assessment	Honesty, integrity Teamwork	Mainly formative, partly summative	Number of observations can be more and frequent	Requires willingness, confidentiality and anonymity
Patient assessment	Empathy Respect for others Duty Commitment	Formative and summative	Credible source of feedback	Patient is not competent to give specific feedback
Multisource feedback 360-degree assessment	All professional qualities	Formative and summative	Credible than any other single tool	Time consuming, costly, and difficult to implement

Assessment by Peers

Assessment of professional behavior can be carried out by peers, using a checklist or a rating scale. Since they are in close contact with each other, their observations can be more in number and frequency. The internal consistency of such measurement is found to be moderate. Peer assessment is therefore recommended for formative assessment. However, the psychometric properties of such a rating scale needs improvement. In addition, bottlenecks such as lack of willingness to rate friends, and the tendency to rate clinical competence rather than professional qualities, need to be addressed.

Assessment by Patients

Patient surveys are effective modalities of assessing satisfaction with professional behavior including students' empathy, listening skills, and sensitivity to cultural issues, besides overall quality of care. They are aided by rating scales (e.g., poor, fair, good, very good, excellent), checklists, questionnaires, or any other kind of feedback on the level of satisfaction experienced by patients during their encounter with the candidate. Reliability estimates have been found higher for the practicing physicians, compared to residents during the training. The surveys mostly yield a group performance data rather than individual data. Hence, they are more useful in improving the system rather than individual performance.

360-Degree Assessment Instrument (Multisource Feedback)

The current trend in assessment greatly supports the use of 360-degree assessment, especially in the context of professional qualities which require constant assessment (Norcini & Burch, 2007). The 360-degree assessment consists of using measurement tools (checklist or rating scales) completed by multiple observers including faculty members, peers, patients, and other health personnel such as nursing or technical staff. The idea is to capture the performance of a candidate in multiple settings so as to arrive at a comprehensive and true picture. The observation is usually recorded with rating scales, mostly the Likert scales for assessing communication skills and professional behavior.

Research shows that the 360-degree assessment is more reliable when the number of observations/ratings increases (Norcini & Burch, 2007). Moreover, the ratings by those who are in constant interaction with the students are more reliable than the ratings given by the faculty. The practical limitations of the 360-degree assessment are the extensive effort involved in the construction and administration of a proper tool uniformly across diverse stakeholders, and further analyzing and interpreting the data collected in taking the final decision.

Several tools and techniques of clinical assessment are also useful in assessing professionalism. While checklists and rating scales are commonly used instruments, OSCE and Standardized Patients (SPs) are becoming more popular in a bid to make such assessment more feasible.

Assessment of Professionalism in the Workplace: Workplace-Based Assessment

The concept of workplace-based assessment has gained a lot of attention (Norcini & Burch, 2007) in the recent years. It has great potential for the assessment of professionalism. Workplace in medicine can be outpatient department (OPD), inpatient ward, clinic, or community. Carrying out assessment in the workplace is akin to the traditional apprenticeship model in which clinical experience is gained and assessed under the guidance of a clinical supervisor. The focus is on the actual performance, not on the knowledge. The supervisor observes the professional behavior directly, for example, how a resident reassures a patient who has to undergo surgery, or counsels members of a bereaved family in an effective manner. The bottomline of workplace-based assessment is therefore on how knowledge and skills are applied to real-life situations. Another major significance of workplace-based assessment is its developmental value through feedback. The supervisor can make useful suggestions for correcting behavior or demonstrate exemplary behavior as a role model which will have a lasting effect on the learner.

Supervisors' Rating

Supervisors' ratings are perhaps more authentic as they are done over time. However, it has some limitations. Firstly, it is difficult to undertake these amidst busy clinical practice. Secondly, the number of observations and the number of raters are important considerations. The more their number, the higher is the reliability. However, standardizing measurement of a behavior becomes problematic especially when different observers are involved.

Supervisors can directly observe and assess expected behavior by global ratings or by using a checklist. While the checklist approach helps to overcome inter-examiner variability, it fails to capture the holistic picture of students' performance. Some studies (Turner et al., 2014) have shown that global ratings are as reliable as the ratings made by using checklists. Finally, not all professional behavior can be broken down into checklist items.

In addition to supervisors' rating, tools like the Mini-Clinical Evaluation Exercise (mini-CEX) have a component of professionalism. It has the advantage of assessing professionalism in the context of the case being presented by the student. This has been discussed in Chapter 13.

Professionalism Mini-Evaluation Exercise

Another tool specifically for the assessment of professionalism is Professionalism Mini-Evaluation Exercise (P-MEX). It has proven value in assessing four essential attributes, viz., (1) reflection, (2) doctor-patient relationship, (3) time management, and (4) interprofessional relationship. These are assessed by 21 items. Each of the items is rated on a 4-point scale. The rating is done as follows: 1—if the performance is unacceptable, 2—if it is below expectations 3—if it meets expectations, and 4—if it exceeds expectations (Cruess et al., 2006). The main advantage of P-MEX is that it allows the supervisor to discuss the lapses in professional behavior with the student and to suggest appropriate remedial measures. Hence it has a formative role to play. A sample format of the recording form can be seen at *https://www.acgme.org/Portals/0/430_Professionalism_MiniCEX.pdf.* Reports of its use are beginning to appear from India (Kaur et al., 2020)

While assessment by single teacher is likely to cause personal 'bias', the introduction of another assessor will add strength provided a consensus is reached on the judgment, to overcome inter-examiner variability. The only way out is to organize rigorous training of examiners before the commencement of the assessment session. Scrutinizing a sample of narratives or video clippings of performance outcome jointly can be helpful exercise in bringing credibility to the assessment.

Narrative-based Approaches to the Assessment of Professionalism

It has been argued that objective approaches are not reliable or suitable for assessing professional qualities. The recent trend is, therefore, to explore the narrative approach to assessment of professionalism (Coulehan, 2005). Reflection of the behavior, or reflective practice is at the heart of professionalism. Narrative-based professionalism consists of immersing the students into the real-life stories of them, and encouraging them to listen, reflect, and connect with the patients, so as to develop and refine their professional behavior. The narrative approach is a movement from objectivity to subjectivity, from quantitative to qualitative, and from 'head' to 'heart'. This approach demands 'role modeling' by a highly committed faculty, contextual learning and problem solving in small groups, connecting to the patients' life stories, and deep engagement in community-based activities. Critical incident technique and portfolios fall under the category of narrative-based approach.

Critical Incident Technique

This consists of writing a short narrative on a challenging situation encountered by the student or resident and how they responded to this in a professional manner or otherwise. These are mostly qualitative reports and submitted by the faculty to the Dean as a part of longitudinal measurements. These observations can be recorded in logbooks or comment cards. While critical incident reports are expected to be more authentic than rating scales, they suffer from deficiencies such as time constraint on the part of the faculty for furnishing data. Some of the professional behaviors may not be amenable for accurate reporting and interpretation.

Portfolios

Portfolio approach consists of continuous documentation by students about their day-to-day experience with patients. A portfolio is a collection of products prepared by a candidate that provides evidence of learning and achievement related to a learning plan. It includes written documents, photographs, audio/video recordings or other form of information. A student during the course of clinical posting writes a portfolio describing his/her personal experience of interaction with the patient and what he/she learnt from the patient. The supervisor examines the portfolio, interacts with the candidate, and provides feedback. The information can be used for the formative and/or summative assessment. The portfolio can be a very effective tool for assessment of professional behaviors, including ethical practice by the students. It is also highly useful in recognizing ones' strengths and limitations which help in monitoring the progress.

The disadvantage of portfolios is that they are not as quick and easy to compile and evaluate, as they involve extensive paperwork. They are also difficult to score, grade or rank the students for summative purposes, as they mostly yield qualitative data. However, considering the importance of longitudinal assessment, portfolio has a great potential for assessing professionalism elements.

Future of Assessment of Professionalism: Professional Identity formation

Recent researches in professionalism have focused on professionalism as a continuous process of forming professional identity (Cruess et al., 2016). Each medical student develops his own professional identity during medical training as a result of collective influence of his previous background, peer influence, influence of role model(s), and encounter with patients and community at large. The concept of professional identity formation has practical implications for teaching and assessment of professionalism based on the Miller's pyramid. After Miller's four level ('knows', 'knows how', 'shows how', and 'does'), a next level 'is' has been proposed. At the highest level, the professional 'is' a self-actualized person. She is a unique physician who acts according to her sum total of experience gained earlier. If we agree with the concept that each professional is unique the approach to the teaching and assessment will be somewhat different. The progress evaluation and the product evaluation will have to be customized instead of shaping everyone to a common mold.

Considering that professionalism is a continuous and incremental process, it is necessary to see that assessment also reflects this process. We need to focus on the assessment of the process of teaching, the progress of learning, and the performance of the product before they are certified as the Indian Medical Graduates (IMGs).

While curricular interventions such as the introduction of Attitude, Ethics and Communication (AETCOM) module (MCI, 2018) are promising initiatives, we need to develop a robust mechanism of faculty development for enabling and empowering faculty to carry forward this movement. Exposure to medical humanities, involving students in community-based, social service activities, fostering over all development of students with a strong component of Co-curricular activities are steps in this direction. The teachers' influence as mentors and role-models will play a key role in this process.

Keeping in mind the time consumed in implementing curricular reforms by the regulatory bodies, what can be done is proactive intervention by teachers to make judicious use of the internal assessment. Additionally, steps taken by the institutions to promote a culture of professionalism will finally decide the contour of an IMG. Admitting fully that professionalism is a resultant product of several factors, every faculty member can contribute his/her best as a part of the cogwheel.

Some Final Thoughts

Though there is a growing consensus that the teaching and the assessment of professionalism are vital components, there are some unresolved issues regarding the tools and the way they should be assessed. There is no unanimity regarding the exact tool or even a toolkit that can be recommended across the board. By and large, multiple methods using quantitative and qualitative tools, over a long period of time assessed by different stakeholders are being preferred.

A major development in the field of professionalism assessment is the work by John McLachlan and colleagues at Durham University. They have come out with the concept of measuring 'Conscientious index' (McLachlan et al., 2009). The index was developed based on the evidence that negative student behavior during undergraduate programs predicted unprofessional behavior leading to disciplinary action by the state board in later career (Reed et al., 2008). However, further research is needed to establish the validity and reliability of the conscientious index.

Should all components be assessed at all levels or can certain components be prioritized at each level, is yet another unresolved issue. Some people think that assessment may be tailored according to the maturity level attained by the medical student during various stages. For example, a medical student may be assessed for knowledge and awareness, a resident for the competencies developed, and a practicing physician for the application of these competencies in real-life settings. This area needs further research. Another key issue is providing an environment conducive to the growth of professionalism. Perhaps the most challenging issue for the medical schools of the future is to foster professionalism in an integrated frame of teaching and assessment.

Cooke et al., (2006) while commenting on the 'American Medical Education 100 years after the Flexner Report' hit the bottom line:

"The groundwork that has been laid by explicit instruction in professionalism, combined with effective role modeling and attention to hidden curriculum of the practice environment, can support the development of a comprehensive and sophisticated understanding of professional education."

"Self-assessment, peer evaluations, portfolio of the learner's work, written assessments of clinical reasoning, standardized patient

examinations, oral examinations, and sophisticated simulations are used increasingly to support the acquisition of appropriate professional values as well as knowledge, reasoning, and skills. Rigorous assessment has the potential to inspire learning, influence values, reinforce competence, and reassure the public."

REFERENCES

Albanese, M.A., Snow, M.H., Skochelak, S.E., Huggett, K.N., & Farrell, P.M. (2003). Assessing personal qualities in medical school admissions. *Academic Medicine, 78(3)*, 313–21.

Arnold, L. (2002). Assessing professional behavior: yesterday, today, and tomorrow. *Academic Medicine, 77(6)*, 502–15.

Brainard, A.H., & Brislen, H.C. (2007). Learning professionalism: a view from the trenches. *Academic Medicine, 82(11)*, 1010–14.

Cooke M., Irby, D.M., Sullivan, W., & Ludmerer, K.M. (2006). American medical education 100 years after the Flexner report. *New England Journal of Medicine, 355(13)*, 1339–44.

Coulehan, J. (2005). Viewpoint: today's professionalism: engaging the mind but not the heart. *Academic Medicine, 80(10)*, 892–8.

Christianson, C.E., McBride, R.B., Vari, R.C., Olson, L., & Wilson, H.D. (2007). From traditional to patient-centered learning: curriculum change as an intervention for changing institutional culture and promoting professionalism in undergraduate medical education. *Academic Medicine, 82(11)*, 1079–88.

Cruess, R.L., Cruess, S.R., & Steinert, Y. (2016). Amending Miller's pyramid to include Professional Identity Formation. *Academic Medicine, 91(2)*, 180–85.

Cruess, R., McLIroy, J.H., Cruess, S., Ginsburg, S., & Steinert, Y. (2006). The professionalism mini-evaluation exercise: a preliminary investigation. *Academic Medicine, 81(10 Suppl)*, S74–8.

Epstein, R.M. (2007). Assessment in medical education. *New England Journal of Medicine, 356(4)*, 387–96.

Epstein, R.M., & Hundert, E.M. (2002). Defining and assessing professional competence. *Journal of the American Medical Association, 287(2)*, 226–35.

Hafferty, F. (2006). Viewpoint: the elephant in medical professionalism's kitchen. *Academic Medicine, 81(10)*, 906–14.

Hilton, S. (2004). Medical professionalism: how can we encourage it in our students? *Clinical Teacher, 1(2)*, 69–73.

Kaur, T., Jain, R., Thomas, A.M., & Singh, T. (2020). Evaluation of Feasibility, Acceptability and Utility of Professionalism Mini Evaluation Exercise (P-MEX) Tool in Dental Students of India: A Preliminary Report. *J Res Med Educ Ethics*, 10, 147–51.

Kirk LM. (2007). Professionalism in medicine: definitions and considerations for teaching. *Proceedings (Baylor University Medical Center). 20(1)*, 13–6.

McLachlan JC, Finn G, & Macnaughton J. (2009). The conscientiousness index: a novel tool to explore students' professionalism. *Academic Medicine, 84(5)*, 559–65.

Medical Council of India. (2018). *AETCOM module*. [online] Available from https://www.mciindia.org/CMS/wp-content/uploads/2020/01/AETCOM_book.pdf [Last accessed August, 2020].

Miller, G.E. (1990). The assessment of clinical skills/competence/performance. *Academic Medicine, 65(9 Suppl)*, S63–7.

Norcini J., & Burch, V. (2007). Workplace-based assessment as an educational tool: AMEE Guide No. 31. *Medical Teacher, 29(9)*, 855–71.

Reed, D.A., West, C.P., Mueller, P.S., Ficalora, R.D., Engstler, G.J., & Beckman, T.J. (2008). Behaviors of highly professional resident physicians. *Journal of the American Medical Association, 300(11)*, 1326–33.

Stern, D.T., & Papadakis, M. (2006). The developing physician—becoming a professional. *New England Journal of Medicine, 355(17)*, 1794–9.

Swing, S., & Bashook, P.G. (2000). Toolbox of *assessment methods*. Evanston, IL: Accreditation Council for Graduate Medical Education (ACGME), and American Board of Medical Specialties (ABMS).

Thistlethwaite, J. & Spencer, J. (2008). *Professionalism in medicine*. Oxford, New York: Radcliffe Publishing.

Whitcomb, M.E. (2005). Medical professionalism: can it be taught? *Academic Medicine, 80(10)*, 883–4.

Chapter 13

Workplace-based Assessment

Upreet Dhaliwal

> **KEY POINTS**
> - Workplace-based assessment (WPBA) provides opportunities for assessing clinical competence in authentic settings.
> - The cornerstone of WPBA is direct observation and immediate feedback.
> - WPBA allows for assessment of competencies generally not assessable by conventional methods.
> - WPBA depends on assessment data generated at the workplace, as well as competencies required for effective functioning in the workplace.

Students direct their learning towards that which is assessed during examinations. Since assessment guides learning, if we wish for our students to acquire competencies in the performance of certain caregiving tasks, we should modify our assessment methods keeping two things in mind—firstly, the assessment should actually measure competencies; secondly, the assessment should be made during the performance of real tasks. In this way, not only will assessment guide learning, but it will also facilitate learning (Singh & Modi, 2013).

There is no better place to assess if a learner is competent than during the performance of an actual healthcare related task that embodies the desired competency. Such assessments, that take place in authentic settings and during real tasks, are collectively called Workplace-Based Assessments (WPBA).

Need for Workplace-based Assessment

The change is driven by the realization that learners, after acquiring credentialed degrees, struggle in real-life situations. The reason for this struggle is that in real life nothing is straightforward or textbook-like; rather, it is unpredictable and multiple factors make it so, such as time constraints, manpower and infrastructural limitations, and situational issues. If training can be as true to real life as possible, learners can learn to juggle multiple responsibilities that require a mix of attributes from attitudinal, knowledge, and skill domains.

Most traditional assessments have some degree of clinical or practical component built into them; however, the emphasis is largely on assessing learners' knowledge. Demonstration of clinical competence involves not only the use of knowledge, but also requires procedural abilities, interpersonal skills, decision-making ability, professionalism, ability to self-assess and reflect, and an ability to continuously improve oneself. Traditional assessments, unfortunately, cannot assess many of these skills (Singh & Sood, 2013).

Workplace-based assessments conform to the highest level of Miller pyramid of clinical competence. They allow an assessment of what the learner 'does'—here the learner actually performs (in an authentic setting) instead of merely 'showing' that he can (in a simulated, test environment). WPBAs are performance-based assessments. With their inherent provisions for feedback and learner reflection, they fulfill all the major roles of an assessment—they drive learning; facilitate further learning due to the provision of feedback and the formative nature of the assessment; measure learning and, therefore, the teaching; and achieve standards, thereby protecting the end-user (the patient) (Liu, 2012).

In the current scenario of competency-based medical education (CBME), we need to collect evidence of learners' competence in the workplace. This can be done if we observe trainees performing all such tasks that they will have to perform independently once they complete their training. **Table 13.1** details how traditional methods of assessment, on their own, are inadequate in assessment of clinical competence.

Prerequisites for an Ideal Workplace-based Assessment

To be valid, assessment should be made while the learner is in the *workplace*, while he is performing healthcare related *tasks*, and while he is under *direct observation* so that feedback can be given. After feedback, the learner should be provided with *opportunities to practice* so that she can improve her performance. Ideally, this cycle of observation, assessment, feedback, and practice should be repeated *multiple times* until *multiple assessors* deem that competence has been achieved.

Terminology in Relation to WPBA

The following terms are critical elements of a WPBA and understanding them will help when we attempt to transition to WPBA in our institutions.

Workplace: The workplace is where the actual work of patient her care is done. It could be one or more places including the ward, the outpatient

TABLE 13.1: Traditional methods of assessment versus workplace-based assessment (WPBA) (Jain et al., 2014; Julyan, 2009; Miller & Archer, 2010; Yanting et al., 2016)

Reality	Impact	Solution (WPBA)
Conventionally, assessment is made of whether a learner has the knowledge and skills to pass an year-end examination; if he passes, competence is presumed	Learner may not be competent in practice at the workplace	At the workplace, competence is demonstrated by learners on a daily basis in the clinical work that they do
Direct observation of the learner-patient encounter is not routinely done	It is difficult to assess the learner's basic clinical skills, her affective domain and her skill in communicating with patients—these are essential components of competence	Competencies can be directly observed by teachers and others associated with the workplace, including patients and caregivers
When clinical skills are assessed, such as during an objective structured clinical examination (OSCE), the learner demonstrates only isolated elements of the clinical encounter	In practice, the learner will have to integrate various competency domains during a clinical encounter for which he is ill-prepared	The learner actually performs in the workplace, and so it is possible to gather evidence in all domains of learning
Traditional assessments are usually made in an artificial, protected environment	The learner may not be able to competently diagnose and manage a legitimate patient in an authentic workplace setting	The workplace is an authentic environment
Most assessments help in making pass-fail decisions	There is no provision of feedback and hence, no opportunity for the learner to improve performance before she moves to practice in the workplace	WPBAs are formative. Feedback on performance and learner reflection are built into the assessments
It is a time-bound, high-stakes system	There is very little that one can do to help a struggling trainee once the time is up, apart from failing her and potentially ruining her career	The most vital aspect of WPBA is the ability to diagnose the learning needs of a trainee and to help her improve performance through constructive feedback

department, operation theater, emergency department, laboratories, and so on. WPBAs should only start once the learner has had at least 10 hours of exposure to the workplace in the form of outpatient visits, ward rounds, theater postings, and emergency rotations.

Healthcare-related tasks: These are the daily activities that are expected to be routinely performed by a practitioner of that discipline during care of patients. Depending on the hierarchy of the learner, the tasks should not be limited to health care in the strict sense, but could also include teamwork, meetings, teaching, research, and mentoring which are important activities for a health care provider.

Direct observation: Direct observation of the learner's performance at the workplace is desirable when we are assessing competence.

Observing a learner as she works is more authentic than any surrogate marker [viva, long case, objective structured clinical examination (OSCE), etc.]. It allows one to make assessments of not only the learner's knowledge and core skills but also of other broad areas like critical thinking, problem-solving ability, teamwork, interpersonal skills and communication. Another advantage of direct observation is that the learner can immediately receive authentic feedback on her performance and can correct whatever she is doing wrong.

Feedback: The educational impact, of constructive feedback cannot be overemphasized. The strength of WBPA lies in the potential for formative feedback which is the backbone of assessment for learning. Assessment of learning, or summative assessment, on the contrary, is sometimes thought to impede learning since it focuses only on outcomes and does not address the difficulties that learners experience during the learning process. Feedback can be provided by any member of the healthcare team and even by patients and their caregivers. Feedback can improve clinical performance and professional competence if it is given by a credible source and learners use it to modify their practice.

Practice: To acquire a competency, learners need to be given multiple opportunities to work, initially under supervision, and later, independently, receiving feedback as they progress. For those learners who feel that they need more practice in certain areas, they must be given the encouragement and time to practice. Although the observer assesses whether the learner has acquired the competency, the learner has the autonomy to decide if he is ready to be assessed. Assessment does not have to be time-bound, according to a predefined schedule.

Multiple methods, tools and assessors: Multiple formative and summative assessment activities should be combined in a coherent manner throughout the period of training so that multiple competencies can be validly assessed. Multiple trainers and multiple assessors drawn from a broad spectrum of workplace stakeholders can bring multiple perspectives and contribute to a more valid judgment of the learner's competence rather than to rely on the judgment of an individual assessor.

The strengths and weaknesses of WPBA have been listed in **Table 13.2**.

Setting-up WPBA in your Discipline

(Barrett et al., 2015; Boker, 2016; Joshi, et al., 2017; Kundra & Singh, 2014; Norcini & Burch, 2007)

The following steps can help you to set-up WPBA in your discipline.

***Step 1*: Define the content to be assessed:** The content should be aligned to the outcomes desired of a competency-based curriculum as defined in the recommendations of the regulatory body (Medical Council of India) and the ordinances of the university. Five domains

TABLE 13.2: Strengths and weaknesses of WPBA

Strengths	Weaknesses
❖ Increases contact time with the supervisors	❖ WPBA demands prior training of the faculty in performance evaluations and providing effective feedback
❖ Effective means of judging the competence since assessments are made by authentic workplace seniors and colleagues who actually observe performance	❖ More time is required per assessment
	❖ Student sensitization is essential
	❖ Students may report that it reduces training time because of the longer time required to complete assessments
❖ Can explore all areas of Miller pyramid of clinical competence	
❖ Formative assessment or assessment for learning provides opportunities and instructions for improving performance	❖ The trainees who perform well in initial encounters may not feel the need for further improvement
	❖ Trainees who are struggling may not seek feedback
❖ Feasible since it is applied during day-to-day routine work at the workplace	❖ Trainees tend to seek assessors who are not very senior and who may provide higher performance ratings that are not truly accurate
❖ Feasible because institutions do not need enhanced infrastructure to establish WPBA	❖ There is a need for rigorous quality assurance to ensure consistently high standards
❖ Identifies learners who are struggling	

of competence or roles have been identified: (1) Clinician, (2) Leader, (3) Communicator, (4) Lifelong learner, and (5) Professional. For new curricula that are competency-based, each specialty has to define the competencies specific to its specialty along with some generic competencies that are common to all specialties. Depending on the tasks that a learner must be able to perform independently after completing training, one can map out the knowledge, skills, attitudes, and behaviors that are necessary performing with competence. One must look at the contexts in which the tasks are to be performed and the natural sequence of events in a workplace so as to plan realistically and make more meaningful content decisions.

Step 2: **Define the purpose of the assessment:** Very often, the purpose of WPBA is formative, but occasionally it may be summative, and this fact should be clarified right at the beginning to avoid conflict or wastage of an assessment opportunity. The purpose will guide the type and combination of instruments that you use, the number of observations that must be made, and how the scores will be used in decision-making. The trainees and trainers/assessors must be helped to understand how important their roles are in achieving the purpose of the assessment.

Assessment from the learner's point of view could serve the purpose of providing feedback to motivate learning, nudging the novice toward mastery, collecting evidence to inform the learner of progression, demonstrating progression over time when the assessment is repeated, and for diagnosing a slow learner.

For the training department, the purpose of assessment could be demonstrating trainee progression across the course, for making summative pass/fail decisions, for identifying slow learners, or collecting evidence to support curricular changes that could help slow learners catch up.

The purpose of assessment for the institution would be to encourage excellence, while for the end-user, it would be to ensure that medical practitioners are competent.

***Step 3*: Blueprint the assessment process:** Make a template that defines the content of the assessment keeping in mind all the competencies required by the curriculum. This is likely to be complex for WPBAs since the delivery of health care in the workplace is complicated and unpredictable and a great deal of teamwork is involved. Thus, no single assessment method can capture all the desired competencies of a learner; instead, different aspects of performance will have to be assessed by different tools, and the global picture will emerge when the results are combined. For example, assessment of communication skills may require direct observation, but assessment of professionalism may be done through multisource feedback (MSF). During blueprinting, it is good to avoid duplication, where two tools measure the same aspect of performance; however, there is sure to be a degree of overlap between the facets assessed by different methods. This overlap can be considered as triangulation or corroboration of evidence and is not necessarily a bad thing to achieve.

Blueprinting should ensure that all the domains or roles of a competent doctor are assessed and that curricular requirements are broadly covered. Each domain should be assessed separately since adequate performance in one domain may not guarantee satisfactory performance in another. As far as the curriculum is concerned, it is not feasible to sample every clinical condition that a clinician may be expected to deal with; nevertheless, the learner should be assessed across an appropriate mix of conditions so as to allow making a broad judgment about competence in performance. The assessment blueprint should include instructions in simple language.

***Step 4*: Choosing appropriate assessment methods** is part of blueprinting. There are numerous WPBA tools as will be shown in the following section and, keeping in mind the purpose of assessment, one may choose a combination thereof. An assessment method is not chosen because it is very reliable but because it is fit for purpose. The assessments should be realistic, logical and with measurable outcomes, and should include opportunities for observation and feedback at regular intervals throughout training (formative assessment or 'assessment for learning'). There should also be inbuilt mechanisms that allow learners to monitor their progress. The data from multiple tools and multiple assessors, including any other information from other sources, are usually collated into an e-portfolio which is accessible to the learner.

Step 5: Training of assessors is critical if WPBAs are to be reliably administered. The medical education units can initiate training for all levels of potential assessors, including medical and non-medical staff, with particular reference to newer concepts that were not used in traditional forms of assessment. This includes training in formative assessment, providing constructive feedback, encouraging learner reflection, and making progress decisions.

Step 6: Setting of standards against which the learner will be assessed. Training of assessors in the standard-setting should be ensured. The standards are criterion-referenced and the criteria on which judgments will be made must be clearly defined. These standards must be defensible, transparent, and fair. Trainers, assessors, and trainees must be aware of the standards.

To avoid a reductionist approach to assessment, the standards of performance need not be very explicitly defined for every competency—some leeway should be given to the expert assessor who can be allowed to use logic and experience in judging learner performance. While performance in many tasks can be referenced against absolute criteria, in some complex or integrated tasks, the assessor may have to compare performance against standards that are based on his own past experience with trainees and that cannot be expressed in terms of clear criteria. Expert assessors tend to develop their own absolute standards of what is expected at a particular stage in training and it is useful in some cases to use such standards.

Step 7: Review the assessment system for quality assurance: It is important to determine if the timelines resources, assessor training, scoring and the standards, mix of assessment methods, documentation, and the outcomes were appropriate.

Tools for Workplace-based Assessment

There are many tools described in literature and departments may choose those that fulfill the purpose of assessment. The purpose of a particular assessment may be to observe a clinical encounter, to initiate discussion on an individual case, or to generate feedback from multiple stakeholders. **Table 13.3** categorizes the tools based on purpose of assessment.

Each assessment tool is context-specific and should be adapted so that it aligns with the curricular objectives of the individual specialty. The same tool may not behave the same way across disciplines since many factors may be different: the number of raters, the content to be assessed, the attributes deemed critical, the performances expected at different stages of progression through the course, and so on.

TABLE 13.3: Categories of tools based on the purpose of assessment

Purpose	WPBA tool
Accumulate and document evidence (Jenkins et al., 2013; Lonka et al., 2001)	Portfolio, Logbook
Sample clinical work (Richards et al., 2007)	Clinical Encounter Cards (CECs)
Observe clinical performance (Norcini & Burch, 2007; Yanting et al., 2016; Beard et al., 2005; Liu, 2012)	Mini-Clinical Evaluation Exercise (Mini-CEX) Direct Observation of Procedural Skills (DOPS) Procedure-based Assessment (PbA)
Discuss clinical cases (Williamson & Osborne, 2012; Boker, 2016; Profanter & Perathoner, 2015)	Case-based Discussion (CbD) Evaluation of Clinical Events (ECEs) Discussion of Correspondence (DOC) Sheffield Assessment Instrument for Letters (SAIL)
Obtain feedback from peers, coworkers, & patients (Barrett et al., 2015; Miller and Archer, 2010; Saedon et al., 2012; Tan, Tengah, Chong, Liew, & Naing, 2015; Guraya, 2015; Lockyer, 2003)	Multisource Feedback (MSF) or 360° assessment Mini-Peer Assessment Tool (Mini-PAT) Team Assessment of Behavior (TAB) Patient satisfaction questionnaire (PSQ)

Figure 13.1 is a pictorial representation of the tools discussed in the preceding paragraphs categorized according to broad purpose, with the caveat that the categories are not water-tight since the tools serve overlapping purposes.

An Overview of Workplace-based Assessment Tools

Tools for Accumulating and Documenting Evidence

(a) Portfolio

Purpose: To accumulate evidence of the learner's journey toward the acquisition of competencies over a long time period; includes critical reflection.

Procedure: Every learning experience and assessment that a learner undergoes during her training is recorded and compiled into a collection that is called portfolio. The portfolio, in the context of WPBA, is usually stored online, and paper-based portfolios can simultaneously be maintained for more traditional assessments. The collection is available to the learner, to the trainer, and to the department, and serves as evidence of the learner's journey toward competence. A portfolio includes every sort of educational experience including professional activities, development, and achievements. The portfolio can store the following— traditional assessment scores, WPBA ratings and feedback

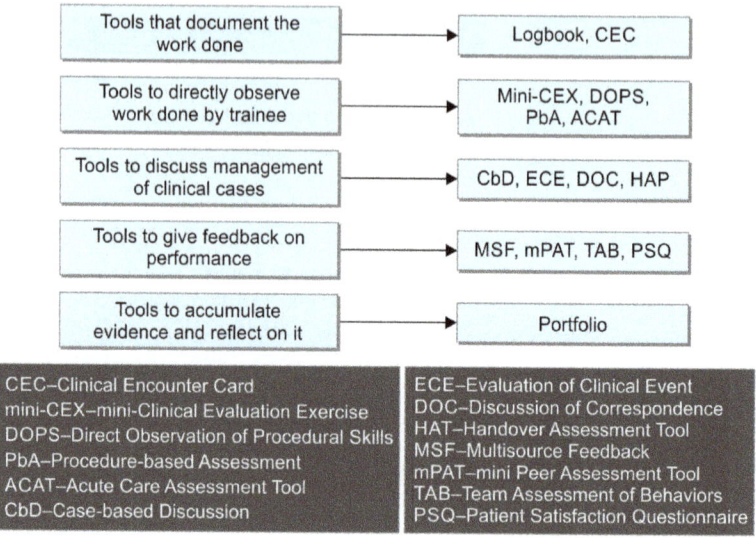

Fig. 13.1: Tools for workplace-based assessment (WPBA). (Singh et al., 2013)

received, logbook records of clinical experience, reflections and plans made for improvement of performance, research activity, teaching activity, critical incidents, letters from patients or their families, personal audits, feedback from peers or team-members, and any other informal record that is related to learning. Each item in the portfolio pertains to a single encounter, but when examined over the period of the entire course, it gives a comprehensive picture of learning (Gilberthorpe et al., 2016, Lonka et al., 2001).

Assessment: Based on the learner's portfolio, assessors make judgments not only about the outcomes of training, but also about the number and nature of educational experiences so as to evaluate both things— the competence of the learner to perform, and the fitness of the assessments. Portfolio allows a broad view of complex and integrated abilities while also considering the level and context of learning. The validity and reliability of a portfolio depend on its content and it is important, to enhance these qualities, for departments to demarcate assessments that are mandatory to include in the portfolio from those that a learner is free to include if she wishes. Portfolios, keeping in mind their reflective component, are best suited to formative assessment since they allow learning from actions. Portfolios have been discussed in detail in Chapter 11.

(b) Logbooks

A discussion of the portfolio is incomplete without a mention of Logbooks. Though they are both collections of work done, the portfolio is more comprehensive in that it includes not just a record of work done through a longer stretch of the course, but also contains evidence of the feedback received; reflections on how the feedback was processed and of the progress made as a result; and details of plans made for the future to continue improving competence. Logbooks are more focused, on the other hand, on helping learners record the learning activities they have undertaken for the acquisition of competencies, and they apply to shorter segments of the course (Sanchez Gómez et al., 2013). The activities required to be completed depend on the objectives of the course and are those that are recommended by departments, institutions, universities and regulatory bodies. They are indicated in the curriculum so that the learner is aware of the work to be done, and she tabulates them according to a prepared framework as and when they are completed. Completion of each task is verified by the trainer in the Logbook, as is the level of competence at which the activity was performed, and a recommendation on whether the learner has satisfactorily completed the task or should receive remedial training. A learner must complete all the tasks outlined in the logbook at a predefined level of competence so as to progress in the course. The trainer gives feedback as required; some logbooks may actively encourage learner reflection.

Logbooks, which are standalone but may form part of the portfolio, are a common tool used to record learning activities undertaken for the acquisition of competencies during a segment of the course (Sanchez Gómez et al., 2013).

Tools that Sample Clinical Work

(a) Clinical Encounter Cards

Purpose: To document the clinical encounters and the feedback provided to trainees.

Procedure: Clinical encounter cards (CECs) get their name from the 5 × 8-inch computer-readable cards that were handed to learners at the beginning of their rotation. They are expected to fill and submit them at the end of their rotations. These have been replaced by computerized cards which are filled online. The list of diagnoses on each card reflects the type of clinical material seen in the discipline and can be tailored if required. The assessment is completed soon after the trainee performs an examination or a procedure on a patient—the encounter should have been observed by an assessor. Both the learner and the assessor complete their portions of the CEC (Richards et al., 2007).

Assessment: The assessor is required to fill up the card indicating the context (inpatient, outpatient) and the chief focus of the encounter in terms of the skills that were performed and observed (one or two out of the following—taking the history, performing a physical examination, professional behavior, technical skill, case presentation, problem formulation, and problem-solving). He then grades the performance on a Likert scale according to the standard expected of the learner (from unsatisfactory to better than satisfactory) and records his comments on what was good. He also gives feedback in the form of suggestions on the aspects that need improvement. The learner fills her segment of the card indicating if it was her first encounter with the patient or not (multiple encounters with the same patient are recorded on the same card), and what she thought was the primary patient problem. Her comments are recorded, and the card submitted to the e-portfolio system. Over time, many such cards can be used by the learner to inform her about and allow her to act on her evolving needs. The program can use the stored documentation to identify matters of concern with respect to quality of trainer feedback; to assess patterns of disease conditions that are seen less often in a particular period and employ ways to improve exposure; and to evaluate learner progress in acquiring clinical competence.

Clinical encounter cards are powerful tools for facilitating timely and effective feedback from trainers. Learners report enhanced quality and quantity of feedback, and trainers find that it prompts them to improve their teaching and their understanding of the benefits of giving contextual feedback. (Richards et al., 2007).

Clinical encounter cards have been modified and are used as Daily Encounter Cards (DECs—useful in contexts where the trainer is available for short periods of time only, or learner rotations are brief); Teacher Encounter Cards (TECs—students provide feedback on clinical teaching); and Oral Case Presentation Encounter Cards (OCP-ECs—to assess oral case presentation skills).

Tools for Observation of Clinical Performance

(a) mini-Clinical Evaluation Exercise

Purpose: To help learners identify their strengths and the areas for improvement in history taking, physical examination, communication and profesiionalism.

Procedure: The mini-Clinical Evaluation Exercise (mini-CEX) is trainee-led with the trainee choosing both the clinical case and the assessor. Occasionally, an assessor, who should be a consultant or a more experienced colleague, can initiate the assessment. The case chosen should be a challenging one that has caused some difficulties for the learner. The assessment may only be concerned with one aspect of the case such as the history-taking or some part of the clinical examination or may be global. It takes place in a clinical setting during an actual learner-patient interaction and lasts about 15 minutes. The patient is informed about the exercise beforehand. The learner conducts a focused history and/or performs a physical examination and suggests a diagnosis and a plan of management. The learner should ideally initiate around six to eight mini-CEX during the year, with a different assessor and a different problem, each time.

Assessment: The assessor observes the clinical encounter and the assessment is recorded on a standard structured format that uses a

9-point Likert scale. The learner is rated in six domains and there is one final rating of clinical competence. Feedback with respect to the learner's strength areas and areas for development is then given by the assessor on skills that are considered essential to the provision of good care. The standard expected at the stage of training is kept as a benchmark. A mutually agreed action plan is drawn up for and by the learner.

mini-CEX has been found to be an acceptable, reliable, and feasible method of providing good quality feedback to learners (Norcini & Burch, 2007; Yanting et al., 2016). More details about mini-CEX can be found in Chapter 9.

(b) Direct Observation of Procedural Skills

Purpose: To help learners identify their strengths and the areas for improvement with respect to their competence in day-to-day, routine practical procedures.

Procedure: Direct Observation of Procedural Skill (DOPS) is trainee-led with the trainee choosing the procedure or laboratory technique and choosing the assessor. If the procedure involves an actual patient, the patient's consent is taken.

Assessment: The assessor evaluates the learner while she is conducting a routine procedure and rates her on a standard proforma against set criteria. The standard of performance is what would be commensurate with the current stage of training. This is followed by an immediate, face-to-face, feedback session during which the learner's strengths are identified and areas for development are highlighted. The trainee will have to repeat the assessment later if the assessor finds him unable to perform with the expected competence. DOPS has been found to be valid, reliable, and feasible in evaluating postgraduate learners. You will find more details about DOPS in Chapter 9.

(c) Procedure-based Assessment

Purpose: To help a surgical trainee understand her strengths, weaknesses and overall ability to perform surgical procedures through a structured form and constructive feedback.

Procedure: The Procedure-based Assessment (PbA) is applicable to all surgical specialties. Each specialty specifies a list of procedures that are either essential to the specialty or are optional procedures. The trainee is observed across six areas of competency where each competency is subdivided into components that are graded as satisfactory, unsatisfactory, or not observed. At the end, the assessor provides a global score that quantifies the ability of the trainee into four levels. Level 1 indicates inability to perform and level 4 indicates that the learner performs competently without supervision. The observer's feedback is recorded, as is the learner's reflection (Guraya, 2015).

Assessment: The six competency areas assessed are: (1) consent, (2) pre-operative planning, (3) pre-operative preparation, (4) exposure and closure, (5) intra-operative technique, and (6) post-operative management. The standard in PbA is invariably the level required at the completion of specialist training. This is unlike other WPBA where the standard is what would be commensurate with the current stage of training. Thus, early in the course, an unsatisfactory grade and a global level of 1 or 2 is only to be expected; the grade and global level should improve over time and should be captured when the PbA for the same procedure is repeated after further training.

The assessor may not be able to observe the learner through all the competency areas for a single case, since consent may be taken a day or two earlier, pre-operative preparation may take place a night before, and aftercare may occur in another setting, like the outpatient department. Nevertheless, observation of performance in all areas should be possible during the completion of the entire operation list for that day. PbAs are found to be reliable and acceptable to both trainers and trainees. In the case that effective feedback is given and received, learners demonstrate improvement in surgical competence (Guraya, 2015).

Tools for Discussion of Clinical Cases

(a) Case-based Discussion

Purpose: To help learners evaluate their Clinical Decision-making and management skills with respect to a patient that they are directly responsible for.

Procedure: While the learner usually initiates a case-based discussion (CbD), the assessor can also initiate one. The cases need not always be routine; rather, they should be challenging and should increase in complexity as the learner progresses in the course. Trainees should seek to be assessed about six times in the year. The trainee chooses a few cases that she has been working up and in which she has recorded her findings; the assessor picks one of the chosen cases a few days before the discussion. The learner and the assessor pre-determine the domains and specific competencies that will be assessed, then the assessor prepares focused questions to elicit responses relevant to the domains.

Assessment: The assessor is a more experienced colleague or a consultant who discusses the case based on the learner's documentation on the case record. The learner is provided with a systematic and structured feedback regarding how her knowledge, skills, and attitudes were applied in the decision-making process. Learner is able to discuss why she made certain decisions, or ordered investigations or interventions, especially in the light of ethical and legal frameworks. CbD assesses trainees based on what they have done in a real-life patient care situation. By using the learner's own cases, their applied knowledge, clinical reasoning, and decision-making skills can be assessed in complex situations, particularly those that involve dilemmas. CbD has significant face and content validity, good reliability, and is a valid method when the assessor is trained in the use of CbD. (Williamson & Osborne, 2012; Boker, 2016).

As can be seen, CbD is not the same as a case presentation. In a case presentation, the learner may hypothetically talk about what she would do next, whereas in CbD, she actually demonstrates the next step by 'doing' it. Each of these techniques fulfill a different assessment need and thus one may not necessarily replace the other. CbD, by observing the learner perform, focuses on how the trainee uses medical knowledge when managing a single case, and assesses for competence in clinical decision-making and problem-solving, while a case presentation tests the learner's knowledge domain, oral communication skills, and some aspects of the clinical examination.

(b) Evaluation of Clinical Events

Purpose: To assess the trainee in the performance of complex tasks that involve teamwork or interprofessional interactions.

Procedure: Evaluation of Clinical Events (ECE) is trainee-driven, with the trainee choosing the event for discussion and choosing the assessor; the latter can be a consultant or any other member of the health care team who is involved in the same area of work. The assessor observes the learner during the activity, which should take about 15–20 minutes, and then takes the next 5–10 minutes to give immediate, constructive feedback.

Assessment: The discussion is structured with the trainee sharing reasons for the actions she took and the assessor highlighting aspects that were good and also those that need improvement. The assessment form is completed soon after in the presence of the trainee; areas for improvement are identified, mutually agreed upon, and recorded on the ECE form. The standard of assessment is what is expected at the end of the trainee's current stage of training. The grading can range from 1 to 6; a score of 3 is considered borderline which means that the learner has not met expectations. A score of less than 3 is an unsatisfactory score and the trainee needs to repeat the assessment (Royal College of Pathologists, 2019).

Over the years of training, the trainee should select events that get more and more complex so that a broad range is covered. The assessor can help with the decision on level of complexity and can base it on the stage of the learner and on curricular requirements. To make an ECE reliable, multiple assessments should be undertaken by different assessors.

Evaluation of clinical events can be used during diagnostic reporting, clinico-pathological evaluations, case presentations at multi-disciplinary meetings, audits, critical incident reporting, quality assurance meetings, patient safety issues, outbreak investigations, root cause analysis, journal club meetings, organizing a departmental seminar or journal club, undertaking a literature review, refereeing an article for a journal, writing an ethics submission or a research paper, and so on.

(c) Discussion of Correspondence

Purpose: To help the trainee improve the quality of written clinical information that she has shared with other professionals and with patients or their family.

Procedure: Discussion of Correspondence (DOC) is an online form and replaces the Sheffield Assessment Instrument for Letters (SAIL) which is a paper form. All types of written communication can be assessed—these include discharge summaries, referral letters, reports to patients, and any other written material that is representative of the work learners do routinely in the workplace. The assessment is done in the presence of the trainee with the correspondence and the patient case sheet being available to the assessor. The assessor may be a consultant or any other member of the team.

Assessment: The assessor looks for three things in the correspondence: (1) its clarity (how easy is it to understand, is it well-structured and has logical flow, and is there any jargon?), (2) the clinical assessment (how accurate is the documentation of details like history, findings, diagnosis, medication, follow-up?), and (3) the communication (have caregiving relatives and other health care professionals associated with the case been sent a copy, and is the plan of action clearly described?). Since the form is structured, the style of writing does not influence the assessment. The assessor discusses the correspondence with the trainee. Immediate feedback is given on the things that have been well documented and the aspects that can be improved. The assessor documents the type of correspondence being assessed, the case summary, and the discussion. She also records any matter of concern and may choose to notify the learner's supervisor if there is a significant concern. The trainee, in her turn, records mutually agreed learning objectives from the issues discussed, and records his reflections on the experience of writing the correspondence (Profanter & Perathoner, 2015).

Tools for Feedback From Peers, Coworkers, and Patients

(a) Multisource Feedback or 360-degree Feedback

Purpose: For the trainee to get structured feedback from multiple members of the health care team and from patients who have observed the trainee during practice and can comment on his professional behavior and clinical performance.

Procedure: Multisource Feedback (MSF) is trainee-driven. The trainee sets up a time frame for the assessment after consultation with the supervisor. Then, she chooses respondents from among medical colleagues (6 or more), other health care colleagues (6 or more), and patients (10 or more) and recruits them to fill the MSF form. The form can be completed online or offline. The respondents should have observed the trainee at the workplace and, as far as possible, must be different individuals from those who rated her during a previous MSF session.

Assessment: The process of MSF is explained to the respondents and they are informed that their responses will be anonymous. They rate the trainee on a standard, structured form against several desirable qualities or behaviors. The trainee is also required to reflect and self-assess on how she thinks she is doing. Once the deadline for the respondents to complete the assessment is over, the results are available for discussion between the trainee and the supervisor where the trainee reflects on the feedback received and draws up an action plan. The discussion is recorded by the trainee in her e-portfolio. (Lockyer, 2003; Barrett et al., 2015; Saedon et al., 2012).

MSF is useful to rate and provide feedback on competence in those situations that the supervisor has not personally witnessed. Several forms are available, like the General Medical Council (GMC) MSF questionnaire and the Colleague Feedback Evaluation Tool (CFET) which focuses on clinical ability, communication, and teamwork. The MSF can be modified to include patient feedback—the SPRAT tool (Sheffield Peer Review Assessment Tool); however, separate specific forms are available: the Doctors' Interpersonal Skills Questionnaire (DISQ), the GMC Patient Questionnaire (PQ). More details about MSF can be found in Chapter 9.

(b) Mini-Peer Assessment Tool

Purpose: For the learner to obtain peer feedback about her performance in a range of competence domains.

Procedure: Confidential feedback is taken from eight peers. Approximately two mini-Peer Assessment Tools (mini-PATs) should be solicited per year.

Assessment: Using mini-PAT, the peers evaluate the learner in the following domains (Norcini & Burch, 2007)—diagnosis and appropriate application of available investigative tools; management of time; management of stress, fatigue, and workload; effective communication; and knowledge of one's own limitations. Mini-PAT is an effective and reliable tool for soliciting peer feedback with respect to a trainee's competence. (Southgate et al.,2001; Salmon & Pugsley, 2017)

(c) Team Assessment of Behaviors

Purpose: To solicit feedback from members of the health care team on the trainee's professional behavior.

Procedure: Team Assessment of Behavior (TAB) is an MSF assessment of four domains of professional behavior: (1) professional relationship with patients, (2) verbal communication, (3) teamwork, and (4) accessibility. The trainee distributes at least 15 TAB forms to peers of her choice, of which at least 10-filled forms must be returned so as to make it a valid and reliable assessment. The assessors should be a mix of doctors (about 3, including a consultant) and allied health care professionals (about 5) and they rate the trainee on a 3-point rating scale: (1) no concern, (2) some concern or (3) major concern. (Olupeliyawa et al., 2014)

Assessment: In addition to indicating concern, the assessors are asked to give specific feedback under each domain. The trainee's supervisor collates the information obtained through the TAB and discusses perceived areas of concern identified by the peers, offers more feedback and helps the trainee formulate learning objectives to address professionalism issues. TAB can be used for formative or summative assessment and has been shown to help improve performance. It is a valid tool for the assessment of professionalism and is reliable when at least ten raters assess the learner. It is feasible, taking 5 minutes to complete and requires no particular training to understand; however, the assessors must be trained in giving feedback.

Newer Additions to Workplace-based Assessment

Change in Perspective

Of late, medical educators have begun to move towards a structure of assessment that is truly formative and is heavily feedback-oriented. The first change in this direction is that the scoring aspect of most WPBAs has been entirely removed and is replaced with boxes for recording feedback and suggestions for further improvement. The second change is that the outcome of the assessment is now considered to be the learning that ensues for the trainee (assessment for learning); thus, WPBAs are now called *Supervised Learning Events* (SLEs) (Massie & Ali, 2016). Likewise, summative assessments (assessment of learning) are now called *Assessment of Performance* (AoP) as they make a judgment about whether a specific competency has been achieved or not.

With this change in perspective, mini-CEX, ECE, PbA, CbD, and DOC have been converted to SLEs by making the following changes: eliminating the scoring, expanding the feedback section, and adding a learner reflection section. DOPS, too, has an SLE-DOPS version that has made it formative instead of summative.

Newer Supervised Learning Events

(i) Acute Care Assessment Tool

Purpose: To assess and provide feedback on a trainee's ability to integrate multiple skills during acute, challenging medical situations.

Procedure: The setting can vary and may be the emergency department, the intensive care unit, or the ward. The Acute Care Assessment Tool

(ACAT) assesses competence in clinical assessment, medical record keeping, investigations and referrals, safe prescribing, management of the acutely unwell patient, time and team management, and decision-making (Johnson et al., 2009).

Assessment: The trainer, who may be a consultant or resident, observes the trainee and gives feedback to the trainee on how she performed in each area with reference to what went well and what the areas for development are. After discussion, the trainee records his reflection on what she has learned from the case and how it will change her practice in the future. Finally, the trainer records her global assessment of the competence of the trainee in managing acute care patients. If she has any serious concerns, she records them for onward transmission to the trainee's supervisor.

(ii) LEADER Case-based Discussion (LEADER CbD)

Purpose: To help trainees develop clinical leadership skills essential for delivering high quality patient care.

Procedure: The structured instrument allows a discussion that focuses less on the clinical aspects of a case and more on the leadership issues identified. The case selected could be one that involves teamwork or multidisciplinary collaboration and in which the trainee has been involved in providing care. Trainees should undertake at least one LEADER CbD every year of training out of the quota of total CbDs mandated. Six broad areas of leadership are assessed: (1) leadership in a team, (2) effective services, (3) acting in a team, (4) direction setting, (5) enabling improvement, and (6) reflection (Royal College of Paediatrics and Child Health, 2019).

Assessment: The trainer, who should be a consultant, discusses one or two domains per case. The trainee identifies and records learning points for the domains discussed and records his reflection. The reflection is mandatory and centers on the leadership issues that came out of the discussion, mentions what went well and highlights what learning accrued. The trainee ends with a plan for improvement in leadership skills which could be in the form of training or the conduct of leadership projects.

(iii) Handover Assessment Tool

Purpose: To help learners assess their ability to effectively and safely transfer the responsibility of care to other health care professionals.

Procedure: Handover Assessment Tool (HAT) allows the trainer, who may be a consultant or a resident, and the trainee to discuss a case in a structured manner from the standpoint of patient safety during handovers. The main areas covered include structure of the handover and organization, safety briefing, ward management, workload, and non-technical skills like time management and prioritization. The trainee receives written feedback in each area that helps him identify areas of strength and those that need further development. The trainer records the discussion and the agreed learning objectives while the trainee records her reflection with respect to what she has learned and how it will change her practice in the future. If the trainer has any concerns, she records them so that the trainee's supervisor can be notified (Royal College of Paediatrics and Child Health, 2019).

(iv) Safeguarding CbD

Purpose: To help the trainee understand her competence in safeguarding during pediatric care where safety concerns are raised.

Procedure: Safeguarding is the action that is taken to promote the welfare of children and protect them from harm. The harm may be physical, sexual, emotional, neglect, or fictitious or induced illness. The discussion centers around a case where such harm is suspected or proven. Pediatric trainees should complete at least one CbD that has significant safeguarding elements out of their entire CbD quota per year of training. The trainee seeks the assessment but must complete some parts of the form before the discussion starts. She must record her safeguarding concerns along with a brief case summary. She must also describe her role in the case: as observer; as responsible for admission; referring to social care; examined the child, and so on (Royal College of Paediatrics and Child Health, 2019).

Assessment: The assessor, who may be any health care professional trained in safeguarding, discusses the case with regard to what the learner has recorded as well as how she responds to questions directed at assessing her knowledge and behavior—risks and protective factors in the child's life, elements in the referral to social services, the agencies involved in child care, other interventions that could have been considered, management of difficulties, if any were experienced, and the outcome of the case. Based on the discussion, the assessor indicates if the trainee is competent for her level of training regarding child protection work. The learner records agreed learning objectives and reflects on what she has learned from the case. She ends with a description of how she expects to change her practice in the future. The final submission loads the form into her e-portfolio.

Roles and Responsibilities in WPBA

We have emphasized it repeatedly that many of the tools of WPBA are to be trainee initiated. We have also emphasized the role of faculty development to make optimum use of this modality of assessment. **Table 13.4** summarizes the roles of assessor and the trainee.

TABLE 13.4: The roles of assessor and the trainee

Assessors	Trainees
❖ Remind trainees to complete the mandated WPBAs in a timely manner ❖ Periodically review to confirm that they are being completed ❖ Offer formative feedback to all levels of trainees all year round ❖ Offer guidance on the areas that trainees need to develop further ❖ Follow up on the feedback and on the learning outcomes that trainees identified ❖ Respond to causes for concern raised by assessors for particular trainees	❖ Complete WPBAs in a timely manner rather than leaving all assessments for the end ❖ Remember to send WPBA forms for completion to the supervisor ❖ Reflect after the assessment, as soon as possible, to avoid recall bias in reflections ❖ Draw up a feasible plan of action to meet learning needs

Quality Parameters of WPBA

Before Choosing a Workplace-based Assessment Tool

The following considerations must be kept in mind before choosing a tool for WPBA (Norcini & Burch, 2007; de Jonge et al., 2017; Govaerts, 2015; Singh & Modi, 2013; Tan et al., 2015; Guraya, 2015).

a. *Validity*: Does the assessment purport to test what we intend to test? Are the criteria being assessed those that are required to perform the task?
b. *Reliability*: Is the assessment known to produce the same results at different times or under different conditions? In other words, how consistent are the results of the assessment expected to be. Consistency applies to both the learner's performance and the assessor's judgment.

   For both the preceding parameters, it is not the assessment tool but the results of the assessment that should be valid and reliable.
c. *Feasibility*: Will the results of the assessment justify the amount of time, money, and effort involved in the development and administration of the assessment tool, and the interpretation or results?
d. *Educational impact*: Has use of the assessment tool resulted in enhanced learning and created opportunities for training?
e. *Acceptability*: In the opinion of assessors and trainees, has the assessment tool been found to be acceptable for practice?

A single tool may not meet all the five criteria for quality in equal measure and some compromise will have to be made in favor of one or the other. For assessment of performance, the need for the tool to produce valid results may be more important than for the outcomes to be reliable. Authenticity adds considerably to validity; since WPBAs are based on observations of actual performance in the workplace, rather than on work done in a simulation laboratory or in an examination hall, the setting is as authentic as it gets. Authenticity alone is not enough and the content of the tools, the standards of assessment, and how the outcomes will be used contribute to validity. As far as reliability is concerned, one cannot be certain that the same tool will be reliable in different settings or contexts, or even with every implementation. Reliability is often an issue in WPBAs since health care workplaces are very likely to be erratic and unpredictable and the activity being observed may pan out differently at different times even in the same setting. Thus, each tool should be re-evaluated when used in a new context, except perhaps MSF and mini-CEX, which have been extensively studied and are found to be reliable not only in different contexts but also in different specialties. Feasibility is important, too, when considering performance assessment in the workplace, since time constraints are a major bugbear for busy clinicians. In that respect, most WPBAs, since they fit into the normal day-to-day work, are good options. Educational impact is as important a parameter as validity and feasibility since the whole purpose of changing from traditional assessments to WPBAs is to use assessment activities as opportunities to improve performance. Assessments with proven educational impact should be included in the blueprint even if their reliability is suspect.

To ensure that most parameters of quality are conformed to, a variety of instruments should be chosen. The advantage of such a move has been discussed earlier, include the benefit that it provides triangulation of evidence.

Things to do After Using a WPBA Tool

To maintain standards in WPBA, it is important to evaluate the quality of the assessments in the contexts that they have been used. The same five parameters are used but the order may be changed a bit: Feasibility comes first—did it prove feasible to use in the new context? If it did not, then the inquiry turns away from quality of the WPBA and moves toward finding ways to make it more feasible especially if it seems to have had an educational impact. On the other hand, if it was found feasible, then the next question is—did it prove to be reliable or do you need to increase the number of observations and the number of observers? It is best not to try and change the content of the tool in an effort to improve reliability since increasing the number of items is not as effective as increasing the number of observations. It is possible to make assessments both valid and reliable, by specifying strict criteria that learners must achieve before they can be said to have demonstrated competence; however, the criteria used must be realistic and vetted by other stakeholders otherwise the acceptability of the tool will be poor and it may be reduced to a tick-box exercise. In any case, as discussed earlier, validity is more critical than reliability in WPBAs. Thus, if a tool is reliable but not valid, it should not be used. Likewise, if one tool has a lower reliability than the other but is more valid in a certain context, then it should be preferred over the more reliable one. Finally, if a tool shows that it has good educational impact, it is still a good idea to find out if the stakeholders find it acceptable.

Faculty Development for WPBA

Training of the people involved in WPBA is important since many concepts are different from what were traditionally followed. Trainers and assessors need to be sensitized to the newer concepts and reinforcement applied now and then. The training should be a multiprofessional faculty development—it should involve not only medical faculty but allied professionals as well keeping in mind MSF and other WPBAs that rely on members of the entire health care team.

Multiprofessional training should particularly focus on areas that are relatively new—assessing clinical competence especially the learner's communication, procedural ability, interpersonal skills, decision-making, and professionalism; how to observe without feeling discomfort and without making the learner uncomfortable; scoring the WPBA tools meaningfully; giving effective feedback one-on-one; helping learners draw up plans of future action to improve performance; encouraging learner reflection and continuous self-improvement; applying criteria to rate performance; self-directed learning; individualized solutions; and transparency and fairness (Daelmans et al., 2016; Tan et al., 2015; Guraya, 2015).

Methods to train faculty should preferably use a hands-on approach with minimal didactic component. Interaction in small groups, assessment exercises using some of the tools that the group is likely to use in practice, and observation of standardized residents and patients would be a useful way to train.

> **Box 13.1:** Improving assessor engagement in WPBA
> - Facilitate their training in WPBA processes
> - Involve them in the planning and execution of WPBA
> - Reward them for excellence in teaching
> - Advocate for systemic changes at departmental, institutional and governmental levels to give teaching the same level of importance as patient care and research

Potential Problem Areas in WPBA

The following issues can be problematic while implementing WPBA (Nair et al., 2015; Nesbitt et al., 2013; Pereira & Dean, 2009)

(a) Changing Perspectives

Trainers may not want to change traditional practices which involve providing knowledge to learners rather than helping them develop performance skills and thus they may have little interest in integrating WPBA into their training programs. For many, soliciting feedback is seen as a sign of insecurity, and they view it as a means to highlight weaknesses in the learner. In fact, the reverse is true, and this perspective needs to change if WPBAs are to become an accepted means to achieve improvement in practice. Involving the faculty in the initial stages of designing the WPBA can give them a sense of ownership so that when the time comes for implementation, they are already converted to the cause.

(b) Persuading Faculty to get Trained in Workplace-based Assessment

Faculty may be overwhelmed by the newer parameters of WPBAs that they are completely unfamiliar with. Training is essential to build confidence and gather acceptance. Training of trainers should include training in the exact competencies that are to be assessed, the art of giving feedback, and standardization of the assessment. Conflict should be addressed early so that assessors who are reluctant to give a score of 'unsatisfactory' can understand how it can improve learner performance provided constructive feedback is also provided to the learner.

(c) Quality of Training for Workplace-based Assessment

If the training programs for WPBA are not rigorously controlled for quality, then the assessors may not be able to perform assessments with competence or give constructive feedback.

(d) Conflict between the Two Roles of the Assessor: Teacher and Clinician

Some clinicians do not find teaching interesting; even if they do, they resent the fact that it takes them away from what they consider are their core duties—clinical care. Perhaps if clinicians get the same respect and recognition for their teaching accomplishments as they get for their clinical ones, they would be happier to contribute to WPBAs.

(e) The Teacher-Student Relationship

The hierarchical difference between faculty and students may be difficult to overcome. This risks the success of WPBAs which depend on greater one-on-one interaction between individual learners and assessors. Assessors need not always be consultants, especially in view of high student-teacher ratio and the overworked clinicians in many places; however, learners find that the feedback that they get from specialist consultants is more beneficial than that from other health care professionals. This outlook can be changed if all professionals involved in the assessment of learners at the workplace are trained in the particular assessment method and in the giving of feedback.

(f) The Doctor-Patient Ratio

The sheer volume of patients that present for routine care or critical care can be an overwhelming roadblock to the implementation of WPBA. Illiteracy and poverty propagate the paternalistic style of practicing medicine where the doctor makes all the decisions. This will not work in WPBA where the emphasis is on observing and rating a partnership style of consultation. Very often, the need to provide timely services to the masses puts workplace teaching-learning activities on to the back burner. This problem requires systemic changes at departmental, institutional, and governmental levels.

(g) Support from Administration and Government

Universities and institutions may not consider WPBA unless the national regulatory body endorses it. A governmental or equivalent regulatory body decision is essential in order to push forward this ethos of competency-based training to ensure patient safety. This is particularly true for medical institutions where the priority is to strengthen service provision rather than improve the training experience of learners. The institution should provide financial and logistical support for those involved in initiating and maintaining WPBA programs.

(h) Maintaining Transparency and Consistency of Assessments

Assessors tend to have a sympathetic view of learners and care for them when they have a positive relationship with them; thus, they may take more trouble to ensure their progress in achieving competency. If the assessor is one who has never worked with the trainee before, the position may be different. Studying how judgments are made by experts on the performance of learners, and modifying assessments based on the findings, may help to make the assessment system more transparent and fairer. Assessors have varying experiences across varying contexts, so to get consistent results from them for the same instrument and on the same task may be difficult. One way to achieve consistency is to define the competencies to be assessed and the standards in narrow terms to avoid ambiguity; however, such assessments would be unauthentic since they would remove the natural complexities of competencies that are a part of an actual workplace activity. The second thing that could be done is to make assessments descriptive instead of judgmental—that is, make them purely formative, which is what is being attempted these days.

(i) Online Process of Workplace-based Assessment

In resource-strapped countries, the degree of electronic networking required for running a WPBA system, including providing workspaces for the same, may be prohibitive. A possible solution is to develop mobile apps so that assessors and learners can connect to the assessment system and the e-portfolio.

(j) Identifying Underperforming Learners

Multisource feedback is well established as a tool to access competencies like communication, professionalism, and interpersonal skills; however, the feedback given by colleagues, and even by patients, tends to highlight the positive aspects of learner performance and may ignore the negative so that underperforming learners are not identified.

(k) Flexible Delivery of Workplace-based Assessment

Trainers and assessors may be uncomfortable with the notion of learners being assessed on a case of their choice and at a time of their choice rather than at preset times. Flexibility is an important component of WPBA and allows learners to request assessments when they consider themselves prepared, and not according to a predefined schedule. Learning is better when the learner has some autonomy and control over the learning and is encouraged to self-assess her need and her readiness for feedback.

Conclusion and Recommendations

Workplace-based assessment is an amalgamation of learning and assessment, which helps trainees identify areas for improvement and is formative in nature. It focuses on self-directed learning principles. Assessors must be trained, and multiple assessments should be made by different assessors to achieve valid and reliable result. Different WPBA instruments should be used in a specialty to test different attributes. All competencies cannot be assessed at each stage of training and no attempt should be made to do so. Assessments should preferably not be numerically scored but should reflect on the learner's strengths and weaknesses; the learner, herself, should reflect on how to improve performance. Poorly performing trainees should be identified and supported. Training excellence should be recognized and rewarded.

Instituting WPBA does not mean that traditional methods of assessment should be discarded. It might be more practicable to continue to use well-established and extensively evaluated traditional methods, and to employ WPBA for all the formative components of assessment. Knowledge and skill assessment provide useful complement to WPBA.

REFERENCES

Barrett, A., Galvin, R., Steinert, Y., Scherpbier, A., O'Shaughnessy, A., Horgan, M., et al. (2015). A BEME (Best Evidence in Medical Education) systematic review of the use of workplace-based assessment in identifying and remediating poor performance among postgraduate medical trainees. *Systematic Reviews, 4*, 65.

Beard, J., Strachan, A., Davies, H., Patterson, F., Stark, P., Ball, S., et al. (2005). Developing an education and assessment framework for the Foundation Programme. *Medical Education, 39(8)*, 841–51.

Boker, A. (2016). Toward competency-based curriculum: application of workplace-based assessment tools in the National Saudi Arabian Anesthesia training program. *Saudi Journal of Anaesthesia, 10(4)*, 417–22.

Daelmans, H.E., Mak-van der Vossen, M.C., Croiset, G., & Kusurkar, R.A. (2016). What difficulties do faculty members face when conducting workplace-based assessments in undergraduate clerkships? *International Journal of Medical Education, 7*, 19–24.

De Jonge, L., Timmerman, A.A., Govaerts, M., Muris, J., Muijtjens, A., Kramer, A., et al. (2017). Stakeholder perspectives on workplace-based performance assessment: towards a better understanding of assessor behaviour. *Advances in Health Sciences Education: Theory and Practice, 22(5)*, 1213–43.

Gilberthorpe, T., Sarfo, M.D., & Lawrence-Smith, G. (2016). Ticking the boxes: a survey of workplace-based assessments. *BJPsych Bulletin, 40(2)*, 89–92.

Govaerts, M. (2015). Workplace-based assessment and assessment for learning: threats to validity. *Journal of Graduate Medical Education, 7(2)*, 265–7.

Guraya, SY. (2015). Workplace-based assessment; applications and educational impact. *Malaysian Journal of Medical Sciences, 22(6)*, 5–10.

Jain, M.D., Tomlinson, G.A., Lam, D., Liu, J., Damaraju, D., Detsky, A.S., et al. (2014). Workplace-based assessment of internal medicine resident diagnostic accuracy. *Journal of Graduate Medical Education, 6(3)*, 532–5.

Jenkins, L., Mash, B.& Derese, A. (2013). The national portfolio of learning for postgraduate family medicine training in South Africa: experiences of registrars and supervisors in clinical practice. *BMC Med Educ 13,* 149. https://doi.org/10.1186/1472-6920-13-149

Johnson, G., Wade, W., Barrett, J, & Jones, M. (2009). The acute care assessment tool: a new assessment in acute medicine. *Clinical Teacher, 6(2)*, 105–9.

Joshi, M., Singh, T., & Badyal, D. (2017). Acceptability and feasibility of mini-clinical evaluation exercise as a formative assessment tool for workplace-based assessment for surgical postgraduate students. *Journal of Postgraduate Medicine, 63(2)*, 100–5.

Julyan, T.E. (2009). Educational supervision and the impact of workplace-based assessments: a survey of psychiatry trainees and their supervisors. *BMC Medical Education, 9*, 51.

Kundra, S., & Singh, T. (2014). Feasibility and acceptability of direct observation of procedural skills to improve procedural skills. *Indian Pediatrics, 51(1)*, 59–60.

Liu, C. (2012). An introduction to workplace-based assessments. *Gastroenterology and Hepatology from Bed to Bench, 5(1)*, 24–8.

Lockyer, J. (2003). Multisource feedback in the assessment of physician competencies. *Journal of Continuing Education in the Health Professions, 23(1)*, 4–12.

Lonka, K., Slotte, V., Halttunen, M., Kurki, T., Tiitinen, A., Vaara, L., et al. (2001). Portfolios as learning tool in obstetrics and gynaecology undergraduate training. *Medical Education, 35(12)*, 1125–30.

Massie, J., & Ali, J.M. (2016). Workplace-based assessment: a review of user perceptions and strategies to address the identified shortcomings. *Advances in Health Sciences Education: Theory and Practice, 21(2)*, 455–73.

Miller, A., & Archer, J. (2010). Impact of workplace-based assessment on doctors' education and performance: a systematic review. *British Medical Journal (Clinical Research Ed.), 341*, c5064.

Nair, B.K., Parvathy, M.S., Wilson, A., Smith, J., & Murphy, B. (2015). Workplace-based assessment; learner and assessor perspectives. *Advances in Medical Education and Practice, 6*, 317–21.

Nesbitt, A., Baird, F., Canning, B., Griffin, A., & Sturrock, A. (2013). Student perception of workplace-based assessment. *Clinical Teacher, 10(6)*, 399–404.

Norcini, J., & Burch, V. (2007). Workplace-based assessment as an educational tool: AMEE Guide No. 31. *Medical Teacher, 29(9)*, 855–71.

Olupeliyawa, A.M., O'Sullivan, A.J., Hughes, C., & Balasooriya, C.D. (2014). The teamwork mini-clinical evaluation exercise (T-MEX): a workplace-based assessment focusing on collaborative competencies in health care. *Academic Medicine, 89(2)*, 359–65.

Pereira, E.A., & Dean, B.J. (2009). British surgeons' experiences of mandatory online workplace-based assessment. *Journal of the Royal Society of Medicine, 102(7)*, 287–93.

Profanter, C., & Perathoner, A. (2015). DOPS (Direct Observation of Procedural Skills) in undergraduate skills-lab: Does it work? Analysis of skills-performance and curricular side effects. *GMS Zeitschrift für Medizinische Ausbildung, 32(4)*, Doc45.

Richards, M.L., Paukert, J.L., Downing, & S.M, Bordage, G. (2007). Reliability and usefulness of clinical encounter cards for a third-year surgical clerkship. *Journal of Surgical Research, 140(1)*, 139–48.

Royal College of Paediatrics and Child Health. (2019). *Assessment guide*. [online] Available from https://www.rcpch.ac.uk/resources/assessment-guide [Last accessed August, 2020].

Royal College of Pathologists. (2019). *Evaluation of clinical events*. [online] Available from https://www.rcpath.org/uploads/assets/6aabdae8-64bc-44da-8ab7d70968eba2ed/Histopathology-ECE-form.pdf [Last accessed August, 2020].

Saedon, H., Salleh, S., Balakrishnan, A., Imray, C.H., & Saedon, M. (2012). The role of feedback in improving the effectiveness of workplace-based assessments: a systematic review. *BMC Medical Education, 12*, 25.

Salmon, G., & Pugsley, L. (2017). The mini-PAT as a multi-source feedback tool for trainees in child and adolescent psychiatry: assessing whether it is fit for purpose. *B J Psych Bulletin, 41(2)*, 115–9.

Sánchez Gómez, S., Ostos, E. M., Solano, J. M.& Salado, T. F. (2013). An electronic portfolio for quantitative assessment of surgical skills in undergraduate medical education. *BMC medical education, 13*, 65. https://doi.org/10.1186/1472-6920-13-65

Singh, T., & Modi, J.N. (2013). Workplace based assessment: a step to promote competency based postgraduate training. *Indian Pediatrics, 50(6)*, 553–9.

Singh, T., & Sood, R. (2013). Workplace-based assessment: measuring and shaping clinical learning. *National Medical Journal of India, 26(1)*, 42–6.

Southgate, L., Cox, T., David, T., Hatch, D., Howes, A., Johnson, N., et al. (2001). The General Medical Council's performance procedures: peer review of performance in the workplace. *Medical Education, 35(Suppl 1)*, 9–19.

Tan, J., Tengah, C., Chong, V.H., Liew, A., & Naing, L. (2015). Workplace based assessment in an Asian context: trainees' and trainers' perception of validity, reliability, feasibility, acceptability, and educational impact. *Journal of Biomedical Education, 2015(615169)*, 1–8.

Williamson, J.M., & Osborne, A.J. (2012). Critical analysis of case-based discussions. *British Journal of Medical Practitioners, 5(2)*, a514.

Yanting, S.L., Sinnathamby, A., Wang, D., Heng, M.T., Hao, J.L., Lee, S.S., et al. (2016). Conceptualizing workplace-based assessment in Singapore: undergraduate mini-clinical evaluation exercise experiences of students and teachers. *Tzu-Chi Medical Journal, 28(3)*, 113–20.

Chapter 14

Competency-based Assessment

Upreet Dhaliwal, Jyoti N Modi, Piyush Gupta, Tejinder Singh

KEY POINTS

- Assessment in competency-based medical education has to be a longitudinal, continuous process since competence is achieved over a continuum.
- Being an assessment for learning, effective formative feedback is paramount to help learners improve their skills.
- It must be conducted in authentic, workplace settings with assessors making direct observation of the performance at frequent intervals, and use this to provide developmental feedback to the learner.

Competency-Based Medical Education (CBME) is the new trend in education which uses competency framework for instruction and assessment. Much more than a different style of teaching, CBME obligates a vastly different perspective on assessment. It mandates greater emphasis on setting up an ongoing assessment so that teachers can diagnose the stage of the learner and identify whether they need further learning opportunities to improve competence. From that outlook, CBME can be considered to be synonymous with 'good' assessment. In this chapter, we will look at the basics of CBME and then examine ways and means to assess competence using a competency framework.

What is a Competency?

For health professionals, the International Competency-Based Medical Education (ICBME) collaborators have defined competency as 'an observable activity that comprises multiple components like knowledge, skill, attitude, behavior, and communication and is habitually performed during a patient-care related task' (Frank et al., 2010). A person is called 'competent' if it is observed that he demonstrates predefined abilities in predefined domains, in specific contexts, and at defined stages of medical education. For optimal patient outcomes, however, being competent also means that individuals apply those abilities appropriately in routine clinical practice while exercising professional judgment.

Competency Frameworks to Facilitate Competency-based Medical Education

Of the many competency frameworks available, the major ones are those proposed by the Accreditation Council for Graduate Medical Education (ACGME) in the United States, the Canadian CanMEDs Consortium, and the United Kingdom's Good Medical Practice, Tomorrow's Doctors, and The Scottish Doctor. Recently, the Medical Council of India (MCI) too has identified prospective roles of the Indian Medical Graduate and condensed them into five competency domains, viz., clinician, leader and member of health care team, professional, communicator, and lifelong learner (MCI Regulations on Graduate Medical Education, 2019). These must be considered while designing CBME curricula and assessment. Using the entrustable professional activities (EPA) framework provides a useful starting point for competency-based assessment (CBA). *Entrustable professional activities* are 'essential' (must be able to do) and 'professional' patient-care activities that learners, after a certain period of training, will be trusted to perform without supervision (Dhaliwal, et al., 2015). They are observable and measurable activities that integrate one or more of the competency domains. Say for example, an EPA for a Pediatrics resident is: Care of a normal neonate.

Each EPA is broken down into incremental steps (called sub-competencies in the MCI framework). These sub-competencies are milestones which are defined to run over an expected timeline, until the learner can be trusted to perform the entire activity competently without supervision. These predefined subcompetencies are the abilities expected of a learner at different stages of training. Have a look at **Table 14.1** to which uses the EPA of care of the neonate to illustrate the concept in greater detail.

TABLE 14.1: The link between EPA competency domains, milestones, and the Dreyfus & Dreyfus model: an example of how EPAs are defined

EPA: *Care of the neonate* Competencies: Clinician, Leader, Professional, Communicator

	Novice learner	Advanced beginner	Competent	Proficient	Expert
Expected timeline	By month-3 of joining the course	By month-6 of joining the course	By the beginning of year-2 of joining the course	By the end of the postgraduate course	By month-6 of joining senior residency
Milestones	Is able to examine the newborn and detect congenital anomalies	Is able to receive and resuscitate term newborns in uncomplicated cases	Is able to manage immunization and common problems in newborns in outpatient settings	Is able to receive and resuscitate the newborn in complicated cases such as preterm, growth restriction, large baby	Is able to manage common problems in the newborns in intensive care settings

Designing Entrustable Professional Activities

The following paragraphs will show how designing EPAs for each specialty can be a useful first step in implementing CBME.

EPAs are 'essential' (must be able to do) and 'professional' patient-care activities that learners, after a certain period of training, will be trusted to perform without supervision (Dhaliwal, et al., 2015). They are observable and measurable activities that integrate one or more of the competency domains. Each EPA, and consequently, each competency being developed, is broken down into incremental steps (sub-competencies). These subcompetencies are defined to run over an expected time line, up to the point where the learner can be trusted to perform the entire activity without supervision, and competently. These predefined subcompetencies are the abilities expected of a learner at different stages of training. In other words, they are milestones on the way to achieving a particular competence.

Dreyfus & Dreyfus (1986) have provided a model of adult skill acquisition which outlines the levels through which competence is acquired **(Fig. 14.1)**. Skill acquisition starts at the level of the novice learner who, through training, becomes an advanced beginner. Further she becomes competent, then proficient, and finally turns into an expert.

To simplify the concept, think of it in this way: Competency is the 'ability' to perform a professional 'activity' (EPA), with this ability being honed over time along a continuum from simple to complex (*milestones*) so the learner moves from novice to competent (or expert) (Carraccio et al., 2017). In yet other terms, EPA can be seen as an activity which the learner can be 'trusted' to perform at a given level of training.

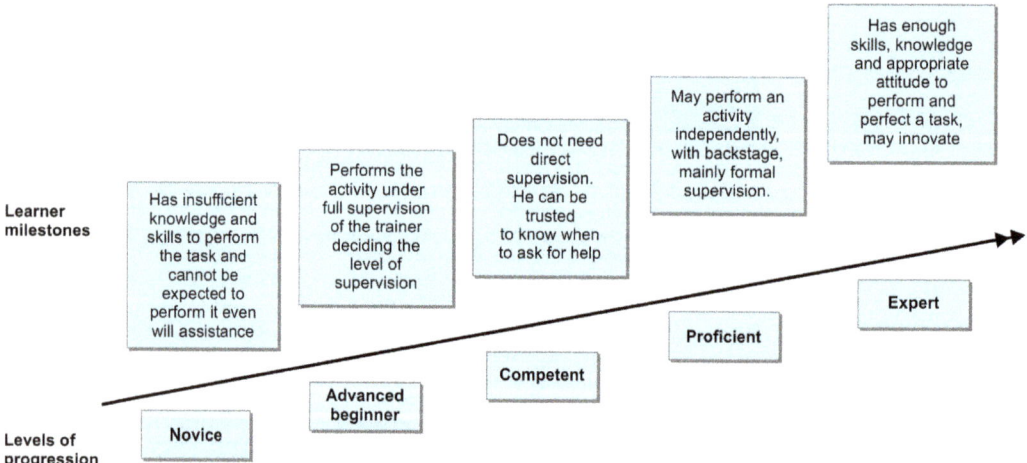

Fig. 14.1: Dreyfus & Dreyfus model depicting learner progression from novice to expert. (Used with kind permission of the Editor, Indian Pediatrics, from Dhaliwal et al., 2015).

Figure 14.2, through a very basic, simplified example, shows the connection between EPAs, competency domains, milestones, and the Dreyfus and Dreyfus model. **Table 14.1** illustrates the concept in greater detail.

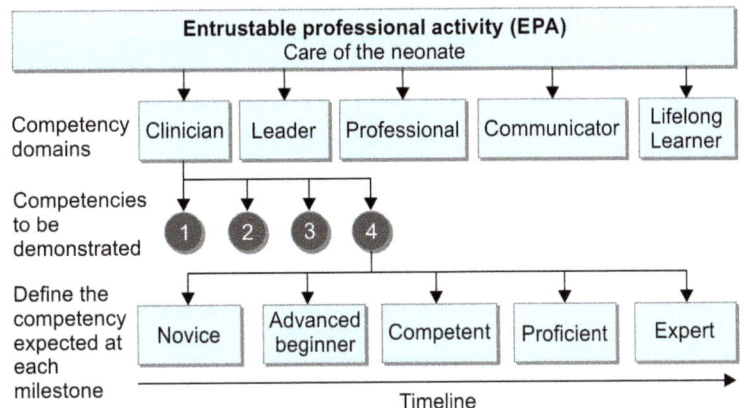

Fig. 14.2: Designing an entrustable professional activity.

These examples show how EPAs can be a useful framework for implementing CBME. They also help to understand how several competencies usually intersect in a single patient-care activity (EPA). An EPA may incorporate as many milestones as needed depending on the complexity of the activity, with each milestone relating to an individual competency.

Further, we see that competence is not a static thing—it is not achieved once and for all. Rather, it is contextual, and competence in one context may not translate into competence in another. Thus, a postgraduate (PG) student who is competent at this task and is therefore entrusted with providing care to uncomplicated neonates, may have to be assessed all over again starting at level 2 (advanced beginner) when he is posted in the intensive care unit and is dealing with very sick neonates.

The Dreyfus and Dreyfus model sees a *competent* learner falling somewhere in the middle of the spectrum. But learning should not stop after achieving competence. Instead, one should aim for further development of expertise to *proficient* and *expert* levels. It is interesting to note that formal training is generally required to bring a learner to competent level, but a deliberate and continued practice is needed to attain the proficient/expert stage. You may also notice that this model looks at the development of a learner as a continuous process from undergraduate (UG) to specialist level, rather than viewing UG and PG education as two separate domains. A learner should be certified competent at the end of UG course and should strive to develop her competency through formal or informal training.

Earlier we used to frame specific learning objectives (SLOs), which may need to be replaced by EPAs. The distinction between SLOs and

EPAs are listed in **Table 14.2**. When contrasted with SLOs, which are generally domain-specific, fairly easy to measure and have the benefit of familiarity, EPAs are complex, integrate various domains, and are relatively more difficult to measure.

TABLE 14.2: Comparison of SLOs and EPAs

Specific learning objectives	*Entrustable professional activities*
They describe what the learner should be able to do at end of instruction	They specify a professional task which the learner will be entrusted to perform after a particular stage of training
The expected outcome is an observable and measurable change in knowledge, skills or attitudes, after which the learner will be assumed to be competent	The expected outcome is the application of requisite knowledge, skills, and attitudes to perform a professional task. With EPAs, the competence is observed and measured and the end result is the learner being trusted to perform the task unsupervised

Not all frameworks use EPAs as part of CBME; however, even in those frameworks which do not use EPAs, the curriculum is organized around expected learner outcomes and advancement in the course depends on the learner having achieved those outcomes.

A recent innovation is to base entrustment decisions on *Observable Practice Activities* (OPAs) instead of on EPAs (Teherani & Chen, 2014). OPAs are discrete work-based skills that are smaller units than EPAs. Several OPAs may be matched to an EPA. Since an EPA integrates several competencies and milestones, and may need to be performed in multiple settings, it can be difficult to assess meaningfully across all settings. For example, assessment of competence for an EPA such as 'Manages care of patients with common acute diseases across multiple care settings' would not be feasible for an assessor who works in an inpatient setting to appraise appropriately, since he would be unable to comment on how the learner performs in an emergency or in a critical care setting. OPAs make the job easier by restricting the activity to a specific posting: 'Manages elevated blood pressure' or 'Initiates enteral and parenteral nutrition' (Warm et al., 2016).

Prerequisites for Assessment in Competency-based Medical Education

Assessment in CBME—*competency based assessment (CBA)*—is a process of collecting and analyzing evidence to decide if a trainee is competent in a pre-defined competency in relation to her stage of training.

The learner is given the opportunity to perform an EPA/OPA multiple times under observation, with feedback being given each time to help the learner improve performance. The endpoint of the EPA/OPA is when the observer finds that he can trust the learner to complete the activity competently without supervision. This is one of the real challenges of assessment in CBME—assessment must be *continuous* and not a one-time event. A single assessment can never be enough to determine competence, since competence is achieved over a continuum and is different in different contexts. Also, it is against a set of predefined criteria, making CBA a criterion-referenced assessment (Modi, et al., 2015).

This concept of assessment for learning is crucial and aligns very well with the basic principles of CBME, viz., active involvement of the learner, creating an authentic environment for learning, direct observation, and provision of formative feedback (Lockyer et al., 2017). For CBA to aid the process of learning, effective feedback is paramount to helping learners improve. CBA is an ongoing process so that any deviation in learning can be recognized early and taken care of by providing formative feedback. CBA requires active participation by the trainee in the form of self-assessment and reflections. Since competencies are integrated into patient care, any approach to competency assessment must focus on performance in the workplace (Singh & Modi, 2013). EPAs and OPAs present attractive assessment frameworks because they focus on day-to-day activities at the workplace.

CBA assesses the ability of a learner to perform, and it includes assessment of skills, attitudes, communication, and other elements of the affective domain. Surrogate markers of competence are no longer tenable, hence logbooks and training records are not taken as proof of competence. Direct observation of how the learner applies discrete behaviors is critical. It might be worth stating here that CBA does not focus on discrete behaviors on their own, but on how the learner integrates discrete behaviors to provide competent care (Holmboe et al., 2010). As mentioned earlier, EPAs and OPAs are useful in this regard as they address multiple competencies at once instead of looking at discrete behaviors. Direct observation also enables the assessor to provide feedback and provides opportunity for course correction. CBA is not so much concerned with looking at incompetence, as it is with helping with the development of competence.

Contrary to the popular belief that 'objectivity is best', CBA very often requires experts to use subjective judgment. Conventional standardized and highly objectivized assessment tools may not be able to do justice to direct observation. As discussed Chapter 26 later, this is not always a bad thing. Expert subjective judgments do not necessarily give results which are less reliable; subjectivity is not synonymous with bias; validity is more important than reliability; and low reliability can be compensated by increasing the sample of assessments, tasks, contexts and assessors.

A mention must also be made of the notional concept of utility of assessment, which is represented by the product of reliability, validity, acceptability, feasibility, and educational impact. We have discussed it in detail in Chapter 1 earlier. It is useful to understand that an assessment low in one element can compensate by being high in another. Assessment of empathy, for example, is very difficult (at least with present state of our knowledge) by objective methods and any such attempt will end up lowering the validity of the assessment. Subjective assessment of empathy, on the other hand, may have some inter-rater variance, but more than makes up for it by being high on validity—and in its educational impact, since it improves learning. Further, objective assessments do not provide data rich enough considering the high stakes of assessment.

Unlike conventional assessments, where the assessment is either diagnostic, formative or summative, in CBA there is an overlap between these aspects so that any assessment moment can also be used as a decision-making moment. When an assessment is used only to decide the progression of learners to the next stage of the course, learners tend to hide their weaknesses, and their learning is from the point of view of passing the summative assessment rather than to develop competencies. CBA uses multiple assessment moments to provide formative feedback to the learners. At the same time, the observer accumulates evidence that helps to decide if the learner can progress to the next stage. Learners, aware of this beforehand, view this form of assessment differently and prepare for it accordingly—not for a pass/fail outcome, but for achievement of competency. To use a metaphor, it can be said that conventional assessment is like a staircase, where the learner must halt at each step, whereas CBA is like an escalator where the learner seamlessly progresses from one stage of competence to another. There is a general agreement that *Programmatic Assessment* is the best approach for a competency-based curriculum. We have discussed this in detail in Chapter 18.

Designing a System of Competency-based Assessment

Designing CBA follows the same processes that are generally used for any assessment design, but with a few important considerations. The first step is to list the competencies and, presuming this has been done, the next important thing is to decide which domains—knowledge, skills, attitudes, and communication—are an essential part of each competency. The next step is to decide what the expected behaviors from a learner who has attained a competency are, and how these are going to be assessed. Simultaneously, benchmarks need to be established for various stages of training (e.g., for the competency of history-taking, what level of performance is expected from a 3rd year student versus a final-year one?). This has been depicted in **Box 14.1**.

> **Box 14.1:** Designing Competency-based Assessment
> - Step 1: Define competencies
> - Step 2: Decide domains involved in each competency
> - Step 3: Decide which activities are to be assessed, when and where, and who will assess
> - Step 4: Decide benchmarks or expected levels of competence or performance for each stage of learning

Competency-based assessment is best designed as a three-dimensional (3D) model **(Fig. 14.3)**. The first dimension is the competency domain and this depends on the competency framework being adopted. For the Indian Medical Graduate, for example, the domains will be clinician, leader, professional, communicator, and lifelong learner. The second dimension will be the level of assessment. Though many models are available, it is expedient to choose Miller's pyramid and assess in terms of knows, knows how, shows how and does. The third dimension is the level of progression using the Dreyfus and Dreyfus model (novice, advanced beginner, competent, proficient, and expert).

Entrustable professional activities provide a convenient way of assigning a learner to one of five levels and **Table 14.3** shows how entrustment levels can be considered to coincide with levels of competence.

TABLE 14.3: Stages of entrustment compared to levels of competence

Stages of entrustment in an entrustable professional activity		Dreyfus and Dreyfus levels of competence
Level 1	Can't be trusted to perform. Can only observe	Novice
Level 2	Can perform under direct supervision	Advanced beginner
Level 3	Ready to perform with supervision under demand	
Level 4	Ready for unsupervised practice	Competent
Level 5	Ready to supervise others	Proficient/Expert

Table 14.4 gives an example of using Dreyfus and Dreyfus model for assessment using EPAs and competencies as the framework to provide a better understanding of the relation of EPAs with competencies.

Let us condense all our learning about EPAs and how they can be implemented in practice in different settings **(Table 14.5)**.

The existing assessment methods are generally usable for CBA as well; however, considering that every method has strengths and weaknesses, it is best to use more than one method to compensate for their inherent limitations. Using multiple methods also increases the sample and thus helps to even out the subjectivity. It is pertinent to mention that 'reliability' in assessment of competencies is dependent

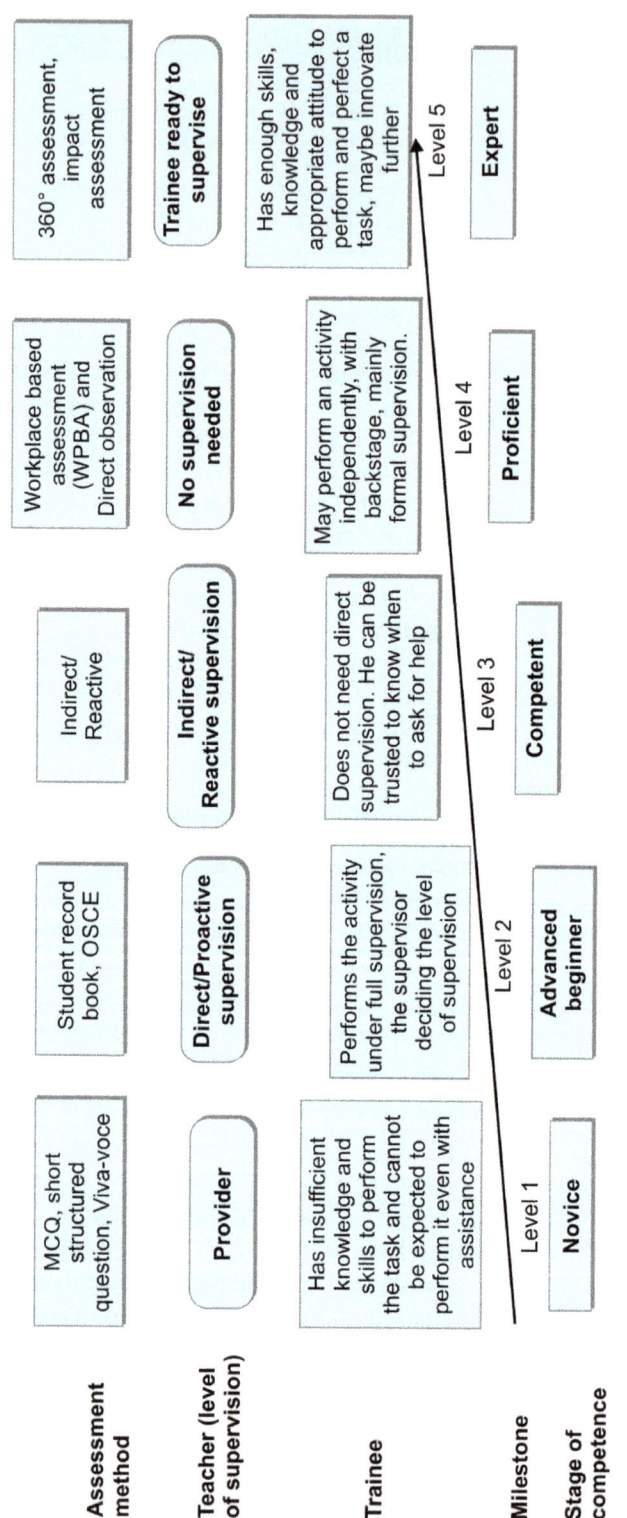

Fig. 14.3: Setting up competency-based assessment.
(Adapted with kind permission of the Editor, Indian Pediatrics, from Dhaliwal et al., 2015;52;591-7.)

Table 14.4: Examples to illustrate application of Dreyfus and Dreyfus model to curricular frameworks of competency-based medical education

Dreyfus and Dreyfus model	Assessment of a 'Competency'		Assessment of an EPA
Developmental steps of skill acquisition as studied in various learning situations ↓	Stepwise achievement of 'milestones' towards acquisition of a competency		Stepwise acquisition and integration of several competencies towards achieving entrustable level of job responsibility (EPA)
	Example 1: Communication with patients (UG to PG years)	**Example 2: Competence in performing delivery by Caesarian Section (CS) (PG training in OBG)**	Example: 'Care of the Neonate' as **an EPA for PG training in Pediatrics** *(This EPA requires an integration of competencies in patient care, procedural skills, communication & counseling skills, teamwork, managerial & leadership skills)*
Novice	Able to talk with the patient so as to take basic medical history according to established framework. (At entry: II-III Semester MBBS student)	❖ Counsels the patient and caregivers, takes written informed consent in presence of the supervisor. ❖ Makes pre-operative preparations by effective communication with the nursing, anaesthesia, OR team ❖ Assists in the surgery as second assistant ❖ Documents surgical notes, and provides postoperative care under supervision.	**Level 1:** Can be entrusted with examination of newborn to look for congenital anomalies
Advanced beginner	Able to establish rapport with the patient and take a medical history for a diagnostic workup. Able to counsel the patient for health practices such as diet, hygiene) (Mid level: IV – VII Sem MBBS)	❖ Counsels and takes consent without supervision. ❖ Assists the superior as first assistant during surgery. ❖ Effectively communicates with other members of the OR team during surgery e.g. scrub nurse ❖ Provides routine postoperative care without supervision	**Level 2:** Can be entrusted to attend deliveries, receive and resuscitate term newborns in uncomplicated cases.

Contd...

Contd...

Competent	In addition to above: able to take a history of delicate personal issues and based on that make a provisional diagnosis. Able to counsel for taking informed consent for surgeries and procedures (UG Exit level: VIII-IX Sem & Internship)	❖ Performs CS in patients with low surgical complexity (simple uncomplicated cases) under direct supervision of a senior who scrubs and assists during the surgery. ❖ Provides postoperative care and counseling in complicated cases	**Level 3:** Can be entrusted with immunization and management of common problems in newborns in outpatient setting.
Proficient	In addition to above: Able to counsel patient and care givers for a newly made diagnosis, diagnosis of serious illness and for seriously ill patients. (I-II Year PG students)	❖ Performs CS in patients with high surgical complexity under indirect supervision e.g. the expert is available and supervises without actually scrubbing for surgery. ❖ Manages minor intraoperative complications independently ❖ Counsels patient and caregivers in adverse outcomes	**Level 4:** Can be entrusted with receiving and resuscitation of the newborn in complicated cases such as preterm, growth restriction, large baby.
Expert	In addition to above: Able to counsel Patient's care givers in the event of death of patient. (III Year PG student)	❖ Performs caesarean section independently in patients with varying surgical and clinical complexity, and effectively manages complications and adverse events. ❖ Maintains effective communication and teamwork with colleagues within and across discipline	**Level 5:** Can be entrusted with management of common problems in the newborns in intensive care setting

*Used with kind permission of the Editor, Indian Pediatrics, from Modi et al., 2015.

TABLE 14.5: Example of an EPA for training and assessment of a resident in pediatrics

Title of the EPA	*Managing a child presenting with diarrhea*
Characteristics of EPA	Executable independently, observable, measurable, essential to profession, reflects competencies, focused tasks
Setting	Outpatient department, emergency care unit, pediatrics ward, community
Description	This EPA includes the following: ❖ Interacting with the child, parents, and team members ❖ Clinical and laboratory evaluation of the child ❖ Interpreting the history, examination, and other evaluation ❖ Making a differential diagnosis and arrive at a working diagnosis ❖ Plan and execute management of the condition and preventing further episodes ❖ Working in team with other medical personal/health care workers ❖ Record keeping
Competencies required	This EPA requires an integration of the following competencies, each further compartmentalized in several milestones:
Medical knowledge	*Ability to demonstrate knowledge of:* ❖ Anatomy, physiology, microbiology of gastrointestinal (GI) tract ❖ Diseases of GI tract ❖ Disorders presenting with diarrhea ❖ Methods and process of evaluation of such patients
Patient care	*Ability to demonstrate skills of:* ❖ Clinical examination ❖ Performing basic laboratory investigations ❖ Making the diagnosis ❖ Planning and executing management ❖ Writing a prescription ❖ Administering fluids and drugs ❖ Identifying complications and managing them ❖ Recognizing when to seek guidance ❖ Customizing care as per preference of patient and availability of resources
Communication skills	*Ability to demonstrate skills of:* ❖ Eliciting history ❖ Counseling the mother and family on immediate management, follow-up and prevention ❖ Interacting appropriately with team members
Professionalism	*Ability to demonstrate the following attributes*: ❖ Behaving appropriately ❖ Ethical and compassionate handling of patient, families ❖ Provide support (physical, psychological, social, and spiritual) for dying patients and their families ❖ Provide leadership ❖ Recognize when it is necessary to advocate and effectively advocate ❖ Treat patients with dignity, civility, and respect
System-based practice	*Ability to demonstrate continued behavior of:* ❖ Practice of rational management ❖ Ethical practice

Contd...

Contd...

	• Understanding unique roles and services provided by local health care delivery systems • Managing and coordinating care and care transitions across delivery systems including ambulatory, subacute, acute rehabilitation, and skilled nursing • Negotiate patient-centered care among multiple care providers				
Practice-based learning	*Ability to demonstrate skills of:* • Identification of areas of deficiency and improvement by self-learning • Constant updating self on recent advances • Identification of new challenges and zest to find their solutions • Identify probable areas of research and conduct the same • Actively seek feedback from all members of the health care team • Maintain awareness of the situation in the moment, and respond to meet situational needs				
Level of achievement of EPA	Level 1 Novice	Level 2 Advanced beginner	Level 3 Competent	Level 4 Proficient	Level 5 Expert
	At the beginning of first year of residency	At the end of first year of residency	At the end of second year of residency	At the end of third and final year of residency	As a practitioner
Assessment	Global evaluations, MSF, direct observation, case-based discussion, written student reflections (portfolio), multiple choice questions (MCQs), short structured questions, viva voce, objective structured clinical examination (OSCE)				

As per ACGME model of competencies.
(Used with kind permission of the Editor, Indian Pediatrics, from Dhaliwal et al., 2015:52;591-7).

more on an adequate and appropriate sampling of content rather than on the type of tool or objectivity involved. Tools used for workplace-based assessment meet many of the criteria that we expect from CBA.

While many of the available tools can be used for CBA, the emphasis must shift from numbers to narratives. As an example, an assessor can grade a learner with 3/5 after observing his history-taking skills or she can say, 'you used appropriate open-ended questions to begin the history-taking and you included all relevant aspects'. The latter is more likely to help the resident learn compared to the former. In other words, it requires a greater emphasis on qualitative assessment methods. Needless to say that a shift to this approach requires extensive faculty training in skills of observation and skills of providing feedback.

A word of caution is necessary when we go about trying to combine the results of multiple assessments. The trend is to combine the scores/marks of assessment tools that have a similar 'format'. Thus, conventionally, marks of all objective structured clinical examination (OSCE) stations are added together because they all test practical/

clinical skills, while the marks of all multiple choice questions (MCQs) are added together since they all test the knowledge component of learning. This is erroneous thinking and it is more appropriate to combine the marks based on the content rather than on the format. For example, the marks scored on questions related to, say, the cardiovascular system should be added to marks scored on OSCE related to the same system. A corollary to this is to organize assessment around content rather than format—this is more likely to give useful information about competency rather than when we club assessments according to the format of the test.

To summarize, CBA must be developmental with emphasis on helping the learner to progress. The learner's competence must be compared with previously laid-down standard criteria, rather than compared with the competence of other learners. These criteria need to be aligned to milestones, so that assessment becomes a part of the learning process, instead of being an add-on accessory. It must be conducted in authentic, workplace settings with assessors making direct observation of the performance at frequent intervals. Direct observation allows provision of effective feedback, and this has been shown to have the single most important influence on learning.

REFERENCES

ACGME outcome project. Accreditation Council for Graduate Medical Education and American Board of Medical Specialties. *Toolbox for assessment methods*. Version 1.1. [online] Available from www.acgme.org/outcomes/assess/toolbox.pdf [Last accessed August, 2020].

Carraccio, C., Englander, R., Gilhooly, J., Mink, R., Hofkosh, D., Barone, M.A., et al. (2017). Building a framework of entrustable professional activities, supported by competencies and milestones, to bridge the educational continuum. *Academic Medicine, 92(3)*, 324–30.

Dhaliwal, U., Gupta, P., & Singh, T. (2015). Entrustable professional activities: teaching and assessing clinical competence. *Indian Pediatrics, 52(7)*, 591–7.

Dreyfus, S.E., & Dreyfus, H.L. (1986). The five-stage model of adult skill acquisition. In: *Mind over machine: The power of human intuition and expertise in the era of the computer*. New York: Free Press.

Frank, J.R., Snell, L.S., Cate, O.T., Holmboe, E.S., Carraccio, C., Swing, S.R., et al. (2010). Competency-based medical education: theory to practice. *Medical Teacher, 32(8)*, 638–45.

Holmboe, E.S., Sherbino, J., Long, D.M., Swing, S.R., & Frank, J.R. (2010). The role of assessment in competency-based medical education. *Medical Teacher, 32(8)*, 676–82.

Lockyer, J., Carraccio, C., Chan, M.K., Hart, D., Smee, S., Touchie, C., et al. (2017). Core principles of assessment in competency-based medical education. *Medical Teacher, 39(6)*, 609–16.

Medical Council of India. (2019). *Graduate medical education regulations.* [online] Available from https://mciindia.org/ActivitiWebClient/open/getDocument?path=/Documents/Public/Portal/Gazette/GME-06.11.2019.pdf [Last accessed August, 2020].

Medical Council of India. (2012). *Regulations on graduate medical education.* [online] Available from http://www.mciindia.org/ tools/announcement/Revised_GME_2012.pdf [Last accessed August, 2020].

Modi, J.N., Gupta, P., & Singh, T. (2015). Competency-based medical education, entrustment and assessment. *Indian Pediatrics, 52(5),* 413–20.

Singh, T., & Modi, J.N. (2013). Workplace based assessment: a step to promote competency based postgraduate training. *Indian Pediatrics, 50(6),* 553–9.

Teherani, A., & Chen, H.C. (2014). The next steps in competency-based medical education: milestones, entrustable professional activities and observable practice activities. *Journal of General Internal Medicine, 29(8),* 1090–2.

Warm, E.J., Held, J.D., Hellmann, M., Kelleher, M., Kinnear, B., Lee, C., et al. (2016). Entrusting observable practice activities and milestones over the 36 months of an internal medicine residency. *Academic Medicine, 91(10),* 1398–405.

FURTHER READING

Baartman, L.K.J., Bastiaens, T.J., Kirschner, P.A., & van der Vleuten, C.P.M. (2006). The wheel of competency assessment: Presenting quality criteria for competency assessment programs. *Studies in Educational Evaluation, 32,* 153–70.

Cook DA, Kuper A, Hatala R, et al. (2017). When assessment data are words: validity evidence for qualitative educational assessments. *Acad Med.* 91(10), 1359–69.

Medical Council of India. Assessment Module for Undergraduate Medical Education Training Program, 2019: pp 1-29.Downloaded from: https://www.nmc.org.in/wp-content/uploads/2020/08/Module_Competence_based_02.09.2019.pdf

Schuwirth, L. & Ash, J. (2013) Assessing tomorrow's learners: In competency-based education only a radically different holistic method of assessment will work. Six things we could forget. *Med Teach,* 35, 555–9.

Ten Cate O, Hart D, Ankel F, et al. (2016). International Competency-Based Medical Education Collaborators. Entrustment decision making in clinical training. *Acad Med,* 91, 191–8.

Chapter 15

Community-based Assessment

Subodh S Gupta, Abhishek V Raut

KEY POINTS

- ☞ The community provides a setting for authentic assessment where students can be observed while performing tasks in actual health care settings.
- ☞ Student assessment in community settings can complement and address gaps in assessment methods.
- ☞ It provides distinct advantages for assessing personal values and professional skills of students.
- ☞ Assessment in the community is apt for using informal methods for student assessment, e.g., portfolios, reflections, and project-based assessment.
- ☞ Multisource feedback or 360° assessment completed by multiple individuals in that person's sphere of influence provides insight into learners' competence, professionalism, work ethics, capacity for teamwork, and interpersonal skills.

It is widely believed that the outcome of any course is determined by its content, method of content delivery and assessment. Medical schools either adapt or remodel these substantially, to suit their needs and preferences. They often work in silos, and teaching remains restricted to their four walls. The *context* in which medical education happens has been identified as the fourth element which determines the outcome of a course. Here, by 'context' we mean not only the physical environment, but also the social climate in which medical schools function, and this is often a neglected element. Medical curricula need to adapt to changing contexts. Advocating medical education that is outside of hospitals and based within the community makes intuitive sense because most illnesses occur there. But it also makes cognitive sense, because we tend to remember our patients' illnesses in context (Lewkonia, 1997).

What is Community-based Medical Education?

The community provides a contextual learning environment for medical education that is relevant to community needs. Community-based medical education (CoBME) consists of activities that use the community extensively as a learning environment in the process of providing medical education that is relevant to community needs (World Health Organization, 1987). In this setting, apart from teachers, a diverse set of stakeholders, including community members and representatives, different cadres of health care providers and professionals from other sectors are actively engaged in providing educational experience throughout the course undertaken by medical students. The distinctive experience and expertise that participants bring from their respective professional fields enriches student learning.

Special Features of Assessment in Community Settings

The word 'assessment' originated from the Latin word '*assidere*', which means "to sit with" (Wiggins, 1993). This perspective which conveys how the teacher needs to sit with students, observing, discussing, and working with them, has unfortunately been lost with the emphasis on standardized tests. This particular image of assessment needs to be retained at least in the settings of authentic student assessment, the community being one of them. If properly designed, student assessment in community settings will complement and could address gaps in the assessment methods routinely used in medical schools.

The community provides a setting for authentic student assessment where students may be observed while performing tasks in actual health care settings. The advantages may include—availability of settings to assess higher level skills in each domain of learning, opportunities for assessment of professional qualities and of student-centered teaching, and obtaining direct evidence of student performance. However, there are also challenges of conducting student assessment in real-life situations, such as, the challenge of assessing students while they work in groups, difficulties in controlling the field conditions, need for better resources, and better planning for workplace-based student assessment (Mueller, 2016).

The settings and objectives for CoBME differ among institutions and, therefore, each institution will require a customized student assessment plan. As students work in the community at different stages in their curriculum, multiple forms of student assessment will be required to match their work during each period (World Health Organization, 1987).

Even within a particular setting, exposure of students may differ from each other depending upon the type of cases/families they encounter or type of tasks assigned to them. Therefore, a system of learning needs analysis and personal learning plan development for individual students could be of extreme help (Kelly et al., 2014). Wherever possible, the student assessment system should have the flexibility to align student assessment with their personal learning plans. Real-life settings in CoBME provide huge opportunities for engaging students in assessment, and through this process, teaching them the art of self-assessment. Self-evaluations are important as they give students a chance to self-regulate their learning. This may be achieved through reflection about professional qualities, portfolios, and other innovative techniques. Multiple assessment methods are necessary to capture all or most aspects of clinical competence and any single method is not sufficient to do the job.

As mentioned earlier, different cadres of health care providers and professionals from other sectors are actively engaged in providing educational experiences to medical students. Integration of medical education with different levels of health care (from primary to tertiary) thus becomes an essential element of CoBME. Multisource feedback (MSF) or 360° assessment, in which more than one individual provides feedback to every learner from his/her circle of influence, including assessment by other members of the team, peer assessment and assessment by community representatives, provides meaningful insight into learners' competence, professionalism, work ethics, capacity for teamwork, and interpersonal skills (Lockyer, 2003).

Worley's Framework for Community-based Medical Education

Worley (2002) in a landmark article gave a framework for articulating important principles in CoBME. In his 4R model, he proposed four axes of relationships, viz., (1) clinical, (2) evidence, (3) social, and (4) personal—each axis representing a relationship. This framework can also be utilized while institutions develop their plans for student assessment in CoBME **(Fig. 15.1)**.

1. *The clinical axis*: This axis represents the doctor-patient relationship. Lots of clinical opportunities are available in community settings, which may act as triggers for learning about disease processes and their management. Further, community settings help in understanding the role of family and social environment, including individual and household practices in the etiology of diseases. Teaching in the community is mostly directed toward the priority health needs, and emphasizes on the acquisition of clinical skills, knowledge, capabilities, and attitudes, as well as on the redistribution of resources to specific populations.
2. *The evidence axis*: This axis represents the relationship between the theory and practice of health sciences. It provides opportunities to students to meaningfully relate the knowledge of health science with clinical decisions.
3. *The social axis*: This axis represents the opportunity given to students in learning about adequacy, quality, and relevance of health services for addressing the health needs of different sections of society. Further, students learn about the intersectoral nature of health and the roles that other sectors, including community networks, play in the health of the people.

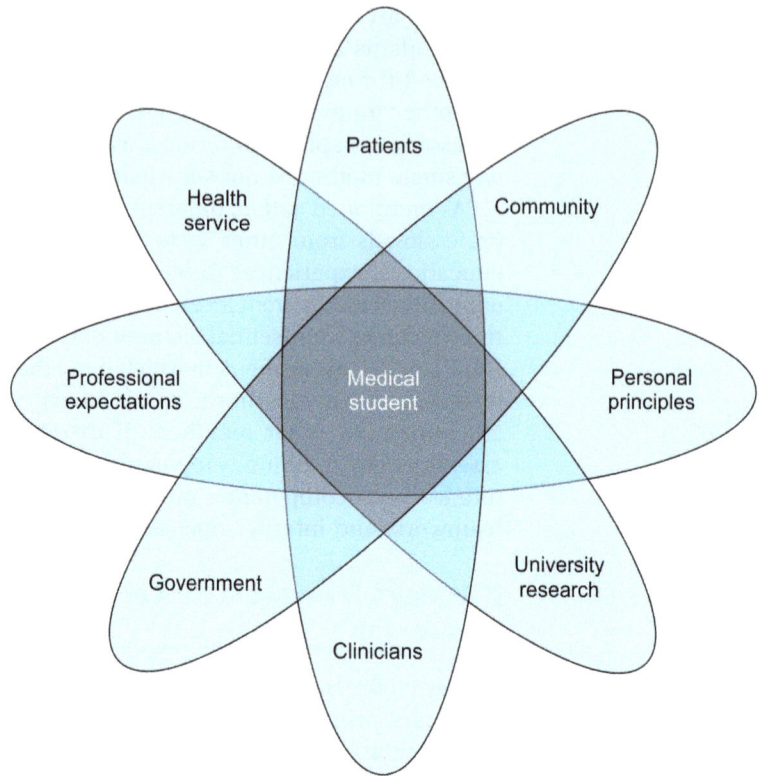

Fig. 15.1: Framework for community-based education.
Reproduced with kind permission from Worley, P. (2002).

4. *The personal axis*: This axis represents the relationship between personal principles and values and professional expectations. Opportunities to interact with community members and know their circumstances, in early years during medical education, provides the much-needed triggers to absorb the intricacies of morals, values, and ethics. It also helps in nurturing students emotionally and helps them in becoming sensitive physicians.

Building Student Assessment for Community-based Medical Education

Table 15.1 lists different assessment methods for the four axes based on Paul Worley's model. Assessment for the first two axes (i.e., clinical and evidence axes) is already part of assessment currently being used in most medical schools. If properly built, assessment in community settings may complement and further enhance student assessment for these axes. In the traditional assessment system, emphasis is usually not given to important issues, such as, screening of apparently healthy individuals, diagnosis and management of common ailments or

TABLE 15.1: Methods for formative and summative assessment in community settings (based on Paul Worley's framework) (Worley, 2002)

Axis as per Paul Worley's framework	What does it mean	Methods for student assessment	
		Formative	**Summative**
Clinical	Being thorough in all communication and procedures; treating patient as a whole person	❖ Mini-CEX (e.g., assessment of nutritional status of family members, use of 24-hour diet recall method) ❖ Direct observation of field skills (e.g., health education skills, counseling skills, collecting survey data)	❖ Multiple choice questions/ Short answer questions/ Long answer questions ❖ Family study assessment ❖ Long case assessment ❖ OSCE—individual or counseling skills
Evidence	Having a sound theoretical underpinning to clinical decision-making	❖ Mini-CEX ❖ Direct observation of procedural skills ❖ Project assessment	❖ Multiple choice questions/ Short answer questions/ Long answer questions ❖ Family study assessment ❖ Long case assessment
Social	Having an upright standing within the community in leadership, understanding, advocacy, and service	❖ Self-assessment through professional qualities reflection and/or portfolio ❖ Direct observation of practical professional skills (e.g., teamwork, advocacy skills) ❖ Project assessment ❖ Observation by community stakeholders ❖ Multisource feedback or 360° assessment	Assessment of student journal or logbook, reflections, portfolios, projects
Personal	Being honest with patients and colleagues, build trust, prepare self for a sustainable career as a clinician	❖ Self-assessment through professional qualities reflection, portfolio ❖ Direct observation of practical professional skills (e.g., teamwork, advocacy skills) ❖ Project assessment ❖ Observation by community stakeholders ❖ Multisource feedback or 360° assessment	Assessment of reflections, portfolios, projects

counseling skills for health promotion, diagnosis and management of illnesses in low-resource settings, or affordability and cost-effectiveness considerations during patient management.

Assessment for these issues could easily be built within community settings. A few examples include:

❖ Mini-Clinical Evaluation Exercise (mini-CEX) for assessment of nutritional status, clinical examination of a pregnant woman, normal newborn or child, assessment during follow-up visits for non-communicable diseases, utilization of opportunities for

screening of common ailments during routine visits to health facilities
- Direct observation of field skills for health education skills, counseling skills, skills for collection of survey data
- Assessment of projects may be utilized to assess students' skills to find out gaps in current evidence base and logical thinking.

In addition, assessment for the knowledge and skills imparted to the students on the clinical and evidence axes may also be built into traditional assessment methods already in use, such as, multiple choice questions, short answer questions, long answer questions or long case assessment.

CoBME provides distinct advantages for assessing students for the other two axes, i.e., social and personal axes. Descriptive methods of student assessment (e.g., portfolios, reflections, project-based assessment) are most apt for this purpose. Apart from these, assessment of student progress may be carried out routinely during performance of tasks. This may also help in timely assessment of student learning and identification of appropriate approaches for learning. Examples include:
- Self-assessment of professional qualities through reflection and/or portfolios
- Direct observation of practical professional skills (e.g., teamwork, advocacy skills) while students are involved in community-based activities and when they are participating in the mock learning exercises prior to the actual tasks
- Assessment while students participate in community-based projects
- Multisource feedback or 360° assessment, integrating information from all important stakeholders.

Box 15.1 provide tools being used at our institute for engaging students in the self-assessment of their personal and professional skills.

As several of the assessment methods have been described in detail elsewhere in this book, we are limiting ourselves to describing a few assessment approaches that are most suited for assessment of students' competence in social and personal axis.

Portfolio Assessment

Portfolio refers to a collection of one's professional and personal goals, achievements, and methods of achieving these goals. Portfolios are an important tool for documentation of student performance in the community. Portfolios also drive student learning, encourage them to take responsibility for their learning and enable them to measure outcomes such as professionalism that are difficult to assess using traditional methods. They facilitate assessment of integrated and complex abilities and take account of the level and context of learning. Portfolios, that sample evidence over time, are a potential and reliable

Chapter 15: Community-based Assessment

Box 15.1: Self-assessment of professional skills within a community setting

The Mahatma Gandhi Institute of Medical Sciences, Sevagram has developed a plan for engaging students in self-assessment of their professional skills. For this purpose, seven domains for personal and professional development were identified based on literature. These include—professional, communicator, manager/collaborator, scholar, health advocate, cultural competence, and self-care. In each of these domains, subdomains were identified. Students are told to self-assess themselves every year for each of these subdomains on a scale of 1–10 and plot it on a spiderweb diagram, as shown below for two of the domains—health advocate and manager/collaborator.

This approach is expected to emphasize the importance for acquiring the professional skills to students.

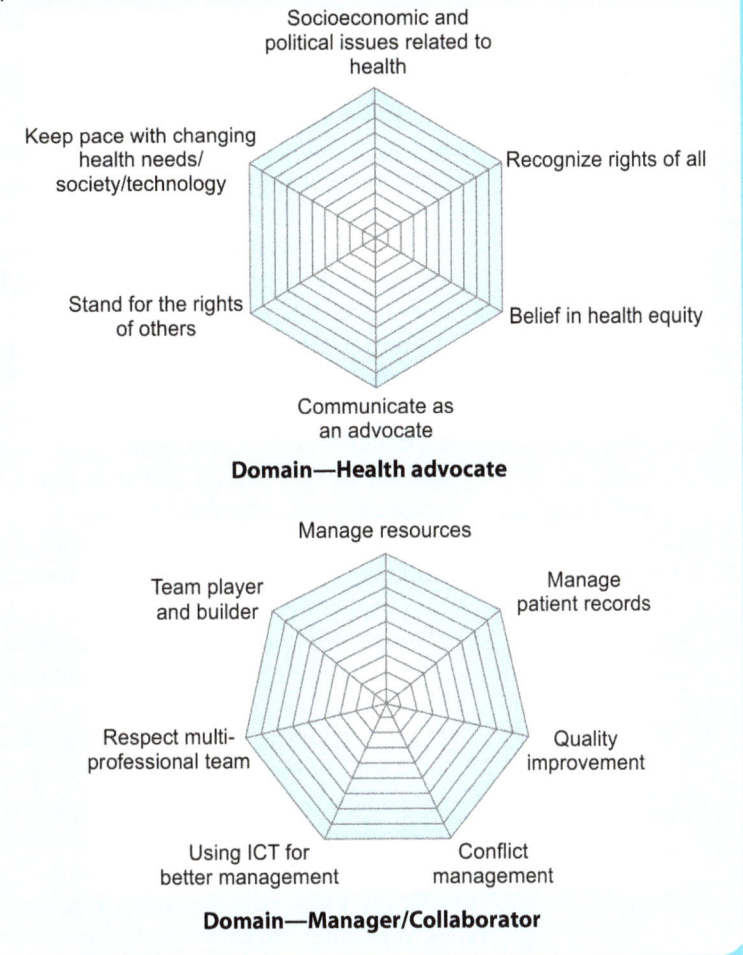

tool for the assessment of acquisition of knowledge, skills, attitudes, understanding, and achievements and 'reflect the current stages of development and activity of the individual'. The sampling of work-related activity reflects the reality or authenticity of an individual's professional clinical practice (Ben-David, 2001). Triangulation of portfolio results with other forms of assessment increases the validity of assessment decisions and guides faculty to the use of the portfolio results.

Assessment of Reflections

Community settings not only provide opportunities for authentic reflection, but actually enhance experiential learning (Brown & Purmensky, 2014). Reflections connect learners cognitively to what they observe or perform. It thus makes lessons that would have been otherwise hidden, explicit. Reflections also help them realize the value of such experiences in their personal and professional growth development (Perry & Martin, 2016).

Assessing reflections can be very challenging, as reflections are meant to be intimately personal in nature. Therefore, altering them simply by defining standards for assessment will make it less personal and an externally imposed process. Further, assessment of reflections usually puts more emphasis on written or spoken language skills, rather than on the students' abilities to engage in reflection. Several models have been given for assessment of reflections (DePaul Teaching Commons, 2020).

A model given by Hatton & Smith (1995) has been utilized frequently for assessment of reflections. This model describes four progressive levels of reflection, with each increasing level indicating more/better reflective processes:

1. *Descriptive writing:* It provides just a basic description and is essentially not reflective.
2. *Descriptive reflection:* This represents a higher level of reflection. Although it is still descriptive, the reasons for experiences become more apparent.
3. *Dialogic reflection:* At this level, several alternative explanations, perspectives, or judgments are considered making reflections more analytical.
4. *Critical reflection:* Considered the peak of reflective writing; at this level, reflections involve multiple perspectives and are discussed in the context of historical and sociopolitical realities.

Another model by Ash & Clayton (2009) uses a guided process for facilitating and assessing reflection. This model was developed specifically for service learning, but it could be applied to other types of learning experiences. Learners have to follow a set of steps in writing reflections:

1. Describe the experience
2. Analyze the experience(s) from multiple perspectives:
   - Personal
   - Academic
   - Civic

3. Identify learning for each perspective
4. Articulate learning by using four guiding questions as a guide:
   - What did I learn?
   - What specific context/approaches helped me learn it?
   - Why does this learning matter?
   - How will I use this learning in future?

Ash & Clayton (2009) suggest several ways to assess students' reflection, including a rubric. **Table 15.2** suggests domains for development of a rubric for assessment of reflection.

TABLE 15.2: Domains for development of a rubric for assessment of reflection

Element	Description
Structure	Writing is clear, concise, and well organized with good sentence/paragraph construction. Thoughts are expressed in a coherent and logical manner
Connection	Clear connection between the experience and the dimension being discussed
Accuracy	Makes statements, which are accurate and supported with evidence; appropriate identification of ideas presented and insights
Clarity	Demonstrate ability to express ideas in alternative ways with appropriate examples
Relevance	Describes relevant learning with specific discussion points
Depth	Adequately addresses the complexity of the problem; answers important question(s) that are raised
Breadth	Presents alternative points of view and interprets meaningfully
Logic and conclusion	Demonstrates a logical line of reasoning with clarity of conclusions

Assessment of Projects

Project-based learning means students are doing work that is real to them—it is authentic to their lives—or the work has a direct impact on or use in the real world (Larmer, 2012).

The community provides an excellent setting for such projects. With good assessment practices, participation in projects can create a culture of excellence for all students and ensure deeper learning for all. Student participation in projects provides a number of opportunities for assessment of learning. Appropriate assessment in such situations requires embedding a system of bilateral feedback between the student and mentor, while the student is supported in the learning process. In addition, self-assessment and peer assessment should form an integral part of such assessment. A number of strategies, such as, rubrics, project assessment maps, reflections by students can be used to scaffold and support these processes to ensure the assessment are constructive (Donnelly & Fitzmaurice, 2005).

The first step in assessment of projects is determining the purpose of assessment (i.e., formative, summative or both) and the content of assessment (i.e., knowledge and general capabilities, such as collaboration, problem solving, and critical thinking). Triangulation of project assessment results with other forms of assessment increases the validity of the decision-making. Results of project assessment could be aggregated as a weighted component toward final graduation scores (Clark, 2017).

Rubrics: Using rubrics makes assessing students much more simplistic and objective and should be used for both individual and group grades. They need to be detailed enough that students understand what is desired of them through the project.

Peer evaluations: A teacher does not always see all that goes on within a group. There are many ways that students can use to grade their group members. Peer evaluations do not need to be done at the completion of a project but also can be effective if conducted throughout the process. Peer rating, peer ranking or peer nominations could be some of the ways to conduct peer evaluations.

Self-evaluations and reflections: These can be done both throughout and at the end of a project. Reflections on the other hand can be done both individually and by groups. Having students reflect on various components of the project can help develop questions students may have and create a more clear vision.

Direct Observation of Learners for Professional Skills

The assessment of professional skills (including medical professionalism) is gradually being considered important; however, its assessment is challenging. If done properly, assessments of professional skills may serve both, formative and summative functions. Formative assessments emphasize the importance of these skills and help students acquire these.

Most common and appropriate assessment method for acquisition of skills (viz., professional skills and procedural skills) is direct observation of learners during mock exercises or real-life setting. The assessment may be based on direct observation of a single or multiple observations over a given time period. However, in real-life settings, opportunity for demonstration of the given skill/s may not arise uniformly for all students. Also, with the awareness that they are is being observed, students' behavior may not necessarily be representative of their typical behavior (Park & Pauls, 2011).

Assessment in community settings provides several opportunities for direct observation:
- Classroom or small group settings for assessing punctuality, responsibility in completing assignments, group collaboration, logical thinking, and articulation of thoughts

- Standardized encounters or mock exercises may be organized for specific skills, e.g., communication skills (for health education or counseling)
- Real-life encounters in home visits, field clinics, community meetings may be utilized for observation of several professional skills, e.g., empathy, respect, responsibility, accountability, communication skills, etc. These settings may also provide opportunities for observation of procedural skills, e.g., assessment of nutritional status, clinical history taking and examination.

Assessment forms developed for specific aspects of professionalism [Professionalism Mini-Evaluation Exercise (P-MEX)] will increase validity and reliability of these observations (Cruess et al., 2006; Tsugawa et al., 2009). Further, training of observers in these exercises along with provision of multiple observers and multiple observations will increase the validity of these ratings.

Multisource Feedback or 360-degree Assessment

Multisource assessment in community settings, apart from perspectives of faculty members, may include the perspectives of students' peers, nurses, other health care professionals and community members. Multisource assessments send across an important message to students regarding the importance of professional attitudes and behaviors and further highlights the importance of teamwork and relationships with community members, and sectors other than health.

Although this kind of student assessment involving peers, other health professionals and community members without any professional certification may not be acceptable from a university standpoint, they may play important role in formative assessment.

Thus, it is evident that assessment in the community provides a setting for assessing learning in the authentic context, and should be used as a useful complement to conventional assessment, to provide learners with skills relevant to actual practice.

REFERENCES

Ash, S.L., & Clayton, P.H. (2009). Generating, deepening, and documenting learning: the power of critical reflection in applied learning. *Journal of Applied Learning in Higher Education, 1(1)*, 25–48.

Brown, A.V., & Purmensky, K. (2014). Spanish L2 students' perceptions of service-learning: a case study from Ecuador. *International Journal of Research on Service-Learning and Community Engagement, 2(1)*, 78–94.

Clark, B.A. (2017). Project based learning: assessing and measuring student participation. *Research and Evaluation in Literacy and Technology, 39*. Downloaded from: https://digitalcommons.unl.edu/cgi/viewcontent.cgi?article=1041&context=cehsgpirw

Clayton, P.H. (2008). Generating, deepening, and documenting learning: the power of critical reflection. In *3rd Annual Conference on Applied Learning in Higher Education, St. Joseph, MO*.

Cruess, R., McIlroy, J.H., Cruess, S., Ginsburg, S., & Steinert, Y. (2006). The professionalism mini-evaluation exercise: a preliminary investigation. *Academic Medicine, 81(10)*, S74–8.

Donnelly, R., & Fitzmaurice, M. (2005). *Collaborative project-based learning and problem-based learning in higher education: a consideration of tutor and student role in learner-focused strategies.* [online] Available from https://arrow.tudublin.ie/cgi/viewcontent.cgi?article=1006&context=ltcbk [Last accessed August, 2020].

DePaul Teaching Commons. (2020). *Assessing reflection.* [online] Available from https://resources.depaul.edu/teaching-commons/teaching-guides/feedback-grading/Pages/assessing-reflection.aspx [Last accessed August, 2020].

Friedman Ben David, M., Davis, M.H., Harden, R.M., Howie, P.W., Ker, J., & Pippard, M.J. (2001). AMEE Medical Education Guide No. 24: portfolios as a method of student assessment. *Medical Teacher, 23(6)*, 535–51.

Hatton, N., & Smith, D. (1995). Reflection in teacher education: towards definition and implementation. *Teaching and Teacher Education, 11(1)*, 33–49.

Kelly, L., Walters, L., & Rosenthal, D. (2014). Community-based medical education: is success a result of meaningful personal learning experiences? *Education for Health (Abingdon), 27(1)*, 47–50.

Larmer, J. (2012). *Project-based Learning (PBL): What does it take for a project to be 'authentic'?* [online] Available from https://www.edutopia.org/blog/authentic-project-based-learning-john-larmer [Last accessed August, 2020].

Lewkonia, R. (1997). Medical education: the fourth element. *The Lancet, 350(9089)*, 1487.

Lockyer, J. (2003). Multisource feedback in the assessment of physician competencies. *Journal of Continuing education in the Health Professions, 23(1)*, 4–12.

Mueller, J. (2016). *Authentic assessment toolbox.* North Central College. [online] Available from http://jfmueller.faculty.noctrl.edu/toolbox/ [Last accessed August, 2020].

Park, J., & Pauls, M. (2011). *The report of curriculum renewal task group #11— professionalism.* [online] Available from http://umanitoba.ca/faculties/health_sciences/medicine/media/Curriculum_Renewal_report_ vFINAL.pdf [Last accessed August, 2020].

Perry, S.L.& Martin, R.A. (2016). Authentic reflection for experiential learning at international schools. *The International Journal of Research on Service-Learning and Community Engagement, 4(1).* Downloaded from: https://journals.sfu.ca/iarslce/index.php/journal/article/view/204

Tsugawa, Y., Tokuda, Y., Ohbu, S., Okubo, T., Cruess, R., Cruess, S., et al. (2009). Professionalism mini-evaluation exercise for medical residents in Japan: a pilot study. *Medical Education, 43(10)*, 968–78.

Van Tartwijk, J., & Driessen, E.W. (2009). Portfolios for assessment and learning: AMEE Guide no. 45. *Medical Teacher, 31(9)*, 790–801.

Wiggins, G.P. (1993). *Assessing student performance: exploring the purpose and limits of testing.* San Francisco: Jossey-Bass Publishers.

World Health Organization. (1987). Community-based education of health personnel: report of a WHO study group [meeting held in Geneva from 4 to 6 November 1985].

Worley, P. (2002). Relationships: a new way to analyse community-based medical education? (Part one). *Education for Health (Abingdon), 15(2)*, 117–28.

Chapter 16

Assessment for Learning

Rajiv Mahajan, Tejinder Singh

KEY POINTS

- ☞ Assessment for learning means learning and improving from assessment opportunities.
- ☞ Feedback is the most important and essential element of assessment for learning.
- ☞ A supportive and conducive educational environment is required to establish a system of 'assessment for learning'.

We have discussed about the formative and summative nature of assessment in Chapter 1 of this book. Formative assessment implies using the assessment to 'form' (build) knowledge and skills of learners, while summative assessment, in a way, could involve assessing the 'sum total' of knowledge and competencies acquired by them. These are two very important uses of assessment, which have also been called the 'improve' and the 'prove' functions respectively. While we use summative function almost every time we assess students, the formative function is highly underutilized in almost every setting. This chapter deals with certain important issues related to use of assessment to improve learning.

Assessments are the cornerstone of learning. It is a common notion that 'assessment drives learning' and 'whatever is not assessed is never possessed by students'. These very notions always prompted the teachers to design learning and assessment activities in a prospective fashion i.e., moving from learning to assessment, thus paving the way to summative assessment or assessment *of* learning (AOL) (Taras, 2005). Without doubt, most visible assessment activities in undergraduate medical education are summative in nature. It is assumed that when students realize that they are going to be assessed at the end of coursework, they will learn. This 'stick-based approach' is considered the most influential factor, which drives students' learning, by medical teachers even in current educational environment. But do AOL activities actually promote students' learning? The truth is far from reality.

Assessment for Learning versus Assessment of Learning

Assessment *for* learning (AFL, also known as formative assessment) takes place during learning. It is distinct from assessment *of* learning (AOL, also known as summative assessment), which takes place after classroom activities to determine whether learning has taken place **(Table 16.1)**. AOL is valuable for documenting student achievement at certain times. AOL data are generally obtained by conducting tests, but these data cannot reflect the full range of the goals of learning. Moreover, evidence that summative assessment improves learning is disputed (Linn, 2000). It is important to point out that although summative assessment has limited learning value, purely formative assessments are not taken seriously by students and teachers alike. There is an increasing trend to merge the two types of assessment so that the *same assessment* can be used to promote as well as quantify learning.

TABLE 16.1: Comparing assessment *of* learning and assessment *for* learning

Assessment of learning (Summative assessment)	Assessment for learning (Formative assessment)
Quantifies learning at the end of a unit of instruction	Provides feedback to teachers and students to make learning better
Focuses on performance	Focuses on progression of learning
Generally norm-referenced	Generally criterion-referenced
High stakes	Low stakes

It is also interesting to note that by *default* all assessments are AOL (literally meaning conducted at the end of something—lecture, chapter, unit, semester or year). They become AFL only when the results are used to provide feedback to the learners and teachers. Thus, it is not the timing (mid-year or end of year) or the type (internal assessments or university examinations) which is used to distinguish them—it is the intended purpose which decides what an assessment should be called. It is good to remember that only very few assessments have formative value.

Detrimental Effects of Summative Assessment

Firstly, summative assessments merely serve 'feed-out' function. While highlighting various issues with summative assessment ranging from contentious reliability, poor predictive validity, cost, and discouraging good learning behaviour, Knight (2002) has very categorically stated that 'summative assessment is in disarray'. Secondly, the retentions in the same class as a consequence of summative assessment have detrimental effect on students' learning. Hattie has highlighted the negative impact of retentions on learning and reported that effect size of retentions on students' learning is −0.15 (Hattie, 1999). Thirdly, summative assessments may promote, what has been described as 'examination-oriented' attitude in the students—converting them from *shiksharthi* to *pariksharthi*, to use a colloquial phrase—thus making them highly vulnerable to negative feedback. Such students, sensing high risk of errors, are more likely to disengage from learning opportunities. In fact, anticipating exposure of their weaknesses, such students will often miss out on curative opportunities, so vital for future success (Chiu et al., 1997). Thus, while summative assessment is important for certification purposes, its influence on students' learning is not unequivocal, and that makes a strong case for the importance of AFL in the coursework.

Strength of Assessment for Learning

The Assessment Reform Group (2002) has defined AFL as: "The process of seeking and interpreting evidence for use by learners and their teachers to decide where the learners are in their learning, where they need to go and how best to get there". The Third International Conference on Assessment for Learning position paper (Klenowski, 2009) has defined AFL as: "Part of everyday practice by students, teachers and peers that seeks, reflects upon and responds to information from dialogue, demonstration and observation in ways that enhance ongoing learning".

These definitions emphasizes five important points:
1. AFL is everyday practice;
2. It is useful to students, teachers, and peers, with students forming the central axis;
3. Students seek, reflect upon, and respond to feedback, thus making it an inquiry-driven process;
4. It involves collection of information from various formal and informal sources using dialogue, demonstration, and observation; and
5. It enhances ongoing learning.

The information thus collected during assessment is used to enhance learning.

The core concept of AFL is based upon educational feedback. Hattie has mentioned the effect size of reinforcement, corrective feedback, and remediation feedback in enhancing students' learning as 1.13, 0.94, and 0.65 respectively, and all these are cornerstones of formative assessment (Hattie, 1992) **(Table 16.2)**. Formative

TABLE 16.2: Effect size of feedback on learning (Hattie, 1992)	
Cues	1.10
Corrective feedback	0.37
Feedback about a task	0.95
Reward	0.31
Reinforcement	0.94
Praise	0.41

assessment opportunities also promote 'learning-oriented' attitude in students.

Formative Assessment—Not Synonymous with AFL

The term 'assessment for learning' is often used synonymously with formative assessment. However, there is a difference between the two. The most important difference between the two approaches is that the traditional formative assessment approach informs only the teacher about students' performance, but AFL also informs the students also about their own learning. AFL is based on the perception that the students are important stakeholders in instructional decision-making. Another difference is that traditional formative theory is more inclined to repeated assessment of learner's excellence of the standards themselves, while AFL lays more stress on progress of a learner along the learning trajectory leading to stated standards (Stiggins, 2005). As such, AFL refers to the collection of approaches and techniques associated with the practice of formative assessment. In other words, AFL is a system, incorporating formative elements, and formative assessment opportunities provide the foundation for AFL. However, due to the strength of familiarity with the term 'formative assessment', both terms have been used in this chapter interchangeably.

Formative assessment is an integral part of the educational system. The components of this system include the learning objectives, teaching-learning methods, and assessment. Being a system, these components are not independent, but are interdependent. Formative assessment is the best example of this interdependence. By providing information about the desired output of the system, it helps regulate the input as well as the processes **(Fig. 16.1)**. Translated to education, it means that students, teachers, and teaching-learning activities form the inputs, while students who have attained desired knowledge, skills, and attitudes become the output. The process of feedback helps us modify both the inputs as well as the process to narrow the gap between desired and actual outcomes.

Cycle of Assessment for Learning

With this unequivocal strength of improving learning and learning outcomes, AFL stands apart; but it must be understood that AFL is

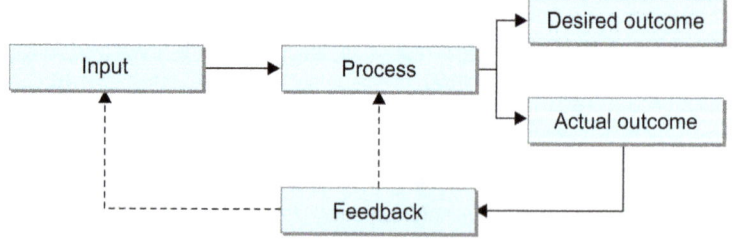

Fig. 16.1: The educational system.

not a single point phenomenon. AFL must be assimilated within the curriculum as an 'iterative program', running in 'cycles' of *learning → assessment → analysis → feedback → learning;* many such cycles run longitudinally over a course of time along the professional development of learner. Any corrective action for midcourse academic rectification is part of the feedback, and not separate from it.

In AFL, any learning experience is followed by an assessment, and the assessment is followed by feedback to the learner. This feedback will be preceded by the analysis of learning and assessment and will lead to defining midcourse corrective measures which are not mutually exclusive of feedback process.

This cyclic occurrence and feedback opportunities are the two characteristic features differentiating AFL from AOL. AFL results in further learning as the inputs are run-in in the form of feedback making it a closed-loop system running in cycles, whereas AOL runs in a horizontal bar fashion, without anything being fed-back into the learning system, resulting in mere certification (**Fig. 16.2**). Though over a period of professional development of the learner, both run in a longitudinal fashion.

Attributes of the Assessment for Learning System

Learners and teachers are the most important stakeholders of the AFL system. Other important attributes in AFL system are the learning process and the learning goals themselves. The five most important attributes of AFL system have been shown in **Figure 16.3** and are being briefly described here.

Learners and teachers: Only willing students who are ready to metamorphose as learners can learn. A learner, open to constructive

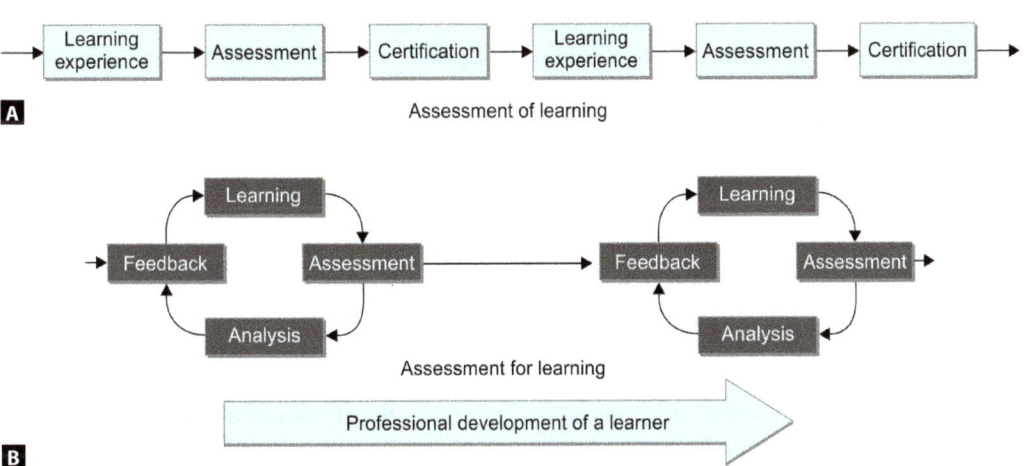

Fig. 16.2: (A) Horizontal process of assessment of learning; (B) Cyclical iterative process of assessment for learning demonstrating progress during professional development.

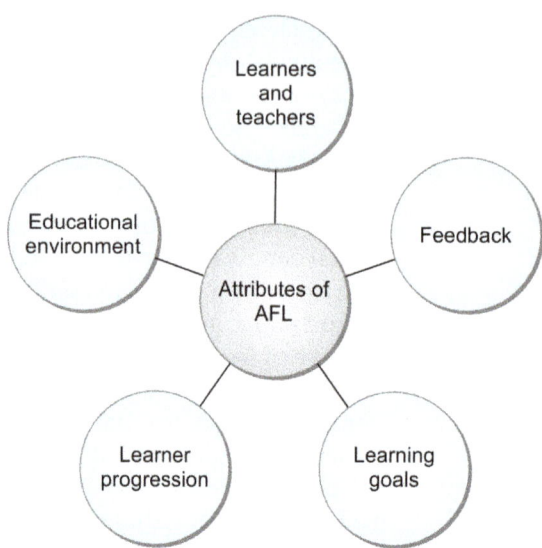

Fig. 16.3: Attributes of the assessment for learning (AFL) system.

feedback, sometimes even criticism, and ready to act upon the feedback given in the form of corrective action, is central to the idea of AFL. Similarly, a teacher who is willing to walk the extra mile, and is ready to dedicate time for providing constructive feedback, suggest actionable remedial educational strategies to the learners and monitor the progress of the learner is the second important attribute of AFL.

Feedback: Constructive feedback is an integral part of the AFL process. Constructive feedback has been documented to improve learning outcomes. The characteristics of effective feedback holds true for feedback in AFL too. For AFL to flourish in any educational institute, the effective feedback must be delivered in an appropriate setting, focusing on the performance of the learners, must be clear, specific, based on direct observation, must be delivered using neutral, non-judgmental language emphasizing the positive aspects, must be descriptive rather than evaluative, and timely.

Typologically, the feedback in formative assessment has been detailed into five phases **(Fig. 16.4)**, extending from 'weaker feedback only' to 'strong formative assessment'. For a sustainable AFL system, students and teachers' should focus on 'strong formative assessment' (William, 2011).

As discussed in detail in Chapter 24, the ultimate goal of formative feedback is to ensure that the a learner comes to hold the concept of quality roughly similar to that held by the teacher, thus fostering self-monitoring skills, leading to development of reflective behavior. AFL helps in fostering metacognitive skills in the learners.

Learning goals: As all AFL activities must culminate in the form of achievement of intended learning goals, teachers must identify and

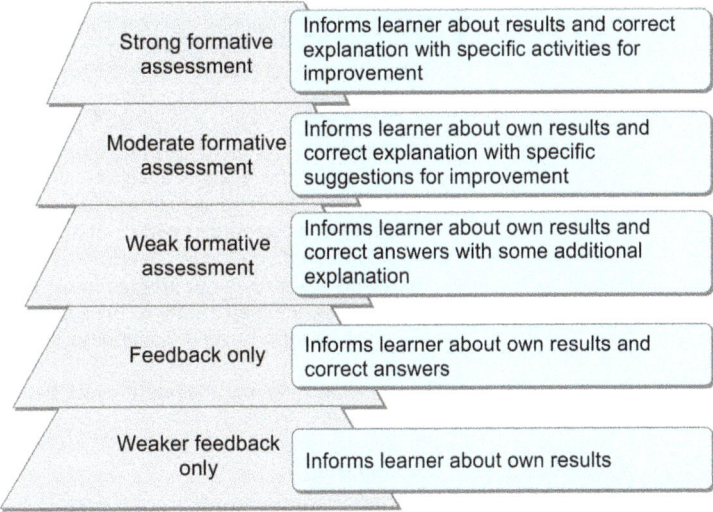

Fig. 16.4: Typology of feedback in formative assessment system (Nyquist, 2003)

communicate intended instructional outcomes and goals to students (McManus, 2008). This should be communicated explicitly and nothing should be left to assumptions. Besides stating the nature of goals, criteria by which the learning will be assessed must also be shared so that students can monitor their progression.

Learning progression: Learning progression shows the trajectory of learning along which the students are expected to progress. Learning progression helps the teachers for planning instruction to meet short-term goals and connect them with formative assessment opportunities to keep track of students' learning (McManus, 2008). Learning progression should clearly express the subgoals of learning goals. Such an articulation helps the teachers to identify learning gaps well in time and devise remedial strategies, so that the progression of the student is not halted.

Educational environment: For active and continuous progression of students' learning, students must feel that they are important stakeholders and equal partners in the learning process. This sort of behavior can be inculcated in students only in a conducive educational environment. Supportive educational environment is required for educational feedback system to progress. An educational environment where teachers share learning goals and criteria for success with students, where students seek feedback actively, where students and teachers provide constructive feedback to each other, is a norm rather than an exception for AFL system to sustain. The characteristics of an institute and institutional educational environment, supportive of AFL system have been detailed in **Box 16.2**.

> **BOX 16.2:** Educational environment supportive of AFL system
> - The institute must have an organizational plan to integrate and coordinate AFL activities.
> - There must be a central control with departmental accountability in place.
> - Educational environment must be competent to provide data and feedback from different stakeholders in variety of ways.
> - Institute must have an in-built mechanism to explicitly share the learning outcomes and assessment criteria of a course.
> - An institutional curriculum development cell, with the responsibility of improving the assessment program must be in place.
> - AFL must be complementary to the summative assessment.
> - AFL must be introduced in continuous fashion longitudinally through the course.
> - Responsibility for improvement must be placed on both learners and teachers.
> - Faculty development programs must be integral part of the educational environment.

Opportunities for Assessment for Learning

Learning from assessment does not require conduct of any special assessment tests. Learning opportunities for AFL can be availed through routine teaching-learning activities like questioning in usual classroom teaching, seminars, tutorials, routine written assessment tests, clinical encounters, bedside teaching, etc. Portfolios, reflections, peer assessment are some other avenues leading to AFL.

Written tests: As discussed in Chapter 24, written comments on written assignments can be a good opportunity of learning from assessment, provided basic rules of providing feedback (no vague comments; giving detailed feedback; providing specific assessment criteria on how the marks are computed, etc.) are followed. When written assessment criteria is provided before-hand and used subsequently for marking, it improves learning. However, one main hurdle in using written assignment as a feedback opportunity is that it is subject to multiple interpretations and more than 50 criteria have been identified in evaluating the quality of written assignments (Sadler, 1989).

Classroom engagement opportunities: Tutorials, seminars, class viva are some of the encounters providing opportunities to learn from assessment. One-to-one verbal feedback may be even more helpful in eliciting the learning gaps and motivating more accurate self-analysis by weaker students (Aggarwal et al., 2016).

Clinical encounters: Clinical case presentations, educational OSCE, mini-CEX and other WPBAs provide opportunities for learning from assessment to the students in clinical skill areas. Such clinical assessment encounters can be used judiciously for learning of clinical skills.

Portfolios: A professional portfolio is a collection of learning materials, assignments and professional work that illustrates individualized learning, skills and competence, and is helpful in assessing professional growth. By using portfolios, students can improve their awareness toward their own learning thus, helping to inculcate the attitude of self-learning and self-improvement. Also self-motivated learning improves with critique on one's professional development, achievement of learning goals, and identification of learning gaps, which are integral to the portfolios (Joshi et al., 2015). Portfolios also support self-assessment behaviors. Portfolios give ample opportunities to the evaluator/facilitator to provide feedback to the students during the course itself. These inherent qualities of portfolios provide learning opportunities for improvement while assessing the student along the course of professional development (Mahajan et al., 2016).

Reflections: These have been referred to as "an important human activity in which people recapture their experience, think about it, mull over and evaluate it, and this working with experience promotes learning" (Boud et al., 1985). Reflections involve critical thinking about the new learning experiences, either during the learning process or after the process is over, and linking prior knowledge and experiences with the new learning experiences to re-establish future learning goals and design future learning strategies (Mahajan et al., 2016). Reflection provides opportunities for self-assessment, learning gap identification, planning future learning strategies, promoting self-directed learning and improving metacognitive skills. Students should be encouraged to reflect on the learning experiences.

Peer assessment: The process, by which a student rates her peers against benchmark set by teachers, can be used for creating learning opportunities. In many instances, students respond better to the feedback received from their peers than from the tutor. It also allows students to interpret where they stand in professional development compared to their peers. Peer feedback when delivered timely promotes deep learning. It improves students' metacognitive skills.

Portfolios, self-reflection, and peer assessment inculcate reflective practice behavior in addition. Key features of reflective practice for 'AFL' are given in **Box 16.3**.

BOX 16.3: Key features of reflective practice for assessment for learning (AFL)

- Reflections, portfolios, and peer assessment improve critical thinking in students and their metacognitive skills.
- Feedback and self-improvement are the key features of these AFL methods.
- It is not the tool or method, but the use of results to improve learning which makes any assessment as AFL.

SWOT Analysis of Assessment for Learning

Strengths, weaknesses, opportunities, and threats (SWOT) analysis is antecedent to any strategic planning, to bring any new intervention in balance with the external environment. SWOT analysis of an AFL system is presented in **Box 16.4**.

BOX 16.4: SWOT analysis of assessment for learning system

Strengths	Weaknesses
- Helps track learning progression - Helps take midcourse corrective measures - Helps make instructional and/or curricular modifications - Helps foster self-monitoring and self-assessment skills in students - Helps foster reflective practice	- Requires continuous monitoring by facilitator too - Can unnerve apprehensive students - Requires lots of time and efforts from facilitators

Opportunities	Threats
- Provides opportunities to foster self-directed learning skills in students - Promotes lifelong learning skills in the students - Makes educational environment learner centered	- Increasing students' strength—colleges admitting 200–250 students per batch - Delays in incorporating innovative curriculum changes, which are already delayed by 3–4 years

---

As evident from **Box 16.4**, the stakes are heavily in favor of AFL system. It has huge advantages and opportunities against minor threats which can be overcome by suitable local adjustments.

Incorporating Assessment for Learning in Undergraduate Medical Training

Though the opportunities of learning, professional development and improving the institutional educational environment are abundant in a system which has assimilated AFL, it has hardly been incorporated in medical colleges across India. Even if sporadically instituted in some colleges, it is performed as a ritual thus undermining the utility of potential benefits to the stakeholders. Four fundamental requirements for incorporating AFL in regular undergraduate medical curriculum have been described in **Figure 16.5**.

Faculty development: The most important intervention is probably the most neglected one. Even if undertaken, often it serves as a 'process compliance activity' and not as a 'skill development opportunity'. Application of skills learnt during medical education technology workshops are mostly restricted to routine teaching. Laboratory to field transition is hardly visible. More importantly, to incorporate the AFL system, we have to move out of our comfort zone of participating in

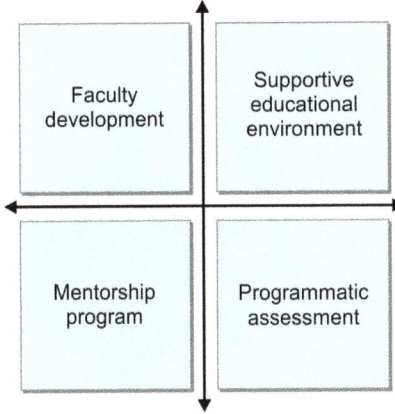

Fig. 16.5: Basic requirements for incorporating assessment for learning.

mandatory programs only and should look beyond. Hands on training workshops on feedback process, interactive teaching, lesson planning blueprinting, mentorship educational leadership must be made part and parcel of institutional faculty development programs.

Educational environment: As discussed above, the educational environment must be conducive and supportive for AFL system to sustain. It must be able to create a culture that supports 'learning orientation' in students and not 'examination orientation'. With learning orientation, students would freely admit their educational mistakes and will seek help and advice to rectify them, while with examination orientation; students will try to hide their mistakes in order to look good! Students must be convinced that institutional educational environment values inquiry seeking behavior, curiosity, and risk taking.

Vygotsky (1962) defined the Zone of Proximal Development (ZPD) as the 'learning edge'. These are the knowledge or skills that are at the limits of a student's competence and they find most challenging, but are achievable through guidance. According to Vygotsky, someone who is a 'knowledgeable other' and has mastered the area already, needs to coach learners in their ZPD. An educational environment where students are helped to master challenging competencies through formative assessment builds the trust of students. This culture shift encourages learning over performance in an examination (Konopasek et al, 2016).

Programmatic assessment: It is an approach of moving away from individual assessment methods and looking at the framework of entire program of assessment (Vleuten & Schuwirth, 2005; Singh, 2016). Any assessment should be a part and parcel of instructional design, and not a mere afterthought activity. A program of assessment at any institute will provide ample opportunities for the conduct of AOL- and AFL-related assessment activities (Mahajan & Singh, 2017) **(Fig. 16.6)**. No standard

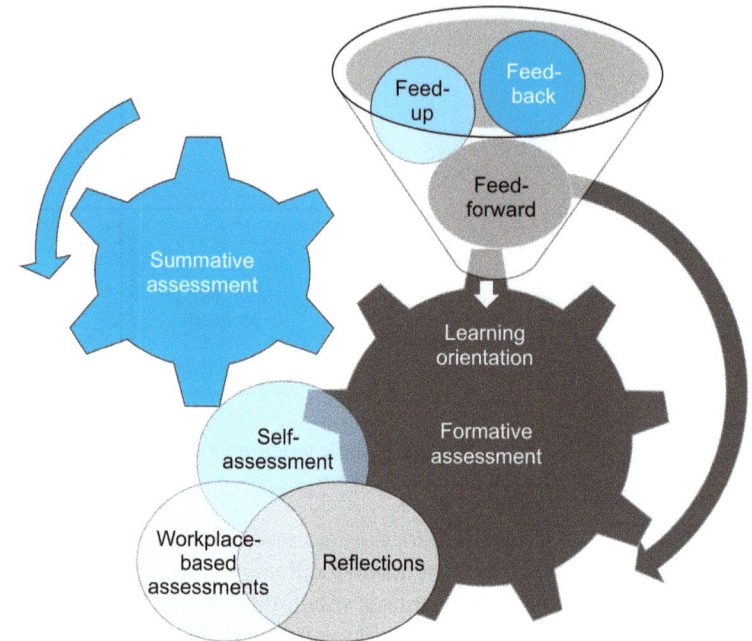

Fig. 16.6: Components of an effective assessment system.
Reproduced with kind permission of the Editor, National Medical Journal of India, Mahajan & Singh,2017,30,275-278

program can be drawn for all institutes. Individual institutes have to make efforts to devise their own program considering students' strength, faculty position, and other local factors. Institutional instructional goals, learning progression, and assessment criteria should be well-designed and made known to all students explicitly.

Programmatic assessment has been discussed in detail in Chapter 18.

Mentorship: Introducing a mentorship program will help build student-teacher trust at the very beginning of the course itself. Students can be better guided about institutional educational environment, education policies, program of assessment, instructional goals, etc., during one-to-one mentor-mentee encounters. At the same time scaffolding, so essentially required during the initial period as medical student, can be better provided by the teacher during mentorship program. The trust so built can subsequently be used for proper implementation of AFL system.

Assessment for learning is not a one-time, stand-alone event; rather it is a continuous process along the professional development of the student. Challenges in incorporating AFL may be manifold, but the unequivocal influence of AFL students and its high educational impact will certainly motivate teachers to leave no stone unturned to implement it in medical institutes.

REFERENCES

Aggarwal, M., Singh, S., Sharma, A., Singh, P., & Bansal, P. (2016). Impact of structured verbal feedback module in medical education: a questionnaire- and test score-based analysis. *International Journal of Applied and Basic Medical Research, 6(3)*, 220–5.

Assessment Reform Group. (2002). *Assessment for learning: 10 principles. Research-based principles to guide classroom practice assessment for learning.* [online] https://www.aaia.org.uk/storage/medialibrary/o_1d8j89n3u1n0u17u91fd d1m4418fh8.pdf. [Last accessed August, 2020].

Boud, D., Keogh, R. & Walker, D. (1985). *Reflection: turning experience into learning.* London: Kogan Page. p. 43.

Hattie, J. (1992). Measuring the effects of schooling. *Australian Journal of Education, 36(1)*, 5–13.

Chiu, C.Y., Hong, Y.Y., & Dweck, C.S. (1997). Lay dispositionism and implicit theories of personality. *Journal of Personality and Social Psychology, 73(1)*, 19–30.

Hattie, J. (1999). *Influences on student learning. Inaugural Lecture, University of Auckland, New Zealand.* [online] Available from https://cdn.auckland.ac.nz/ assets/education/hattie/docs/influences-on-student-learning.pdf [Last accessed August, 2020].

Joshi, M.K., Gupta, P., & Singh, T. (2015). Portfolio-based learning and assessment. *Indian Pediatrics, 52(3)*, 231–5.

Klenowski, V. (2009). Assessment for learning revisited: an Asia-Pacific perspective. *Assessment in Education: Principles, Policy, and Practice, 16(3)*, 263–8.

Knight, P.T. (2002). Summative assessment in higher education: practices in disarray. *Studies in Higher Education, 27(3)*, 275–86.

Konopasek, L., Norcini, J., & Krupat, E. (2016). Focusing on the formative: building an assessment system aimed at student growth and development. *Academic Medicine, 91(11)*, 1492–7.

Linn, R.L. (2000). Assessments and accountability. *Educational Researcher, 29(2)*, 4–16.

Mahajan, R., Badyal, D.K., Gupta, P., & Singh, T. (2016). Cultivating lifelong learning skills during graduate medical training. *Indian Pediatrics, 53(9)*, 797–804.

Mahajan, R., & Singh, T. (2017). The national licentiate examination: pros and cons. *National Medical Journal of India, 30(5)*, 275–8.

Nyquist, J. B. (2003). *The benefits of reconstruing feedback as a larger system of formative assessment: A meta-analysis.* Master of Science thesis, Vanderbilt University.

McManus, S. (2008). *Attributes of effective formative assessment.* Washington DC: Council of Chief State School Officers. [online] Available from https:// schoolturnaroundsupport.org/resources/attributes-effective-formative [Last accessed August, 2020].

Sadler, D.R. (1989). Formative assessment and the design of instructional systems. *Instructional Science, 18(2)*, 119–44.

Singh, T. (2016). Student assessment: moving over to programmatic assessment. *International Journal of Applied and Basic Medical Research, 6(3)*, 149–50.

Stiggins, R. (2005). From formative assessment to assessment for learning: a path to success in standards-based schools. *Phi Delta Kappan, 87(4)*, 324–8.

Taras, M. (2005). Assessment—summative and formative—some theoretical reflections. *British Journal of Educational Studies, 53(4)*, 466–78.

van der Vleuten, C.P.M., & Schuwirth, L.W. (2005). Assessing professional competence: from methods to programmes. *Medical Education, 39(3)*, 309–17.

Vygotsky, L. (1962). *Thought and Language.* Cambridge, Mass: MIT Press.

Wiliam, D. (2011). What is assessment for learning? *Studies in Educational Evaluation, 37(1)*, 3–14.

Chapter 17

Assessment for Selection*

Tejinder Singh, Jyoti N Modi, Vinay Kumar, Upreet Dhaliwal, Piyush Gupta, Rita Sood

KEY POINTS

- ☞ The purpose of assessment must guide the design of assessment.
- ☞ It is most desirable that such selection processes utilize a combination of cognitive and non-cognitive testing (soft skills such as interpersonal communication, ethical reasoning, etc.) along with aptitude testing.
- ☞ A single high-stakes national level examination for selection to undergraduate and postgraduate medical course in terms of its educational impact.
- ☞ While such an examination has benefits in terms of resource efficiency and standardization, it can adversely affect the learning priorities of student.
- ☞ Some of its limitations can be counterbalanced by giving due attention to designing of questions, duration of testing, strengthening of the University final examination, and by making the in-training assessment more robust.

Selection of students to medical schools is a matter of worldwide discussion and debate (Powis, 2015; Prideaux et al., 2011; Siu & Reiter, 2009). A major reason for this is the gap between medical training and societal health needs. India is at the threshold of a national-level policy change in the procedure of admissions to medical courses. A single examination at the national level has been introduced for selecting students to Undergraduate (UG) and Postgraduate (PG) medical courses. There is a raging debate, involving educationists, policymakers, and the judiciary, on what is most suitable in terms of logistics, transparency, effectiveness, fitness to purpose, and acceptability. A consolidated opinion of medical educationists is yet unexpressed.

Only when there is a clear purpose to the selection, linked to orientation, can the most appropriate process for admission to medical

---

* *This write-up was initially published as Singh, T., Modi, J.N., Kumar, V., Dhaliwal, U., Gupta, P. & Sood, R. (2017). Admission to undergraduate and postgraduate medical courses: looking beyond single entrance examinations. Indian Pediatrics, 54, 231–8. Is being reproduced with the kind permission of the Editor. Minor modifications made to bring it up to date to the current context.*

schools be evolved. The obvious purpose of selection to UG courses is the identification of the most suitable candidates for a future physician role. The selection process must also weed out the applicants who may harm the community. The purpose of selection to PG courses is to identify the most appropriate among the medical graduates, who have the ability to carry out specialty practice.

Working backward, a good admission process must involve procedures and criteria that subserve both, the desired purpose and outcome. It is therefore crucial to know which selection procedures contribute, and to what extent, toward achieving them.

What Works and to What Extent?

Motivation, aptitude, and ability are the three pillars that enable a person to perform well in any profession. 'Motivation' is assumed when a student applies for admission to a medical school. 'Aptitude' pertains to natural flair and plays a key role in deciding how comfortable the person will be in functioning as a physician. 'Ability' decides whether the student has the potential to go through the academic rigors of medical training, and subsequently fulfill the demanding roles of a physician. Therefore, the optimal admission process must consider both 'academic' and 'non-academic' criteria. **Table 17.1** compares the processes followed for admission to UG medical courses in India with that of some other countries.

Academic evaluation for selection: Academic evaluation is universally applied for selecting students to medical courses **(Table 17.1)**. Academic performance prior to admission to the medical school has a moderate influence on performance during medical school explaining about 13% of the variance (Cleland et al., 2012; Mercer & Puddey, 2011). This suggests that prior academic performance is not adequate on its own for predicting performance in medical school or in later professional life. For this reason, countries such as the United States, the United Kingdom, and Australia utilize a combination of end-of-school examination scores, a medical admission/entrance test score, and also additional criteria for the suitability for admission to UG courses (Cleland et al., 2012; Julian, 2005; McGaghie, 2002; McManus et al., 2005; Mercer & Puddey, 2011; Prideaux et al., 2011; Wilson et al., 2012; Wright & Bradley, 2010).

In India, academic performance in the end-of-school examination scores is used almost exclusively to determine eligibility for appearing in the medical entrance examination; it is not used for admission decisions save in the state of Tamil Nadu* (Selection Committee, Directorate of Medical Education, Government of Tamil Nadu, 2016). For admission to PG courses, the term 'prior academic performance' would refer to the performance during UG medical training. While

---

* Since modified

TABLE 17.1: Comparison of processes followed for admission to undergraduate medical courses in the United States of America (USA), Canada, the United Kingdom (UK), and India*

Parameter	USA and Canada (Siu & Reiter, 2009)	UK (Cleland et al., 2012; McManus et al., 2005; Mercer and Puddey, 2011; Wright and Bradley, 2010)	India
Basis of admission decisions	A combination of cognitive and non-academic methods	A combination of cognitive and non-academic methods	Usually a single cognitive method[†]
Eligibility	After 3 years of graduate college education	Soon after school education	Soon after school education
Methods used	Medical College Aptitude Test (MCAT) scores supplemented by undergraduate Grade Point Average (uGPA), an interview or Multiple Mini-Interviews (MMIs), personal statements, and letters of reference	End-of-school scores (A Level) supplemented by personal interviews or letters from referees for assessing noncognitive attributes, and aptitude testing by the UK Clinical Aptitude Test (UKCAT)	An MCQ-based written entrance test across almost all states[†]

*Nearly 60,000 students appeared for MCAT in 2015; approximately 475,000 students registered for the reintroduced NEET-UG in India in 2016.
[†]Exceptions:
1. In the state of Tamil Nadu, 85% medical admissions are based on class 12 marks in science subjects (Selection Committee, Directorate of Medical Education, Government of Tamil Nadu, 2016).*
2. The Armed Forces Medical College, Pune (2016), and the Christian Medical College (2016), Vellore, shortlist applicants on the basis of cognitive test scores (the All India Entrance Examination); the former institution then supplements the scores with a separate Test of English Language, Comprehension, Logic and Reasoning (ToELR), a psychological test, and an interview, while the latter adds on scores based on an online aptitude assessment.

the United States of America utilizes the scores of the United States Medical Licensing Examination (USMLE) in selection decisions, no such procedure is followed in India and many other countries.

Evaluation of non-academic attributes: It is ironic that while selecting entrants to medical schools, the greatest emphasis is on academic performance/potential whereas at the user end (when visiting a doctor for consultation), the patient can discern only the professional, ethical, and interpersonal behavior of the physician. A higher compliance with treatment, better satisfaction, and less litigation has been found to be associated with such soft skills of the physician (Laidlaw & Hart, 2011; Tamblyn et al., 2007, Urlings-Strop et al., 2013). The intention in bringing these facts to the fore is not to de-emphasize academic and cognitive attributes, but to throw light on soft skills/non-academic attributes.

Evaluation of non-academic attributes can cover a wide range of attitudinal and behavioral characteristics, and skills such as interpersonal communication, professionalism, ethical reasoning, team-work and stress coping ability (Powis et al., 2007; Urlings-Strop et al., 2013). All of these, being complex constructs of many human qualities, are not amenable to easy evaluation by a single test. Also, it is not feasible to evaluate all of these; thus, for selection purposes, only some of the most important may be assessed (Powis et al., 2007). The popular methods utilized are aptitude tests, personal interviews, personal statements or essays by applicants, Multiple Mini-Interviews (MMIs), letters of reference, Situational Judgment Tests (SJTs), and other tests such as personality assessment and emotional intelligence (Cleland et al., 2012; Powis et al., 2007; Urlings-Strop et al., 2013). A few key aspects of some of the methods are discussed here.

Personal statements and letters of reference, though extensively used, have been found to lack reliability, and have limited validity and overall utility as a predictors of future performance (Cleland et al., 2012; Siu & Reiter, 2009). They are prone to contamination by way of plagiarism and third-party inputs. Also, they are resource intensive, as they have to be individually assessed by subject experts. Reference letters have also failed as predictors of future performance perhaps because of the inherent bias on the part of the self-selected referees (Siu & Reiter, 2009).

The interview is a versatile though resource and time-intensive method. The way it is conducted, its content, and the interviewer all have a bearing on its reliability and validity. Selection interviews are best conducted in a structured manner, with standardized questions, via a trained panel of interviewers and by using validated scoring criteria (Cleland et al., 2012; Kreiter et al., 2004; Wilson et al., 2012). Increasing the number of assessors can minimize interviewer bias. MMI offer a further improvement; the predictive validity of MMI is found to be higher (0.4–0.45) than that of traditional interviews (<0.2) (Cleland et al., 2012; Eva et al., 2004).

Aptitude may be tested separately or incorporated as a separately evaluated and weighted section in the cognitive test. The Medical College Aptitude Test (MCAT) in the United States of America and the UK Clinical Aptitude Test (UKCAT) in the United Kingdom are some examples. While the UKCAT is predominantly an aptitude test, the MCAT, in addition to aptitude, also tests biological and physical science knowledge base, writing skills, and problem-solving skills. The evidence for predictive validity of aptitude testing is positive but widely variable (0.14–0.6) with respect to performance in medical school (Cleland et al., 2012; Julian, 2005). In India, testing for aptitude is non-existent at present except for Christian Medical College, Vellore (2016) where an online aptitude test is conducted.

Need for Change in the Selection Procedures for Medical Courses in India

Lessons from other countries: Most universities and medical schools in the United States of America and Canada utilize a combination of methods for ranking and admission decisions (Siu & Reiter, 2009). Three years of graduate college education is a prerequisite for entry into medical school. The undergraduate Grade Point Average (uGPA) score from college education is included, and usually supplemented with MCAT, along with additional methods such as interviews, personal statements, and letters of reference. McMaster University, Canada, is credited with the introduction of MMIs that has remarkably improved the personal interviews and has replaced traditional interviews at many universities (Eva et al., 2004).

It is important to note that the United States of America does not use a single high-stakes examination such as MCAT (for UG admissions) or USMLE (for PG admissions). It is a common misconception that scores at such standardized tests are the major determinants of acceptance. In addition to these being used as one of several measures of suitability for admissions, they are utilized to compare applicants from diverse universities that have different degrees of rigor in how they award grades that eventually determine the GPA. The MCAT and undergraduate GPA are used less as a ranking tool and more to determine who should be invited for personal interviews. Data from the written examinations is integrated with several other modes of assessment for the admission decisions including selection interviews. Interviews do not test content knowledge but critical thinking and communication skills. Due attention is also paid to the life experiences of the applicants and their ability to evaluate such experiences in their essays. The weightage given to each of the above components varies widely in different universities.

Similarly, countries such as the United Kingdom, Australia, and the Netherlands use a combination of prior academic performance, some form of cognitive testing, aptitude testing, and additional methods of non-academic assessment for deciding suitability of the candidates for admission to medical schools (Cleland et al., 2012; Powis et al., 2007; McManus et al., 2005; Mercer & Puddey, 2011; Wilson et al., 2012; Wright & Bradley, 2010; Urlings-Strop et al., 2013).

Lessons from the past: Initially, the end-of-school, i.e., Higher Secondary Examination (HSE) scores alone were used for creating a rank list and selecting students to medical schools; no other input was considered necessary. Variations in standards of school-leaving examinations and unfair practices creeping into the selection process prompted the introduction of entrance examinations as a common platform for entry to medical schools. However, there were multiple examinations, some conducted by individual states, others by institutions, and one national level examination, the All India Pre-Medical Test (AIPMT). The State examination was used to fill 85% of the medical seats in a given state, while the remaining 15% seats were filled through the AIPMT; aspirants ended up preparing for and giving several entrance examinations, and as a result often traveled across the country multiple times in the admission year.

The next major change: Single, nationwide entrance examination: In order to improve selection processes, the Medical Council of India (MCI), in 2009, proposed doing away with entrance examinations conducted by states and institutions and replacing them with a single national level examination from 2013 onward. The Government of India (2010, 2012) passed the proposal in December 2010. The proposed examination was called the National Eligibility cum Entrance Test (NEET) for admission to UG (NEET-UG) and PG (NEET-PG) courses. However, it was widely challenged in the courts and after being struck down initially, the Supreme Court of India recalled its judgment on April 11, 2016 for reconsideration and finally NEET was reintroduced in 2017.

The policy-makers and conducting authorities debated largely about administration logistics, cost, the value of a common standard of examination nationwide, and containment of corrupt practices. Medical educationists, on the other hand, deliberated the utility of a single entrance examination—a debate that still stays *sans* consensus (Ananthakrishnan, 2013; Gupta et al., 2013; Pardeshi et al., 2012; Singh, 2014). The NEET may seem like the end of the discussion for students, parents, and conducting authorities, but for medical educationists it is only the beginning of a mammoth challenge. It is a challenge to decide the appropriate modality, content, assessment tool(s), duration of such high-stakes examination, weight given to various aspects, and how to use the scores to make ranking decisions.

Pardeshi et al., (2012) explored the thoughts of the most important stakeholders—the students—when NEET was first announced. Though they focused on the NEET-PG, it is interesting to note that only about half the interns felt the need for a single entrance examination. This is ironic since one of the bases for introducing NEET was student convenience in appearing for only a single examination. More interesting were the reasons that students shared for not wanting a single examination: they felt that, being their only chance that year, it would be a single high-stakes opportunity; if one was sick on that day or, unable to appear for other legitimate reasons, there would be no second chance or alternative. They also voiced concerns about having a single uniform examination that did not take into account variation in the quality of training in different states.

Single Entrance Examination for Selection Decisions—A Critique

While NEET appears to be a solution for many ills in the existing selection procedures, it also creates problems because of its unidimensional approach to admissions for medical colleges. Nonetheless, for medical educators, NEET need not be just a challenge but also an opportunity to think about all aspects of medical education in India.

The likely benefits and limitations of using a single high-stakes examination for admission to PG courses are summarized in **Table 17.2** along with suggestions to counterbalance the limitations. Some of the major limitations deserve further analysis and discussion:

Prior academic performance is ignored: Prior academic performance in the form of school-leaving examination scores has been reduced to an eligibility criterion and that too at a meager cutoff score of

TABLE 17.2: Single admission test for Postgraduate (PG) courses: Benefits, limitations, and suggestions for improvement

Benefits of a single admission test such as NEET

- Brings down the cost and efforts for students
- Resource-efficient
- Potential to curtail financial malpractices in admission
- Seemingly, a 'standardized' and 'objectivized' national level platform

Limitations	Possible Remediation
❖ Raises the stakes on a single examination leading to negative educational impact. ❖ Limits options for students who are not selected ❖ Suboptimal assessment of knowledge ❖ Students likely to indulge in examination-oriented learning or 'to crack' MCQs rather than to acquire clinical skills. ❖ Does not assess clinical or soft skills, essential for further medical training and practice ❖ No testing for ethical judgment, professionalism, teamwork, etc. ❖ Students may skip some content with smaller representation (e.g., Anesthesia, Psychiatry, etc.). ❖ Performance depends on many factors in addition to knowledge, thus bringing 'construct irrelevance'.	❖ Give credit/weightage to performance in certifying courses, as a qualifying criterion, e.g., Higher Secondary Examination for selection to UG courses and MBBS for selection to PG courses. ❖ Stop the drift toward MCQ-oriented learning. A robust system of formative, on-going, in-training assessment (Internal Assessment) as well as strengthening of the certifying assessment will retain the focus of students on learning contextually, and acquiring clinical and soft skills toward becoming a competent physician. ❖ Knowledge assessment can be improved by changing the format to a longer examination with MCQs that are context-based and test clinical reasoning. ❖ Other tools for testing higher-order thinking skills, aptitude and ethical judgment may be included.

50 percent (even lower for accommodating special categories of applicants as a welfare effort). The adverse educational impact of this type of assessment can be readily seen—school students have shifted their focus from school studies and concept building to preparing for the Multiple-Choice Questions (MCQs) for the medical entrance examinations. To the students, it makes sense since the HSE scores are devalued. This devaluation of prior academic performance has weighty consequences. Studies from around the globe, including a relatively recent one from Delhi, demonstrate that past performance can predict performance in medical school (Cleland et al., 2012; Gupta et al., 2013; Mercer & Puddey, 2011). A similar pattern of entrance examinations exists in selection to medical PG courses. The performance in MBBS—which is assessed by 56 examiners (14 subjects with 2 internal and 2 external examiners)—is not given any importance, and students spend their internship preparing for the MCQs that comprise the PG entrance examination. Acquiring competency to practice as a physician is not the focus of UG medical students, nor are these competencies assessed while making admission decisions to PG courses. This unintended consequence of not adopting the systems approach deserves debate and alleviation.

Students become MCQ solvers instead of exploratory learners: NEET has an MCQ-based format and is a knowledge test, whereas the purpose of a selection/admission test should be to assess the overall suitability for further medical training and not just the level of knowledge. This diverts the students to 'selection examination'-oriented learning focused solely on solving MCQs. Further, such a test has the potential of discouraging students from exploring other learning experiences thus distorting their learning priorities (Gliatto et al., 2016). This misalignment in purpose and action needs to be addressed and redressed.

The 3-hour 200-question format of entrance tests fails to test higher cognition: Traditionally, most entrance examinations follow the '3-hour-200-question' format, leaving little option for paper setters to go beyond assessing recall of knowledge. Since it becomes difficult to stratify thousands of students on the basis of recall type questions, the examiners resort to adding some 'difficult' questions about rare diseases or single case reports that have no relevance to the objectives of the entrance examination (Anand, 2011). Although NEET being a computer-based test provides a unique opportunity for incorporating videos, recorded patient encounters, and other methods to even test affective domain, the same has not been utilized. Very few efforts have been made to scientifically understand the impact of such large-scale examinations. We allude to the earlier study from Delhi that demonstrated that the entrance examination scores do not predict performance in medical school (Gupta et al., 2013). This is in agreement with the findings from other countries; no similar study could be identified pertaining to PG entrance examinations. Clearly, more research is needed, along with changes in MCQs so that they test higher-order thinking rather than recall, as is the case with most questions in the USMLE examinations (Case & Swanson, 2002).

Clinical skills are not assessed: The PG-NEET does not test clinical competence, yet the implication is that the applicant has the competence to start PG studies. An improvement in the end-of-course MBBS examination as well as the in-training formative assessment and feedback, is perhaps the key in justifying this presumption.

In-training formative assessment has been regarded synonymous with Internal Assessment (IA) in the Graduate Medical Education Regulations (GMER) of MCI (1997) though there is a fine difference (Singh & Anshu, 2009). It has the potential of redirecting students from examination-oriented learning toward in-depth, conceptual, contextual, and experiential learning. Much flexibility has been provided in the regulations for planning and implementing IA in Indian medical schools and every medical teacher has the potential to make the best of it. Hence, this aspect is discussed in some depth.

Can Strengthening Internal Assessment Offset Negative Consequences of PG Entrance Examination?

The basic tenet of understanding the utility of IA in improving selection to PG courses lies in the fact that contrary to the obvious, UG and PG medical training must be viewed as a learning continuum rather than as two different courses separated by the selection examination. Hence, the learning process and competencies mastered during UG training are an important foundation for undergoing further specialty training. Its importance is well elucidated by experts in a recent article wherein they write, 'a formative focus in undergraduate medical education better prepares the students for residency training....' (Konopasek et al., 2016).

The essence of IA lies in its 'formative' role for monitoring and positively influencing the process of learning by way of timely feedback during the course. Further, the competencies that can be assessed during training by direct observation at workplace such as communication, professionalism, procedural skills, etc., are not amenable to assessment in the final end-of-training examination. Hence, the educational information provided by IA and final examination complement each other rather than merely being two numerical scores. This requires careful drafting of a longitudinal assessment program that covers the entire period of study (Singh et al., 2012). The 1997 regulations of MCI (1997) made a beginning in this regard by making it mandatory to pass in IA to be eligible for the final university examination and also giving weightage (20% at present) to IA toward final results. However, the full potential and formative function of IA remains largely untapped in our country (Singh & Anshu, 2009). In most institutions, it is reduced to sporadic assessments during MBBS course rather than deliberately linked assessments of developmental attainment of competencies. An effective IA must be based on multiple observations made by multiple examiners over a period of time and, preferably, all faculties in the department should be involved (Singh & Anshu, 2009; Singh et al., 2012). This can also compensate for any individual examiner's bias.

In the United States of America, an ongoing comprehensive, multimodal, in-training assessment is done over the four years of UG training and these are detailed in a document called the 'Dean's letter'. This is an integral and important part of the application for PG training, along with USMLE scores, personal statements, reference letters, and on-campus interviews. The Dean's letter also includes previous education/accomplishments (prior to medical school entrance), family background (if relevant), extracurricular accomplishments, etc. The idea is to provide a synopsis of the personal attributes of the applicant. In clinical subjects, there is a more extensive write-up that takes into account narratives provided by attending physicians and senior residents as well as standardized subject examinations provided by the National Boards. Most schools end by stating 'On the basis of the overall performance we rate this student as Outstanding/Excellent/Very good, etc.' Usually each institution has certain academic criteria for these adjectives (typically percentiles). Recognizing the utility of the information provided by this comprehensive document in making selection decisions for residency positions, the Association of American Medical Colleges (AAMC) refined it to a standard format referred to as the Medical Student Performance Evaluation (MSPE) (Andolsek, 2016; Katsufrakis et al., 2016). Further modifications to it are now suggested such as the focus on the core competencies, details on professionalism, and evaluation of clinical clerkships (clinical postings) (Association of American Medical Colleges - Medical Student Performance Evaluation Task Force, 2016).

Whether an identical system is appropriate for India can be debated; it is reasonable to say that, in the United States of America, in-training assessment has been accorded importance during planning, implementation, and utilization—not only as a steering force for learning process and skills acquisition in UG education, but also as a measure of suitability for admission to PG training. Further, a subjective description of performance in addition to 'objective' scores is also given importance.

Some Suggestions for Alleviating Limitations of a Single Entrance Examination

i. Duration of test: It is well known that reliability increases with testing time. Increasing the testing time will contribute to building validity as well as reliability. In addition, increasing the time available per question will allow inclusion of application-oriented and problem-solving questions rather than only recall and recognition questions.

ii. Do not disregard the assessment of crucial non-academic components: A conscious effort must be made to overcome the tendency to discard the assessment of communication skills, ethics, professionalism that are not easily amenable to 'objective' assessment methods, but are *the sine qua non* for good medical practice. We are perhaps missing out on the merits of subjective assessment by equating it with bias. While MCQs are labeled as objective, they are not truly so, as the one who designs them does so based on subjective thought. Isolated objective testing can be likened to the story of blind men describing only parts individually (and perfectly), but no one having the correct picture. Subjective assessment also permits a better assessment of soft skills. This could be in the form of an essay, discussion of a situation for judgment analysis, interview, etc., depending on feasibility.
iii. A limitation not discussed further in this paper but definitely worth a thought and mention, is that a single high-stakes examination has led to a culture of students attending expensive preparatory courses and coaching classes. The financially/socially disadvantaged students may find themselves to be further disadvantaged by way of not being able to afford/find time for the same. If the examination is designed to largely test for aptitude, thinking process, and application rather than recall, this may reduce to some extent.

In conclusion, we welcome the move to have a common national examination in the form of NEET that will help standardization and uniformity of admission process. However, we propose in this paper, several other considerations and improvements, if we are to raise the standard of medical education that is desired by the individual and the society. It should be a well-planned test conforming to the principles of assessment as discussed above and subjected to the rigors of evaluation. Some of the likely drawbacks of a single entrance examination can be counterbalanced by strengthening the MBBS final examination, and by making the in-training formative assessment program/IA of MBBS course more robust. The students can be kept on a desirable course of learning with acquisition of necessary skills rather than them drifting to only test-oriented learning.

The concept of golden alignment between curricular components, viz., objectives, teaching methodology and assessment is well accepted. Gliatto et al. (2016) have rightly pointed out that a proper balance be maintained between the various curricular components to provide a working space for innovations in medical education to make it relevant to the health needs of the society. However, putting too many stakes on any one component—single assessment for career trajectories, in this case—is likely to take away any degree of freedom that we have to innovate. They lucidly express it in the American context as quoted here, and it is easy to draw parallels to Indian context:

'If we want our assessments to reflect our values and societal priorities, we need to break free of the self-imposed constraints of using MCAT and USMLE scores to determine who advances into medical school and residency.'

REFERENCES

Anand, A.C. (2011). PG entrance for dummies (Are you looking for a postgraduate seat?). *National Medical Journal of India, 24(1)*, 38–42.

Ananthakrishnan, N. (2013). Saying no to NEET is certainly not neat. *National Medical Journal of India, 26(4)*, 250–51

Andolsek, K.M. (2016). Improving the medical student performance evaluation to facilitate resident selection. *Academic Medicine, 91(11)*, 1475–9.

Armed Forces Medical College, Pune. (2016). *MBBS admissions-2016.* [online] Available from http://afmc.nic.in/PDFfiles/MBBS%202016%20interview%20list.pdf [Last accessed August, 2020].

Association of American Medical Colleges-Medical Student Performance Evaluation Task Force. (2016). *Recommendations for revising the Medical Student Performance Evaluation (MSPE).* [online] Available from https://www.aamc.org/system/files/c/2/470400-mspe-recommendations.pdf [Last accessed August, 2020].

Case, S.M., & Swanson, D.B. (2002). *Constructing written test questions for the basic and clinical sciences.* (3rd ed). Philadelphia: National Board of Medical Examiners. [online] Available from http://www.nbme.org/PDF/ItemWriting_2003/2003IWGwhole.pdf [Last accessed August, 2012].

Christian Medical College. (2016). *Revised supplementary bulletin MBBS admissions.* Vellore. [online] Available from http://admissions.cmcvellore.ac.in/linkeddata/uploads/MBBS%20BULLETIN%202016%20Dated%2015%20Aug%202016.pdf [Last accessed August, 2020].

Cleland, J., Dowell, J., McLachlan, J., Nicholson, S., & Patterson, F. (2012). *Identifying the best practice in the selection of medical students (literature review and interview survey).* [online] Available from http://www.gmc-uk.org/Identifying_best_practice_in_the_selection_of_medical_students.pdf_51119804.pdf [Last accessed August, 2020].

Eva, K.W., Rosenfeld, J., Reiter, H.I., & Norman, G.R. (2004). An admissions OSCE: the multiple mini-interview. *Medical Education, 38(3)*, 314–26.

Gliatto, P., Leitman, IM., & Muller, D. (2016). Scylla, and Charybdis: The MCAT, USMLE, and degrees of freedom in undergraduate medical education. *Academic Medicine, 91(11)*, 1498–500.

Government of India. (2010). *The Gazette of India, Extraordinary Part III, Section 4, 27 December 2010, 342.* New Delhi. [online] Available from http://www.mciindia.org/tools/announcement/2010Dec27_49068_Gazette_Notification_NEET-UG.pdf [Last accessed August, 2020].

Government of India. (2012). *The Gazette of India, Extraordinary Part III, Section 4, 27 February 2012; 41.* New Delhi. [online] Available from http://www.mciindia.org/tools/announcement/2012Feb27_62051_Gazette_Notification_NEET-UG.PDF [Last accessed August, 2020].

Gupta, N., Nagpal, G., & Dhaliwal, U. (2013). Student performance during the medical course: role of pre-admission eligibility and selection criteria. *National Medical Journal of India, 26(4)*, 223–6.

Julian, E.R. (2005). Validity of medical college admission test for predicting medical school performance. *Academic Medicine, 80(10)*, 910–7.

Katsufrakis, P.J., Uhler, T.A., & Jones, L.D. (2016). The residency application process: pursuing improved outcomes through better understanding of issues. *Academic Medicine, 91(11)*, 1483–7.

Konopasek, L., Norcini, J., & Krupat, E. (2016). Focusing on the formative: building an assessment system aimed at student growth and development. *Academic Medicine, 91(11),* 1492–7.

Kreiter, C.D., Yin, P., Solow, C., & Brennan, R.L. (2004). Investigating the reliability of the medical school admissions interview. *Advances in Health Sciences Education, 9(2),* 147–59.

Laidlaw, A., & Hart, J. (2011). Communication skills: an essential component of medical curricula. Part I: Assessment of clinical communication: AMEE Guide No.51. *Medical Teacher, 33(1),* 6–8.

McGaghie, W.C. (2002). Assessing readiness for medical education: evolution of the medical college admission test. *Journal of the American Medical Association, 288(9),* 1085–90.

McManus, I.C., Powis, D.A., Wakeford, R., Ferguson, E., James, D., & Richards, P. (2005). Intellectual aptitude tests and A levels for selecting UK school leaver entrants for medical school. *British Medical Journal, 331(7516),* 555–9.

Medical Council of India. (1997). *Regulations on graduate medical education 1997.* [online] Available from https://www.latestlaws.com/bare-acts/central-acts-rules/medical-health-laws/indian-medical-council-act1956/medical-council-of-india-regulations-on-graduate-medical-education-1997/ [Last accessed August, 2020].

Medical Council of India. (2013). *Final schedule for All India Quota (NEET) UG counseling 2013 (Annexure to letter No. V.11017/1/2009-MEP-1 dated 24th June 2013).* [online] Available from http://www.mciindia.org/tools/announcement/2011_FinalCoreSyllabus_NEET-UG/NEET_UG_Counselling.pdf [Last accessed August, 2020].

Mercer, A., & Puddey, I.B. (2011). Admission selection criteria as predictors of outcomes in an undergraduate medical course: a prospective study. *Medical Teacher, 33(12),* 997–1004.

Pardeshi, G., Lakade, R., & Adhav, P. (2012). MCI and NEET-PG: understanding the point of view of medical graduates. *National Medical Journal of India, 25(5),* 314–5.

Powis, D. (2015). Selecting medical students: an unresolved challenge. *Medical Teacher, 37(3),* 252–60.

Powis, D., Hamilton, J., & McManus, I.C. (2007). Widening access by changing the criteria for selecting medical students. *Teaching and Teacher Education, 23(8),* 1235–45.

Prideaux, D., Roberts, C., Eva, K., Centeno, A., McCrorie, P., McManus, C., et al. (2011). Assessment for selection for the health care professions and specialty training: consensus statement and recommendations from the Ottawa 2010 conference. *Medical Teacher, 33(3),* 215–23.

Selection committee, Directorate of Medical Education, Government of Tamil Nadu. (2016). *Prospectus for admission to MBBS/BDS courses 2016-2017 session.* Government of Tamil Nadu. Chennai. [online] Available from http://www.tnhealth.org/online_notification/notification/N1605308.pdf [Last accessed August, 2020].

Siu, E., & Reiter, H.I. (2009). Overview: what's worked and what hasn't as a guide towards predictive admissions tool development. *Advances in Health Sciences Education: Theory and Practice, 14(5),* 759–75.

Singh, T. (2014). Was it wrong to discard NEET? *National Medical Journal of India, 27(2),* 119–20.

Singh, T., & Anshu. (2009). Internal assessment revisited. *National Medical Journal of India, 22(2)*, 82–4.

Singh, T., Anshu, & Modi, J.N. (2012). The Quarter model: a proposed approach for in-training assessment of undergraduate students in Indian medical schools. *Indian Pediatrics, 49(11)*, 871–6.

Tamblyn, R., Abrhamowicz, M., Dauphinee, D., Wenghover, E., Jacques, A., Klass, D., et al. (2007). Physician scores on a national clinical skills examination as predictors of complaints to medical regulatory authorities. *Journal of the American Medical Association, 298(9)*, 993–1001.

Urlings-Strop, L.C., Stegers-Jager, K.M., Stijnen, T., & Themmen, A.P. (2013). Academic and non-academic selection criteria in predicting medical school performance. *Medical Teacher, 35(6)*, 497–502.

Wilson, I.G., Roberts, C., Flynn, E.M., & Griffin, B. (2012). Only the best: medical student selection in Australia. *Medical Journal of Australia, 196(5)*, 357–61.

Wright, S.R., & Bradley, P.M., (2010). Has the UK Clinical Aptitude Test improved medical student selection? *Medical Education, 44(11)*, 1069–76.

Chapter 18

Programmatic Assessment

Tejinder Singh, Jyoti N Modi, Rajiv Mahajan

KEY POINTS

- Programmatic assessment (PA) is a conceptual model of an assessment plan that is longitudinal, continues through the entire duration of the/phase, and lays emphasis on using assessment *for* learning.
- The stakes on individual assessment event is lowered such that no individual assessment has the pass/fail decisive function, but is used liberally for formative purposes.
- The high-stakes pass/fail decision process is based on the collective integrated picture presented by these low-stakes assessments. Hence, each assessment serves as a data point toward the final decision.
- The psychometric properties of the entire assessment program is of key importance rather than that of each individual method. In this program, it is possible to compensate for the psychometric deficiencies of individual methods.
- The concept of PA is well-aligned with the principles of competency-based education and hence is perhaps ideal for such curricula.

Programmatic assessment (PA) is a conceptual model that harnesses the power of assessment for learning by integrating it with the learning process. Originally proposed by van der Vleuten and Schuwirth (2005), it can be viewed as a logical consequence of the following three evolutionary aspects of medical education:

1. **The concept of utility of assessment:** 'Utility of assessment' began to be viewed as a product of various criteria used for evaluating assessment methods. This coupled with a better understanding of validity and reliability helped in our choice of assessment tools.
2. **An improved understanding of the dynamics of assessment and learning:** Resulting in the shift from 'assessment of learning' to 'assessment for learning' and 'assessment as learning'.
3. **Movement towards competency-based medical education (CBME):** Here the curriculum is driven by the desired outcome competencies that are larger whole professional tasks, rather than just a set of skills.

Rationale for Programmatic Assessment

The above three aspects are discussed in some detail to establish the rationale for introducing PA in institutes, before discussing the key components and principles of PA, steps in its implementation, and challenges thereof.

Utility of Assessment

Utility and psychometrics of assessment have been discussed in depth in this book in Chapter 1, and only some aspects relevant to PA are recapitulated here.

The seminal concept of utility of assessment proposed by Vleuten (1996) presents utility as a product of validity, reliability, feasibility, acceptability, and educational impact. The model emphasizes the contextualization of assessment because these criteria vary with the setting, and the way a tool is used or interpreted. A better understanding of validity, reliability, and educational impact has contributed to this understanding.

Validity refers to the appropriateness of the interpretation from assessment data, meaning thereby that validity is not an innate property of a tool but depends on its use. Alignment with the purpose/curricular goals, testing in appropriate contexts, use of expert judgment, and conduction in authentic settings are some of the things that contribute to the validity of the conclusions drawn from an assessment. For example, results from a written test with 10 highly standardized MCQs at the end of a 3-year training in Medicine cannot be considered to adequately inform about the clinical competence of the student.

Reliability is no longer viewed as mere consistency or reproducibility of results. It is perhaps better read as 'rely-ability' because it conveys how much one can rely on the results. The undue emphasis on standardization, objectivity, and concerns about marker variation are misplaced. It is in fact the multiple, wide (contexts, tasks), and representative sampling of curricular content that contributes to building the reliability of an assessment method. For example, a mini-CEX despite having inter-rater variation is more reliable on inter-task variation. Expert judgment (subjective) about student performance has inappropriately been equated to bias in the past. Use of multiple assessors compensates for the issue of any possible bias that may have crept in. Further, global ratings and narrative reporting on student performance by subject experts have been demonstrated to be as reliable as checklist-based scoring, and with the added benefits.

Educational impact is a crucial attribute for assessment. It is important to factor in the effect an assessment will have on the students' learning behavior. A glaring and unfortunate example is the introduction of an MCQ-based examination for selection to postgraduate courses in India. With the strong focus on future medical training and career, students tend to neglect and ignore the practical hands-on training during internship. This is an immense loss to students and to society at large. At the same time, it is important to be aware that using tools with high educational impact requires more time, effort, and availability of expert assessors. A good strategy to maximize educational impact is to have congruence between what is taught and what is assessed.

At the heart of Vleuten's model (1996) is the concept of compromises and trade-offs. It provides grounds for inclusion of assessment methods that may be relatively low in reliability, but have a high educational impact, and/ or are easy to carry out with available resources, e.g., mini-clinical evaluation exercise (mini-CEX). This is to say that trade-offs between these criteria are possible while retaining the overall utility of assessment.

The concept of utility allows for compensating for the shortcomings of some methods by using assessment methods with complementary psychometric characteristics, in a judicious combination aligned to purpose. As a corollary, it would be unwise to include only methods that are similar to each other in psychometric properties of their component criteria, e.g., including only assessment methods that are high in structure/standardization (e.g., objective methods) but low in educational impact. The combinations are better evaluated as a whole, i.e., utility of the entire programme of assessment rather than individual methods.

Changing Dynamics between Assessment and Learning

While the dynamic relationship between assessment and learning has been dealt with in detail in Chapter 2, some points relevant to the basis of PA are highlighted here.

The traditional concept of assessment is as a measure of learning, i.e., assessment *of* learning. This is essentially its decision-making and summative use, and unfortunately it can foster examination-taking behavior at the cost of learning (Cilliers et al., 2010). The power of assessment as a tool for learning is realized in its formative use, that is, when assessment is carried out with the purpose of helping the learner to improve (Schuwirth & Vleuten, 2011). This is aptly referred to as 'assessment *for* learning'. This is possible only when an assessment is followed by an effective feedback to the learner. Feedback works as a catalyst for learning when the learner is motivated to reflect upon it and act based on it, i.e., the catalytic effect (Norcini et al., 2018). Sometimes assessment activity can simultaneously be utilized as a learning activity referred to as assessment *as* learning.

Assessment *per se* is not summative and formative but it is its purpose and use that make it so. Ideally, a blend of both is needed in a training program. It is desirable that in-training assessment is carried out frequently with provision of feedback. These should be low-stakes examinations which do not place examinees under the undue stress of a pass/fail decision. However, intermittent and summative high-stakes pass/fail, or certification assessments are essential as well. Therefore, for an optimal learning outcome, there is a need for a judiciously worked out longitudinal plan of assessment that has a combination of low-stake learning-assessments and high-stake decisive assessments in appropriate proportions and times (Lockyer et al., 2017). PA addresses this need.

Global Movement towards Competency-Based Medical Education (CBME)

With the global shift toward CBME, the assessment system also needs to be suitably realigned. Traditionally, a reductionist approach had been adopted in assessment i.e., assessment of individual skills rather than focusing on the whole task. It is often erroneously presumed that if a trainee can perform individual skills well, she will also be able to perform a whole task well. However, if this was true, then there was no need for a competency-based model of education! Habitual and consistent integration of several skills judiciously so as to be able to perform a task responsibly defines competence in that area. Hence, assessment needs to be reoriented toward testing complex and meaningfully integrated learning task ideally in authentic settings.

Integration and authenticity are two key contributors to validity of assessment in CBME. Competencies are developmental and their acquisition progresses through learning stages. It is crucial that frequent guidance and modulation of learning occurs as the learner progresses through these stages. Vleuten et al., (2012) emphasized aptly that the primary purpose of assessment in CBME is to drive learning. Optimization of assessment in CBME requires the use of multiple methods, multiple assessors, training of assessors, reconceptualization of the role of psychometrics, and utilization of group processes in taking critical decisions about competence (Lockyer et al., 2017). A longitudinal assessment program as conceptualized in PA includes many of these elements, and is perhaps an ideal fit for a competency-based training. Hence, a transition to CBME calls for a shift toward PA.

It is interesting to draw a parallel between the concepts of PA and the *gurukul* system of education. In *gurukul*, the trainees were observed longitudinally over a period of time by the *guru (expert subjective judgment)*. Such assessments individually did not make a high-stake decision but helped in forming an overall picture about the trainee. In-between, there used to be high-stakes assessments as well with a final certification.

In view of this background that establishes the rationale for change in assessment, the principles and components of PA, as well as the issues surrounding its implementation, are discussed further.

Programmatic Assessment: Principles and Components

Programmatic assessment is a conceptual model best understood in terms of its key principles that govern its planning and implementation. PA uses multiple assessment opportunities with multiple methods suited to different purposes at various times, and weaves them meaningfully to create a robust fabric of assessment that has properties unique and superior to its individual constituent parts. This fabric of assessment has to be evaluated as a whole to draw valid interpretations. The concept of PA has sound logic and is well grounded in educational and learning theories (Torre et al., 2020).

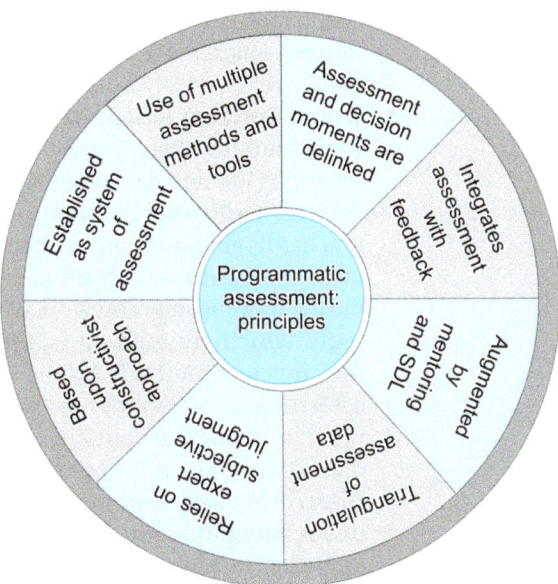

Fig. 18.1: Principles underlying Programmatic Assessment.

The underlying principles in PA have been outlined in **Figure 18.1** and are discussed in detail here.

a. **Delinking of assessment and decision moments:** An important principle governing PA is that no single assessment contributes solely to, or in a significant proportion to high-stakes pass/fail decisions. Each assessment event is made low-stakes and is not decisive on its own, but it serves as a data point contributing towards the overall high-stakes decision. So, multiple low-stakes assessments (with feedback) during training for improvement and modulation of learning, in a relatively stress-free fashion are included in the program, in addition to the traditional intermittent and final summative assessments. The final pass/fail decision considers the information from *all* of these assessments in a holistic integrated manner. Vleuten & Heeneman (2016) metaphorically suggest that each single assessment is like a pixel, which does not tell what the picture is but with aggregation of pixels, transforms into a meaningful whole. It also stands to reason that higher the pixel density, clearer is the picture. Individually, the formative assessments are used to help the learner improve; collectively, they become summative. Schuwirth et al. (2017) suggest the concept of proportionality i.e., depending on the stakes, the number of data points increases. For example, a case for jumping a red light does not require many witnesses in the court, but in a case of homicide, even self-confession is not enough, and it must be supported by multiple evidences. Generally, the police does not stop at minimal evidences; rather it collects as many evidences as possible to support its case. This concept of *proportionality* is the heart of PA. While the terms summative and formative have been used in the chapter for ease of familiarity, the boundary between summative and formative blurs in PA. All assessments contribute to the final decision, and therefore these terms become redundant.

b. **Use of different assessment methods and tools in a judicious combination:** There is general agreement that *one measure is no measure* (Vleuten & Heeneman, 2016), howsoever well-executed because it will never be able to pick all aspects of competence. Each tool has its strengths and limitations and needs to be coupled with other tools purposefully for meaningful interpretation. Therefore, during training, one can work with subjective or less standardized tools, which are high on validity and educational impact. But the choice of methods for the intermittent and final summative assessments commands high validity and reliability. A well-worked out framework that combines various methods purposefully in an optimal time-space is necessary in PA.

c. **Integrating assessment and feedback:** In PA, the key intent of dissociating individual assessment from decision-making is to optimize learning, that is, to move from assessment *of* learning to assessment *for* learning (Schuwirth & Vleuten, 2011). PA mandates establishing a culture of feedback, and training faculty and students in giving and receiving feedback. In fact, some assessment methods such as mini-CEX have feedback built-in as a part of the method itself, while others have time for feedback such as a part of an OSCE. Since competencies are developmental, and progress through stages of expertise; modulation of course of learning (for well-charted milestones attainment) is crucial rather than just assessing for competence at the end of training. With greater emphasis on feedback, marks or grades have a very limited utility to the student unless a narrative on the performance and suggestions for improvement are provided (Ginsburg, et al., 2013). This is particularly true of complex skills, such as clinical decision-making, professionalism or communication.

d. **Effective mentoring and supporting self-directed learning:** With the new competency-based curricula being rolled out in India, the importance of reflections and self-directed learning (SDL) was never greater. For feedback to bring about an improvement in the learner, there must be reflection upon it followed by action for self-improvement. Individual assessments provide an opportunity for students to engage in reflective practice (Sargeant et al., 2009). However, these opportunities for reflection may go unutilized unless a guide or a mentor motivates and encourages further plan of action for improvement (Driessen & Overeem, 2013). PA hinges on effective feedback and therefore needs students support systems in the form of effective mentoring programs. In fact, in PA, it is preferable that the mentor is not involved in the final decision-making process. In view of human resource constraints, faculty involved in low-stakes assessments with feedback may double up as mentors. This also facilitates early recognition of any deviations from the expected course. In our settings, for example, it allows a student with poor internal assessment scores to be picked up early and corrective action taken rather than telling him at the end of the year that he cannot appear for the final examinations.

e. **Triangulation of assessment data:** The assessment system in India has traditionally used a compensatory approach by aggregating unrelated data. For instance, a poor performance in physical examination may be compensated by a satisfactory presentation. Scores in a central nervous system (CNS) case are compensated by viva on a cardiovascular system (CVS) case. At times, even formats are inappropriately aggregated. It is not uncommon to see MCQ marks added to essay questions and OSCE marks added to case presentation. It may make more sense to aggregate the performance in theory, case presentation, viva, and OSCE related to a CNS case than aggregating across cases. PA allows for triangulating information from various sources on specific aspects. One such example is communication skills assessment wherein data from a communication skills station in OSCE may be collated with the data from Multisource Feedback (MSF), or peer feedback for a meaningful interpretation.

f. **Expert judgment forms the cornerstone for decision-making:** PA relies heavily on the expert subjective judgment for in-training low-stakes assessment as well as for the final pass/fail decision. The final pass/fail decision in PA also mandates a subjective assessment by expert committees since a large amount of assessment data needs to be collated for making meaningful conclusions about pass/fail or certification. It is a very rich data from multiple points throughout the course and simple mathematical treatment of the summative scores would not give a true picture of the trainee's competence.

g. **Shift from behaviorist to constructivist approach:** Traditional education views clinical competence as stacking of components and presumes that the learner will be able to integrate and make a meaningful whole. This modular approach is basically flawed and does not go well with constructivist approach to learning. Authentic learning tasks require the learner to go beyond knowledge of individual disciplines to integrating various components within and across disciplines. From the current paradigm of "assessment drives learning", there is a need to shift to "learning drives assessment" (Vleuten & Heeneman, 2016).

h. **Programmatic assessment as a system of assessment:** A more recently presented view of PA is in the form of a system of assessment (Norcini et al., 2018). This does not alter the essential components and guiding principles of PA discussed above. The assessment system must be purpose driven besides being coherent, continuous, comprehensive, feasible, acceptable, and transparent or free from bias (Norcini et al., 2018).

For better conceptualization, a comparison of salient features of PA and traditional assessment is summarized in **Table 18.1**.

A detailed comparison is provided in **Table 18.2**.

TABLE 18.1: Comparison of traditional approach to assessment and programmatic assessment

Traditional assessment	Programmatic assessment
Reductionist approach: Testing of smaller individual skills	Holistic approach: Emphasis on integrated use of skills in performing whole tasks, preferably in authentic settings
Mastery of a module is often presumed as competency attainment	Developmental assessment of student progression through stages of competency attainment
Is not a good fit for purpose in competency-based education since student progression through competency development is suboptimal or not monitored	Is a good fit for purpose in competency-based education since competencies are developmental, and require frequent monitoring and modulation of learning, PA places higher emphasis on this
Assessment is considered extrinsic to teaching-learning activities; assessment of learning takes precedence	Assessment is integrated with the teaching-learning activities by making it more frequent and with feedback for improvement
Psychometric properties of individual assessment methods/tools are considered in isolation (stand-alone approach)	Psychometric characteristics of the entire combination of methods/tools in the program as a whole are important rather than its parts or the sum of its parts (integrated approach)
Mostly very limited assessment tools used	Multiple tools chosen, aligned to the purpose

TABLE 18.2: Comparison of traditional approach to assessment and programmatic assessment

Sl. No.	Aspects compared	Traditional assessment	Programmatic assessment
1.	What is tested?	❖ Reductionist approach ❖ Testing of smaller individual skills ❖ Compartmentalized ❖ Mastery of a module is often presumed as competency attainment.	❖ Holistic approach ❖ Emphasis on integrated use of skills in performing whole tasks, preferably in authentic settings. ❖ Developmental assessment of student progression through stages of competency attainment.
2.	Dynamics of assessment and learning: Assessment *of* learning versus assessment *for* learning	❖ Assessment is considered extrinsic to teaching-learning activities. ❖ Predominant use of assessment is to measure the achievements, and as a judgment on outcome of educational process (Assessment *of* learning takes precedence).	❖ Assessment is integrated with the teaching-learning activities by making it more frequent and with feedback for improvement. ❖ Predominant use of assessment is as a driver for learning, and it is a part of the educational process itself (Assessment *for* learning takes precedence).
3.	Decision-making process: Stakes on individual assessment, and information from assessment	❖ Focuses on summative use of assessment. ❖ The promotion or pass/fail decision depends on additive scores of final and intermittent summative examinations. ❖ Does not take into account the course of learning and development.	❖ Focuses on formative use of assessment with frequent feedback. ❖ Delinking of assessment from high-stakes decision during training (lowers stress during learning). ❖ Individual in-training assessments are low stakes but each one is a data gathering point that contributes to the final decision. They provide a longitudinal view of learning course and competency acquisition.

Contd...

Contd...

Sl. No.	Aspects compared	Traditional assessment	Programmatic assessment
		❖ A lot of information generated from assessment process is discarded to be able to reach a dichotomous decision.	❖ Final high stakes pass/fail decision based on composite interpretation of inputs from multitude of low-stakes assessments by expert subjective judgment usually of a committee. ❖ Assessment is information-rich, and it is used for improving learning, as well as to draw a holistic picture of student competence over time.
4.	Utility of assessment and psychometric properties	❖ Psychometric properties of individual assessment methods/tools are considered in isolation (stand alone approach). ❖ There is a risk of using tools with similar properties, e.g., all high reliability tools, and no tools with high educational impact.	❖ Psychometric characteristics of the entire combination of methods/tools in the program as a whole are important rather than its parts or sum of parts (integrated approach). ❖ Multiple tools with variable psychometric properties (complementary, chosen deliberately, and suited for purpose).
5.	Number of tools and Number of assessors	❖ Mostly very limited assessment tools used for reasons of feasibility sometimes at the cost of compromising the validity. ❖ Even if multiple tools are used, each tool is included on its own merit rather than as a complement to other tools being used. ❖ Hardly any scope for assessment of soft skills such as communication, professionalism, ethics	❖ Multiple tools chosen aligned to the purpose. ❖ Tools that may have low reliability, but high educational impact are suitable for formative use (reliability can be improved by increasing the number of assessments and contexts). ❖ Those that can have a high reliability are used in summative assessments. ❖ Comprehensive formative assessment has the potential for assessing these soft skills and providing developmental feedback. ❖ Increased number of assessment opportunities allows for multiple assessors.
6.	Alignment with curricular goals in competency-based education	❖ Is not a good fit for purpose in competency-based education since student progression through competency development is suboptimally or not monitored.	❖ Is a good fit for purpose in competency-based education since competencies are developmental and require frequent monitoring and modulation of learning. PA places higher emphasis on this.
7.	Type of learning process expected	❖ Behaviorist: Transfer of learning and integration into practice is left to the learner, or is presumed after testing of achievements.	❖ Constructivist: The learner is encouraged and supported to build on prior knowledge and skills.
8.	Student achievement goal	❖ Achievement and certification of acquisition of minimum passing standards for promotion is the overriding goal.	❖ Individual excellence is the overarching goal, and this rests heavily on motivation through coaching/mentoring throughout the program, reflective practice, and SDL.

Contd...

Contd...

Sl. No.	Aspects compared	Traditional assessment	Programmatic assessment
9.	Role of mentoring	❖ Mentoring will have some expected positive effect on learning, but it is not meaningfully intertwined with the educational process.	❖ Mentoring has a key role in encouraging students to reflect upon the feedback received and feel motivated to take action for improvement. It is an essential component for success of PA.
10.	Standardization, objectivity, marking, grading	❖ Undue emphasis on marks and grades given in the in-training assessment. ❖ Subjectivity often misconstrued as bias. So, standardization and objectivity are stressed upon.	❖ Expert subjective judgment is utilized for providing comments, rich narratives during formative assessments so that students have a meaningful feedback for improvement.
11.	Evaluation of assessment	❖ Evaluation of the assessment plan of training would rest mostly on outcome evaluation. Process evaluation is likely to lack.	❖ Program evaluation akin to curricular evaluation is possible in PA. This opens avenues for making changes in the assessment program for better alignment.

The practical implications of PA that conform to the requirements of assessment, especially in the setting of CBME, are summarized in **Box 18.1**.

> **BOX 18.1:** Practical implications of programmatic assessment with respect to competency-based medical education
>
> - Designing assessment as a program gives it as much importance and planning as curriculum design. This makes it amenable to evaluation and further improvement.
> - Assessment is integrated with learning, and is therefore congruent with intended learning outcomes.
> - Designing assessment programs builds in authenticity at all levels of Miller's framework, including assessment in real-life settings.
> - Multiple tools are used in multiple settings and contexts based on the need at that point in training. This allows for mindful and purposeful compensation of deficiencies of some assessment tools by others.
> - Blending assessment and feedback with teaching-learning in a continuous and developmental manner makes it a good fit for competency development.
> - Individual assessment events are used as building blocks to assess overall competence. No single assessment determines the pass/fail decision.
> - Using low-stakes (and hence low stress) assessment fosters reflective practice and self-directed learning, thereby providing far more learning opportunities than decision and judgment events. This is desirable in competency-based training.
> - PA requires enhanced student support in the form of mentoring and coaching to facilitate reflective action, closer monitoring and modulation of learning.
> - Excellence of the individual student is the goal rather than minimum level of achievement by students. Individual mentoring is the key.
> - PA places emphasis on expert subjective judgment. It is therefore crucial to develop examiner expertise in grading performance with narratives and comments that are more helpful to guide learning than only giving marks.
> - This calls for culture change with reorientation to the role of assessment, its planning and implementation. Student sensitization and faculty training essential for success of this model.

Implementing Programmatic Assessment

Since PA is a relatively new concept for most, many lessons in implementation have been derived from the institutions where it has been introduced (Vleuten et al., 2012; Vleuten, 2016; Bok et al., 2013). Framework and steps for implementing PA have been suggested (Dijkstra et al., 2010; Vleuten et al., 2012, 2015; Kwan et al., 2015; Ellis & Hogard, 2016), as discussed here.

Create a Master Plan of Assessment with the Following Elements

- *Goal*: Clearly articulate the program goals that must be in alignment with the curricular goals. This is a prerequisite for the assessment program to be fit for purpose.
- *Framework*: Identify frameworks for assessment planning, e.g., Miller's framework represented as developmental levels, learning outcomes as competency framework, and Dreyfus and Dreyfus model based milestones as progression levels.
- *Longitudinal plan*: Create a longitudinal plan of multiple assessment activities interspersed with teaching-learning activities. These could be end-of-block assessments, but a developmental continuity must be maintained. Keep these assessments low stakes and avoid granting pass/fail function or summative credit to these activities. In fact, do not label assessments as formative or summative. Each assessment represents a data point, which is a part of the whole but not for making a pass/fail decision.
- *Choice of assessment methods and tools using a blueprint*: Use multiple tools, multiple assessors, and multiple contexts to cover a representative sample of the content. The choice of method at any point of time will depend on the purpose at that point and how it fits into the larger plan of assessment (discussed earlier). PA per se does not dictate a preference in assessment method (Vleuten, 2016). If using competencies as building blocks, every competency has to be assessed preferably using "one method for many integrated competencies" approach. Encourage use of narratives of acceptable performance rather than providing only grades/marks.
- *Feedback*: Each assessment must be used for providing feedback, encouraging reflections, and action for improvement. A blending of assessment with feedback is highly desirable (Watling & Ginsburg, 2019).
- *High-stakes pass/fail decision-making*: Define and lay down the process of high-stakes decision-making based on these low-stakes assessment data points. Collect data points commensurate with the stakes of assessment. Thus, a sessional test and university examination will have different number of data points.
- *Articulate the logistics of data gathering, storage, and interpretation*: This includes the information that will be contained therein

(qualitative—narratives, quantitative—numeric/grades), data storage (e.g., e-portfolios), the committee that will take decisions, etc.
- *Meaningfully combine information from data points*: Combine data points based on the domain rather than on the format of assessment. Thus, it is better to combine the marks on communication in OSCE stations with similar grades on mini-CEX, rather than combining them with marks on resuscitation.
- *Support the final decision-making with intermediate decision-making* so that the final summative decision is not a surprise to the student and teachers.
- *Rules and regulations clearly stated*: These must be communicated to the students and faculty at the beginning of the program. These must include details and logistics of assessment, examinations, pass/fail decision process, remediation measures, appeals procedure, etc.
- *Develop an evaluation plan* for the assessment program in measurable terms with scope of gap identification, suggestions, and improvement. This may involve external review, cost-effectiveness, accountability, etc.
- *Document the program.*

Draw a Plan for Supporting Activities

- *Change management*: Most institutions will be migrating from the traditional system of assessment to PA and will require change in management strategies for bringing about this change with maximum acceptance. It calls for a change in the mindset and can be challenging. Involving faculty as stakeholders in the planning process is important.
- *Resource reallocation*: Redistribution of resources for carrying out PA will be required with increased emphasis on collected information over time, as well as ongoing multiple assessments.
- *Environment*: A culture of frequent assessments with frequent feedback has to be created so that the stress of assessments is reduced. Giving and receiving feedback must be encouraged as a habit. Watling & Ginburg (2019) aptly express this as a "culture of improvement rather than a culture of performance".
- *Mentoring*: A robust student mentoring and support program will greatly enhance the success of PA. The effectiveness of feedback depends greatly on the motivation and guidance from a mentor that encourages reflection and action. Individualized mentoring of students for the entire duration of course is recommended (Vleuten, 2016). Ideally, the mentor does not play a role in the final decision-making process but stays as an influential support during the learning process.
- *Faculty training and student sensitization*: Prior to implementing PA, faculty will need to be sensitized to this relatively novel perspective

on assessment. It is also imperative that faculty is trained to appropriately use the various assessment tools, to provide effective feedback, as well as use mentoring skills. The faculty must also be trained in providing narratives and improvement suggestions rather than only grades and marks.

- *Logistics support*: Although in principle PA does not depend on use of technology, but newer technology has the potential to make the process easier. Data generation, storage, retrieval, interpretation may be facilitated by online platforms such as the e-portfolios, or learning management systems, etc.

Most of the above aspects individually represent good practices in assessment, which are orchestrated together into a program of assessment. PA is best seen as an approach to assessment design deeply ingrained into the educational process so as to maximize use of assessment for learning, optimize decision-making and ensure quality assurance (Ellis & Hogard, 2016).

Challenges to Implementation of Programmatic Assessment

It is said that logic and feasibility may be inversely related. So while PA has a sound theoretical logic, its implementation may not, and often does not follow completely (Ellis & Hogard, 2016). There is a relative paucity of literature on experience of implementation of PA. Most research efforts focus on individual methods or methods in combinations that are not truly in form of PA. However, some challenges that have been identified, or are potentially expected, are shared.

A change in assessment culture and reorienting the mindset of the faculty is perhaps one of the biggest challenges. In addition to the faculty development efforts mentioned earlier, it is crucial to make efforts to reinstate the faith in goodness of expert subjective judgment, and not let it be mistaken for bias (Vleuten & Heeneman, 2016). Bok et al. (2013) from their experience of implementing PA felt that faculty training in providing narratives and feedback was crucial, and a single workshop for the same was perhaps inadequate.

Reallocation of resources (costs or human resources) poses another challenge. Vleuten et al. (2012) suggest use of the "less is more" principle to reduce the costs. Use of assessment activities also as learning activities and the use of one method to assess many competencies are some of the ways of doing so. Use of peer assessment and involving residents in undergraduate assessments can help deal with requirement of having multiple assessors.

Heeneman et al. (2015) explored the perception and determinants of student learning when exposed to PA in the medical undergraduate program. It was surprising that students did not view the formative nature of assessment activities in the same spirit. They still regarded these as high-stakes contributing to final decisions, and hence the stress of the summative remained. Many students could not view feedback-rich tools such as the mini-CEX as an improvement exercise. They regarded it as a tick box activity. Grading and scoring strongly influenced student behavior. Many students perceived remediation measures as hurdles to end-of-block assessment. However, oral examinations in PA had a positive learning influence. The students also viewed the reflective activities in the portfolio positively as a motivating factor. Similarly, elements such as frequency of feedback, access to mentors, transparency in assessment procedures, communication regarding decision process were some of the key factors that influenced student behavior.

These challenges bring to fore the gaps in theory and practice of PA, though many of them are possibly due to the newness of concept, and the time for adjustment has not been factored in. It is heartening that partial implementation of PA in terms of its key components (such as longitudinal program, more feedback, and mentoring) has been suggested as a way of meeting these challenges, and drawing some benefit rather than losing all (Vleuten & Heeneman, 2016). The challenges will vary with the setting, contexts, regulations, and therefore, implementation also calls for adaptation of PA for local situations with an effort at maximizing the benefit within constraints.

Adaptation of Programmatic Assessment to the Indian Context

The recent transition in undergraduate medical education in India to competency-based training (Medical Council of India, 2018; Government of India, 2019) makes the concept and practice of PA very relevant. Making assessment a part of the instruction and linking it as a *program to the curriculum* can potentially ensure that no aspect of clinical competence is left unassessed (Singh, 2016).

Some of the elements of PA have been incorporated in the proposed assessment plan of the new curriculum as is depicted schematically in **Figure 18.2**.

The plan of assessment is longitudinal and continuous and extends through the phases of training. The framework of in-training assessment has been made more elaborate with emphasis on frequent assessment and feedback to augment its formative function. The regulations mandate a minimum number of three internal assessment (IA) examinations in each phase as is seen in **Figure 18.2**, and colleges can conduct more as well. Planning and implementing of frequent formative assessment activities based on a well-worked out blueprint is an initiative that the colleges must take to derive the learning benefits of PA. The **Figure 18.2** also depicts several assessment events (formal and informal) interspersed with teaching-learning activities. All these assessments are followed mandatorily by feedback to students. These assessments, though frequent and spread over the course, do not

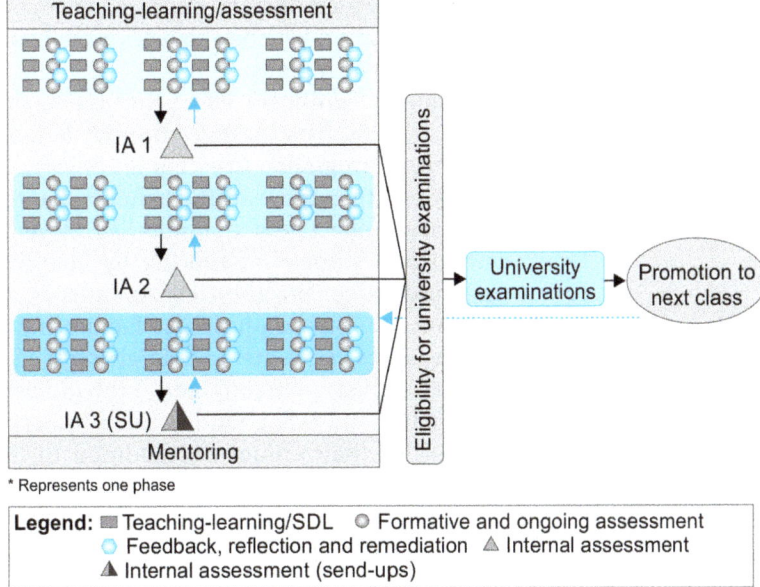

Fig. 18.2: Elements of Programmatic Assessment as applied to the Competency-based Medical Education in the Indian context.

(Adapted from Vleuten et al., 2012)

directly contribute to the pass/fail decision. However, they contribute as a whole to the eligibility of the students to be able to appear in the final summative or university examinations. So individual assessment events have low stakes, but as a whole they contribute to the eligibility for the high-stakes university examination.

The regulations call for use of multiple tools, multiple contexts, and multiple assessors. The colleges must judiciously choose the tools suited for various phases of training and purpose besides considering psychometrics. An important consideration often overlooked is that the methods chosen must aim at assessing more than one competency in an integrated manner. In fact, the unit of assessment in competency-based training must ideally be the milestones leading to full Entrustable Professional Activities (EPAs). The new curriculum document enlists detailed competency statements and details the process of deriving learning objectives and aligning assessments to these objectives. However, a word of caution is warranted here since it is easy to fall into the trap of reductionism. In trying to match assessment method or tool to individual objectives, the larger picture of competencies or whole tasks may be missed. Hence, it is suggested that while competencies (and stacked learning objectives) in the document are taken into cognizance for making a blueprint of assessment, the choice of method should be such that authenticity and integration in competencies is not compromised.

Remedial measures and improvement opportunities have also been provided and universities/colleges have been given the flexibility to devise their own plans.

Another significant effort that universities/colleges can make toward PA is by creating support activities, such as student mentoring programs. Creating an environment of mentoring will greatly enhance the learning benefits that the students derive from feedback. Reflective action and SDL develop and thrive well with one-to-one student mentoring by faculty. Faculty development and student sensitization efforts must be instituted according to regulations. The emphasis on faculty training in optimal use of various assessment methods in giving feedback, and in mentoring students, must be maintained. Individual colleges must work out how many and what kind of faculty development activities are needed for their context, in addition to the minimum that have been prescribed. Vleuten et al., (2012) rightly point out "... all actors in PA must know what they are doing, why they are doing it, and why they are doing it this way."

At present, our system partially conforms to PA and there is scope to include more elements. While the essential minimum framework of assessment has been prescribed, the universities and colleges have been allowed a lot of flexibility in implementation, and this would perhaps be best utilized in efforts toward closing this gap.

REFERENCES

Bok, H.G., Teunissen, P.W., Favier, R.P., Rietbroek, N.J., Theyse, L.F., Brommer, H., et al. (2013). Programmatic assessment of competency-based workplace learning: when theory meets practice. *BMC Medical Education*, 13, 123.

Cilliers, F.J., Schuwirth, L.W., Adendorff, H.J., Herman, N., & van der Vleuten, C.P.M., (2010). The mechanism of impact of summative assessment on medical students' learning. *Advances in Health Sciences Education: Theory and Practice*, 15(5), 695–715.

Dijkstra, J., van der Vleuten, C.P.M., & Schuwirth, L.W. (2010). A new framework for designing programmes of assessment. *Advances in Health Sciences Education: Theory and Practice*, 15(3), 379–93.

Driessen, E.W. & Overeem, K. Mentoring. In: Walsh, K. (Ed). (2013). *Oxford textbook of medical education*. Oxford: Oxford University Press. pp. 265–84.

Ellis, R., & Hogard, E. (2016). Programmatic assessment: a paradigm shift in medical education. *All Ireland Journal of Teaching and Learning in Higher Education*, 8(3), 2951–62.

Ginsburg, S., Eva, K., & Regehr, G. (2013). Do in-training evaluation reports deserve their bad reputations? A study of the reliability and predictive ability of ITER scores and narrative comments. *Academic Medicine*, 88(10), 1539–44.

Government of India. (2019). *The Gazette of India, extraordinary*. [online] Available from https://mciindia.org/ActivitiWebClient/open/getDocument?path=/Documents/Public/Portal/Gazette/GME-06.11.2019.pdf [Last accessed August, 2020].

Heeneman, S., Pool, A.O., Schuwirth, L.W., van der Vleuten, C.P.M., & Driessen, E.W. (2015). The impact of programmatic assessment on student learning: theory versus practice. *Medical Education, 49(5),* 487–98.

Kwan, J., Jouriles, N., Singer, A., Anantharaman, V., Bodiwala, G., Cameron, P., et al. (2015). Designing assessment programmes for the model curriculum from Emergency Medicine specialists. *Canadian Journal of Emergency Medicine,* 1–6.

Lockyer, J., Carracio, C., Chan, M., Hart, D., Smee, S., Touchie, C., et al. (2017). Core principles of assessment in competency-based medical education. *Medical Teacher, 39(6),* 609–16.

Medical Council of India. (2018). Competency based undergraduate curriculum for the Indian medical graduate. [online] Available from https://www.mciindia.org/CMS/wp-content/uploads/2019/01/UG-Curriculum-Vol-I.pdf [Last accessed August, 2020].

Norcini, J., Anderson, M.B., Bollela, V., Burch, V., Costa, M.J., Duvivier, R., et al. (2018). 2018 Consensus framework for good assessment. *Medical Teacher, 40(11),* 1102–9.

Sargeant, J.M., Mann, K.V., van der Vleuten, C.P.M., & Metsemakers, J.F. (2009). Reflection: a link between receiving and using assessment feedback. *Advances in Health Sciences Education: Theory and Practice, 14(3),* 399–410.

Schuwirth, L.W., & van der Vleuten, C.P.M., (2011). Programmatic assessment: from assessment of learning to assessment for learning. *Medical Teacher, 33(6),* 478–85.

Schuwirth, L., Valentine, N., & Dilena, P. (2017) An application of programmatic assessment for learning (PAL) system for general practice training. *GMS Journal for Medical Education, 34(5),* Doc56.

Singh, T. (2016). Student assessment: moving over to programmatic assessment. *International Journal of Applied and Basic Medical Research, 6(3),* 149–50.

Torre, D.M., Schuwirth, L.W., & van der Vleuten, C.P.M., (2020). Theoretical considerations on programmatic assessment. *Medical Teacher, 42(2),* 213–20.

van der Vleuten, C.P.M., (1996). The assessment of professional competence: developments, research, and practical implications. *Advances in Health Sciences Education: Theory and Practice,* 1(1), 41–67.

van der Vleuten, C.P.M., (2016). A programmatic approach to assessment. *Medical Science Educator, 26,* 9–10.

van der Vleuten, C.P.M., & Schuwirth, L.W. (2005). Assessing professional competence: from methods to programmes. *Medical Education, 39(3),* 309–17.

van der Vleuten, C.P.M., Schuwirth, L.W., Driessen, E.W., Govaerts, M.J., & Heeneman, S. (2015). Twelve tips for programmatic assessment. *Medical Teacher, 37(7),* 641–6.

van der Vleuten, C.P.M., Schuwirth, L.W., Driessen, E.W., Dijkstra, J., Tigelaar, D., & Baartman, L.K. (2012). A model for programmatic assessment fit for purpose. *Medical Teacher, 34(3),* 205–14.

van der Vleuten, C.P.M., & Heeneman, S. (2016). A new holistic way of assessment: programmatic assessment. *Fundación Educación Médica, 19(6),* 275–9.

Watling, C.J., & Ginsburg, S. (2019). Assessment, feedback and the alchemy of learning. *Medical Education, 53(1),* 76–85.

Chapter 19

Internal Assessment: Basic Principles*

Tejinder Singh, Anshu

KEY POINTS

- Internal assessment (IA) is useful to assess competencies which are important but which are not usually testable by conventional term end examinations.
- Provision of feedback makes IA a highly useful tool for learning.
- Multiple tests by multiple examiners on multiple content areas provide valid and reliable results.

In 1997, the Medical Council of India (MCI) made an important change regarding the assessment pattern of medical graduates. In a significant departure from earlier regulations, the 1997 MCI Regulations on Graduate Medical Education (GME) (Medical Council of India, 1997) made it mandatory for undergraduate students to pass their internal assessment (IA), before they could appear for their final university examinations.

These MCI regulations specified that IA shall be based on day-to-day assessment, evaluation of student assignment, preparation for seminar, clinical case presentation, etc. They went on to say that 'regular periodical examinations shall be conducted throughout the course'. The question of number of examinations was left to the concerned institution. These regulations specified that day-to-day records should be given importance during IA. Further, IA should relate to different ways in which students' participation in learning process during semesters is evaluated. Some examples being: preparation of

---

*This is an updated version of our paper, Internal Assessment Revisited, which was first published in 2009 in the National Medical Journal of India, 22: 82-84. Reprinted with the kind permission of the Editor. Certain modifications have been made (and newer references added) to bring it in sync with the MCI Graduate Medical Education Regulations, 2019.

the subject for students' seminar, preparation of a clinical case for discussion, clinical case study/problem-solving exercise, participation in project for health care in the community, proficiency in carrying out a practical or a skill in a small research project, multiple choice questions (MCQ) test after completion of a system/teaching.

A cursory perusal of these guidelines makes it clear that the intention was to have a different paradigm of assessment, where the focus was not primarily on knowledge, but on the way the knowledge is acquired. IA was not viewed as another examination without an external examiner. It had been designed to look at a different set of competencies. The importance of day-to-day observations (in contrast to snapshot observations) had also been emphasized. This was a significant amendment in the assessment procedure as it brought the process of learning into focus, in addition to the final product of learning.

However, until 2019, IA had not been implemented the way it seems to have been visualized and legislated. Further, the guidelines given by the MCI were only suggestive and not prescriptive—therefore, a lot of variation has been noted in the pattern of IA followed by various Universities, especially regarding the competencies assessed. The only consensus seems to be regarding the weightage given and the cutoff criteria. Worse, IA was frequently viewed as an examination without external regulation and therefore highly prone to abuse. Several academic frauds specifically related to IA have been reported both in the media as well as in scientific literature (Gitanjali, 2004; Arora report, 2008).

{In 2019, the MCI (Medical Council of India, 2019a) rolled out a new competency-based undergraduate curriculum for Indian medical graduates. This curriculum, like its predecessor in 1997, places emphasis on IA to supplement the final university examinations. It has also been proposed to make certain amendments, notably of not adding the marks of IA to the final score. IA remains an eligibility criterion to appear for the final examinations (Medical Council of India, 2019b). This move appears to have been included to curb unfair practices surrounding the conduct of IA in many colleges}.

Even in the best of settings, the conventional final summative examination (with external examiners) is fraught with several limitations, some of which are:

- It limits the assessment process to only the 'end of the course' setting, with chance and 'luck' of the student playing major roles. Marker reliability becomes an important consideration, especially with essay type questions. A variability of 6–15 marks has been reported even between the *same* examiners marking the *same* script twice (Natu et al., 1999).
- A clever student can bluff the examiner into believing that he knows the subject matter, even when he does not.

❖ The whole emphasis is on the product of learning. It fails to make any distinction between a student who is very studious and regular from one who reads only a month before the examination.
❖ Practical skills (giving an injection, inserting a nasogastric tube, communicating with a patient, etc.) cannot be evaluated for want of time, material, and other logistics.
❖ There is no emphasis on assessment of attitudes, communication skills, ethics, and interpersonal skills. Even where they are assessed, the setting is very artificial and has no way of eliminating 'masquerading' by the students.

Against this background, IA provides us with a very useful tool, which can compensate for several weaknesses of the year-end examinations and provide significant inputs in the assessment process. Our reluctance to exploit the potential of IA is related largely to ignorance about the various facets of IA.

Let us take a closer look at some of the myths surrounding the mechanics of IA and see how this can be used to make learning better. As already mentioned, we have tried to make a case from the MCI guidelines in the light of published literature. However, the interpretation is still ours with the intention to evolve a discussion and consensus on the dynamics and implementation of IA. We are not proposing any schedule/logistics for IA, which has already been done by the MCI expert group (Medical Council of India, 2019b).

Is Internal Assessment Formative or Summative?

Many teachers get entangled in the formative versus summative debate. Strictly going by the textbook definition, IA must be classified as summative because the results are used to make a pass-fail decision. If so, should it be called formative, for it must be used to effect improvement in learning? Further, it is argued that since it is a part of summative examination, the results cannot be made known to the student before the final declaration of results. These arguments prevent us from using the formative value of IA. Formative assessment is known to promote deep learning in the students (Rushton, 2005). The contemporary thinking in assessment is to blur the boundary between formative and summative tests. There is no reason, why a test cannot be used for both—providing feedback and for providing grades for final pass-fail decision (Wijnen, 1981). This argument is therefore unfounded that IA cannot be used for formative purposes and that its results should be kept confidential till the final declaration of results.

Is Internal Assessment a Pre-university Examination?

Internal assessment is a continuous process rather than a snapshot observation. The key features of IA are its ongoing nature and the use of multiple examiners, both of which help to attenuate subjectivity in the assessment procedure. The entire faculty of a department should preferably be involved in the process and the process ought to include multiple observations in multiple contexts. This is essential to overcome any subjectivity which may creep into the process. The results of IA should be transparent, i.e., they should be available to the students to enable them to improve their performance. In effect, the features which are perceived as weaknesses of IA are in fact its biggest strengths.

To ensure that the process is fair and is seen as fair by the students as well as the teachers, meticulous record-keeping is mandatory. A model for IA has been proposed earlier (Singh et al., 1998). This model involves all teachers in the department in assessment of the students and encourages sharing the results with students as soon as possible. To further improve the validity and reliability of IA, we proposed another 'Quarter model', which limits the contribution of individual test, tool or teacher to less than 25%, taking away the effect of subjectivity to a large extent (Singh et al., 2012). Students should be provided an opportunity to discuss their results with the concerned teachers. This discussion should focus both on their strengths and weaknesses, so that students can foster their strengths and improve performances in weaker areas (Natu et al., 1995). Encouragement and constructive criticism can always improve performance.

Should Internal Assessment be Based on Theory and Practical Tests Only?

While acquisition of knowledge and skills is an important focus of IA, it also encompasses other competencies, which are difficult to be assessed by the year-end examination. Regularity, participation in learning activities, seminars, case presentations, community projects, research projects, (e.g., short-term ICMR projects), quiz programs related to subjects, etc. are some of the examples, which need to be recognized and given credit for. Similarly, communication skills, professionalism, ethics, academic honesty, and interpersonal skills are other examples of skills which do not lend themselves to assessment at the term-end examination (Singh & Natu, 1997). While there may be some concerns regarding objectivity of such assessments, the multiplicity of examiners and observations takes care of examiner biases. It is also important to remember that most of the student learning is test-driven. What is not assessed is not learnt. By providing weightage—howsoever small it may be—to the skills mentioned above, we convey a subtle message to the students about the importance of these abilities.

Is Internal Assessment Reliable?

This belief often stems from confusion between the terms 'objectivity' and 'reliability'. Objectivity refers to the consistency of marking between different examiners and is therefore a measurement issue. Reliability, on the other hand, refers to the confidence that we can place on the judgments that we make and is therefore a decision-making issue. Medical educators are placing increasing emphasis on reliability, even though it may be less objective, as the essential attribute of assessment. Even for tools like objective structured clinical examination (OSCE), the current thinking is more in favor of a global rating compared to a detailed checklist (Vleuten & Schuwirth, 2005). IA is a more reliable way of predicting the future performance of the student as a clinician for various reasons, notably the longitudinal nature of observations. We all do classify our students as good or poor—IA tries to make that process evidence-based rather than hunch-based. Correlation between the scores at IA and at term-end examinations has been reported (Gunasekaran & Jayanthi, 1980; Badyal et al., 2018). IA scores, however, tend to be overmarked (Nath, 1980). It is not fair to cast aspersions on the utility of IA, especially, when we accept the results of year-end examinations, which usually have more problems in terms of validity and reliability.

Is Internal Assessment Valid?

Validity relates to the relation between what we intend to measure and what is actually measured. Research indicates high predictive utility and construct validity of IA (Badyal et al., 2018). We need to identify the competencies that we want to assess during IA and then use appropriate tools to assess them. MCI guidelines have given detailed description of competencies in addition to knowledge—which should be included in IA. To this extent, IA is a valid measure of listed competencies. It would, however, be worthwhile, for all subject experts to explicitly define the list of practical skills and professional behaviors, so that a uniform pattern can be followed (Awasthi & Bhandari, 2006).

Should Internal Assessment be an Aggregate of All Tests?

All coursework need not be graded to generate learning. Periodic peer assessments and other forms of engaging the learner have been shown to be as effective even in absence of providing marks to such coursework (Forbes & Spence, 1991). A meta-analysis of meta-analytic studies has brought out feedback as the single most important factor in promoting learning (Hattie, 1987). Another review (Gibbs & Simpson, 2004) has enumerated a few studies showing the utility of feedback in promoting learning. Feedback should be available to students, when it still matters to them and when they still have time to improve their performance by acting on that feedback. It has been aptly argued that the prime concern, especially for formative assessment, should be to enhance the quality and quantity of learning, rather than better measurement of limited learning (Gibbs & Simpson, 2004). Students have been reported to be more receptive to feedback in absence of marks (Black & Wiliam, 1998)—this 'grade-less' assessment is an accepted practice at many institutions. More important than the product of assessment is the framework that the assessment task provides to structured learning. Many of these have specifically been discussed in Chapter 18.

Then what are the implications for us? A perusal of what has been discussed above brings out the following issues for successful use of IA as a tool for promoting learning.

- Internal assessment must be based on day-to-day observation of the student.
- It should focus on the process of learning as much as it does on the amount of learning.
- Internal assessment looks at competencies, which are difficult to be assessed at the term-end examinations.
- All teachers of the department should be involved in the assessment process to even out the problem of reliability.
- The results should be used not only to document the progress of the student but also to provide feedback at a time, when it still matters to the student.
- Meticulous record-keeping is essential to retain faith of the students, teachers, and society in the process.

REFERENCES

Awasthi, S., & Bhandari, M. (2006). Identification and prioritisation of barriers to quality performance in medical education and patient care in medical university in India. *Journal of Social Sciences, 13(2)*, 157–62.

Badyal, D.K., Singh, S., & Singh, T. (2017). Construct validity and predictive utility of internal assessment in undergraduate medical education. *National Medical Journal of India, 30(3)*, 151–4.

Badyal, D.K., & Singh, T. (2018). Internal assessment for medical graduates in India: concept and application. *CHRISMED Journal of Health and Research, 5(4)*, 253–8.

Black, P., & Wiliam, D. (1998). Inside the black box: raising standards through classroom assessment. *Phi Delta Kappan, 80(2)*, 139–48.

Forbes, D., & Spence, J. (1991). An experiment in assessment for a large class. In: Smith, R. (Ed). *Innovations in engineering education*. London: Ellis Horwood.

Gibbs, G., & Simpson, C. (2004). Conditions under which assessment supports students' learning. *Learning and Teaching in Higher Education, 1*, 1–31.

Gitanjali, B. (2004). Academic dishonesty in Indian medical colleges. *Journal of Postgraduate Medicine, 50(4)*, 281–4.

Gunasekaran, K., & Jayanthi, P. (1980). A study of the continuous internal assessment and the university examination marks of the undergraduate semester courses (1976–77 batch), Examination Reform Unit, Madras University.

Hattie, J.A. (1987). Identifying the salient facets of a model of student learning: a synthesis of meta-analyses. *International Journal of Educational Research, 11*, 187–212.

Medical Council of India. (2019a). *Graduate medical education regulations, 2019*. [online] Available from https://mciindia.org/ActivitiWebClient/open/getDocument?path=/Documents/Public/Portal/Gazette/GME-06.11.2019.pdf [Last accessed August, 2020].

Medical Council of India. (2019b). *Module on assessment in undergraduate education: competency based undergraduate curriculum for the Indian medical graduate.* [online] Available from https://www.nmc.org.in/wp-content/uploads/2020/08/Module_Competence_based_02.09.2019.pdf (Last accessed March 2021).

Nath, B. (1980). University examination—an analytical study of the conduct of pre-university degree and master degree examinations of Gauhati University, Ph.D. Edu., Gauhati University.

Natu, M.V., Aggarwal, A., & Singh, T. (1999). Marker reliability correlates of essay type questions. *University News, 37,* 4–6.

Natu, M.V., Thomas, A.G., & Singh, T. (1995). Continuous internal assessment: concepts and application in medical education. *Trends in Medical Education, 2,* 16–7.

Probe into RGUHS marks scandal: Arora report. (2008). [online] Available from http://www.expressbuzz.com/edition/story.aspx?artid=BLrxPX6B3ek=andt [Last accessed August, 2020].

Rushton, A. (2005). Formative assessment: a key to deep learning? *Medical Teacher, 27(6),* 509–13.

Singh, T., Anshu, & Modi, J.N. (2012). The quarter model: a proposed approach to in-training assessment of undergraduate medical students in Indian medical schools. *Indian Pediatrics, 49(11),* 871–6.

Singh, T., Gupta, P. & Singh, D. (2009). Continuous internal assessment. In: *Principles of medical education,* (3rd ed). New Delhi, India: Jaypee Brothers Medical Publishers (P) Ltd. pp. 107–12.

Singh, T., & Natu, M.V. (1997). Examination reforms at the grassroots: teacher as the change agent. *Indian Pediatrics, 34(11),* 1015–9.

Singh, T., Singh, D., & Natu, M.V. (1998). A suggested model for internal assessment as per MCI guidelines on graduate medical education, 1997. Medical Council of India. *Indian Pediatrics,* 35(4), 345–7.

Van der Vleuten, C.P.M., & Schuwirth, L. (2005). Assessing professional competence: from methods to programmes. *Medical Education, 39(3),* 309–17.

Wijnen, W.H. (1981). Formative use of assessment. In: Metz, J.C., Moll, J. and Walton, H.J. (Eds). *Examinations in medical education.* Utrecht: Bunge. pp. 116–31.

Chapter 20

The Quarter Model

Tejinder Singh, Anshu, Jyoti N Modi

KEY POINTS

- In-training assessment has the potential to test a wide range of competencies which are not testable by the year-end examination. However, despite high validity, educational impact, and feasibility; its implementation is flawed.
- This paper proposes a "Quarter model of in-training assessment" for implementation in the undergraduate medical curriculum in India.
- The model proposes that assessments be carried out at least quarterly; no teacher should contribute more than 25% of the marks for any student; no single assessment tool should contribute more than 25% marks, and no assessment should contribute to more than 25% of the total marks.
- Structuring the implementation using multiple tests on multiple content areas by multiple examiners using multiple tools in multiple settings in the proposed quarter model will not only improve the reliability and validity of internal assessment, but also its acceptability.

Internal assessment (IA) provides a valuable opportunity for using assessment for learning. It allows assessment of many competencies which are not assessable during term-end examinations. In 2019, the Medical Council of India released a module on competency-based assessment for undergraduate education which gave detailed guidelines to plan IA in the light of the new curriculum, which are suggestive rather than prescriptive.

We are reproducing here a paper where we had suggested a model for IA called the quarter model. Though there are some modifications in the MCI-2019 regulations, we believe that the concept and the

---

*This is an updated version of our paper, The Quarter Model: A proposed approach to in-training assessment for undergraduate students in Indian Medical Schools, which was first published in 2012 in Indian Pediatrics, 49:871-76. Reprinted with the kind permission of the Editor. Certain modifications have been made and some references added to bring it in sync with the MCI Graduate Medical Education Regulations, 2019.

logistics that we proposed in 2012 remain the same. We hope, readers will notice many concepts of Programmatic Assessment incorporated in the model.

Formative assessment has a major influence on learning (Rushton, 2005). The educational utility of a summative or year-end examination is limited since it usually involves a single encounter with assessment of a limited number of competencies, mostly knowledge-based, with no opportunity for feedback and improvement. IA provides a very useful opportunity to not only test acquisition of knowledge but also provides feedback to make learning better.

The strengths of IA are threefold. One, there is an opportunity to provide timely corrective feedback to students. Feedback is recognized as the single-most effective tool to promote learning (Hattie, 1987). Two, IA can be designed to test a range of competencies, such as, skill in performing routine clinical procedures (giving injections, suturing wounds, performing intubation, etc.), professionalism, ethics, communication, and interpersonal skills, which are hardly assessed in the final examinations (Singh & Natu, 1997). Three, the continuous nature of this assessment throughout the training period has the potential to steer the students' learning in the desired direction over time. The focus is on the process, as much as on the final product of learning.

The concept of IA is not new. The University Grants Commission (2012) recommends that we need to "... move to a system which emphasizes continuous IA and reduces dependence on external examinations to a reasonable extent." Similarly, the National Accreditation and Assessment Council (NAAC) (2012) encourages the use of IA to guide the learning.

The draft of the 2012 revised Regulations on Graduate Medical Education (GME) released by the Medical Council of India (MCI) stipulates that undergraduate students should have passed in their IA to be eligible to appear in the final university examinations. The recommendation is for IA to be based on day-to-day records. Also, regular assessments conducted throughout the course shall relate to assignments, preparation for seminars, clinical case presentations, participation in community health care, proficiency and skills required for small research projects, etc. Further, electives and skills should be assessed as part of IA (Medical Council of India, 2012).

Problems with Internal Assessment in India

Despite its obvious strengths, IA has not been used to its full potential in India. Often trivialized as a replica of the final examination, IA is restricted only to theory and practical tests, while its potential to test other competencies is seldom exploited. The major issues with IA in India are improper implementation, lack of faculty training, misuse or abuse, lack of acceptability among all stakeholders, and perceived lack of reliability (Singh & Anshu, 2009).

Improper implementation: Implementation has a strong bearing on any assessment and its educational utility. The earlier 1997 guidelines (Medical Council of India, 1997) did not carry any mention of how the IA was to be implemented. Institutions were left to design their own plan of IA leading to considerable variation in the methods of assessment and the competencies assessed. Practical guidelines have not been provided for implementation of IA in the 2012 revised regulations on GME (Medical Council of India, 2012) either, giving rise to a sense of *déjà vu.***

Lack of faculty training: Faculty development is prerequisite to proper implementation of any assessment method. Lack of training is often the reason for poor implementation, lack of transparency, and inadequate or no provision of feedback to students. By not providing timely and appropriate feedback, the biggest strength of IA is nullified. When teachers do not give competencies such as communication skills, professionalism, ethics, interpersonal skills, ability to work in a team, etc., enough weightage in the IA due to the fear that these cannot be precisely measured, they indirectly convey to students that these qualities are not important in medicine. While the faculty do gain experience of teaching and research, there is no opportunity for them to get a hands-on experience on student assessment.

Misuse/Abuse: IA is often misused as an examination without external controls (Gitanjali, 2004; RGUHS, 2012). The 2012 draft regulations (Medical Council of India, 2012) have proposed some variations from the 1997 regulations (Medical Council of India, 1997). Marks of IA are no longer to be added to the final scores for making pass/fail decisions. Although not expressly stated, fear of abuse of IA to inflate marks seems to have prompted this change. However, this opens new opportunities to use IA to assess competencies hitherto left unassessed.

Lack of acceptability: The issues that lower the acceptability of IA from all its stakeholders are: assessment in marking by institutions, too much 'power' bestowed to single individuals (often departmental heads), too much weightage to single tests, and a perceived lack of reliability. Reliability (also sometimes described as reproducibility) is commonly seen as 'consistency of marking'. Here, it may be pertinent to clarify that reliability should be seen as consistency or reproducibility of student performance rather than consistency of marking by examiners. Assessing a student in one clinical situation is

---

** The 2019 Amendment to MCI Graduate Medical Education Regulations & the 2019 MCI Competency Based Assessment Module for Undergraduate Medical Education have now given detailed mandates and guidelines.

not predictive of her performance in another clinical situation. Also, it is uncertain that a physician will encounter the same conditions in actual practice under which she was assessed. Therefore, if reliability has to contribute toward prediction of a student's future performance in real situations, the true meaning of reliability should be 'consistency of performance' rather than 'consistency of scoring' (Feldt & Brennan, 1989). Marker variability in IA is often cited as a reason for lack of reliability. Research has consistently shown that increasing the number of assessors and increasing the sample of the content being assessed improves reliability (Vleuten et al., 2000). Even with rather subjective assessments, having different assessors for different parts of a test can neutralize an incompetent/biased assessor's influence (Vleuten et al., 1991). By increasing the number of clinical situations in which a student is assessed, the reliability of the assessment can be improved more than by merely making more objective tests.

The utility of any assessment is dependent upon interplay of its validity, reliability, acceptability, feasibility, and educational impact (Vleuten & Schuwirth, 2005). Although each one of these attributes is important, there is always some trade-off between them. For example, an assessment which is apparently low on reliability can still be useful by virtue its positive educational impact (Vleuten et al., 1991). Where combinations of different assessments alleviate drawbacks of individual methods, use of the programmatic approach to assessment is advocated, thereby rendering the total more than the sum of its parts (Vleuten et al., 2012).

When properly implemented, IA scores over the year-end examination in terms of its validity, reliability (consistency of performance), feasibility, and educational impact (Singh & Anshu, 2009). To ensure that students are not denied the benefit of this extremely useful modality, efforts need to be made to improve its implementation and acceptability.

In this paper, we propose a model for IA, which tries to overcome some of the issues that teachers and students face. We call it the *'In-Training Assessment* (ITA)' as it reflects the philosophy and intent of this assessment better. The ITA is designed to not only test knowledge and skills, but also to provide an opportunity to assess competencies which are not assessable by conventional year-end examinations. The purpose of ITA is to provide feedback to students and teachers, and to improve student learning. It is proposed to be a longitudinal program spread throughout the MBBS training. ITA is expected to be complementary to the *End-of-Training Assessment* (ETA) carried out by the affiliating universities to test for attainment of intended competencies.

Proposed Quarter Model

The salient features of this model are outlined in **Box 20.1**.

> **Box 20.1:** The Quarter Model of in-training assessment
>
> 1. At least one assessment every quarter
> 2. No teacher to contribute more than a quarter (25%) of the marks for any student.
> 3. No single tool to contribute more than a quarter (25%) of the marks.
> 4. No single assessment to contribute more than a quarter (25%) of the total marks.

Format: We propose that students be periodically assessed during their training by the faculty of their parent institutes. Passing separately in ITA and ETA, in both theory and practical/clinical components should be mandatory. As proposed in the GME Regulations 2012 (Medical Council of India, 2012), while passing in ITA will be an eligibility criterion for appearing in the university examinations, marks obtained in ITA will not be added to the marks obtained in ETA.* The scores can be converted to grades using a 7-point scale (using absolute grading criteria) and shown separately on the marksheet issued by the universities.

Organization and Conduct: To allow greater spread of marks, each subject may be assessed out of a maximum of 100 marks (50% for theory and 50% for practical/clinical component) in the ITA. ITA should make use of several assessment tools.* For theory: essay questions, Short Answer Questions (SAQ), Multiple Choice Questions (MCQ), Extended Matching Questions, and Oral Examinations should be used. For practical/clinical assessment: experiments, long cases, short cases, spots, Objective Structured Practical/Clinical examinations (OSPE/OSCE), mini-Clinical Evaluation Exercise (mini-CEX), and Objective Structured Long Examination Record (OSLER) should be used. Viva in practical/clinical assessment should focus on the experiments actually performed or cases actually seen rather than being a general viva. Colleges can add more tools depending on the local expertise available.

The planning and assessment for ITA should involve all teachers of each department to ensure that no single teacher contributes to more than 25% of the marks to the total marks and no single assessment tool contributes to more than 25% marks to the total ITA. For this purpose, teachers would mean all those working as tutors/senior residents and upwards. The proportion of 25% marks should be calculated from the assessments spread over the entire year. For example, the departments should be at liberty to have four assessments with one having only essay type questions, another having only MCQs, the third having only

---

* The 2019 Amendment to MCI Graduate Medical Education Regulations & the 2019 MCI Competency Based Assessment Module for Undergraduate Medical Education have now given detailed mandates and guidelines.

oral examination, and a fourth one with a mix of all. Or they could have four assessments with a mix of essays, SAQs, MCQs, and oral examinations. The same applies to practical/clinical examinations. However, for subjects like radiodiagnosis, pulmonology, dermatology, emergency medicine and dentistry, each teacher and each tool may contribute 50% to the assessment in that subject. In effect, it means that to maintain the 25% limit, at least four teachers and four different assessment tools, should be used for ITA. For subjects with the 50% limit, at least two teachers and two tools will be required.

The division of marks for ITA in one subject is shown in **Table 20.1**. To illustrate application of Quarter model, two examples, one from a preclinical (Physiology) and another from a clinical (Pediatrics) department are provided **(Tables 20.2 and 20.3)**. Utilization of end-of-posting assessment for the practical component of ITA in clinical subjects may contribute toward time efficiency of the ITA program by using same assessments for formative as well as summative purposes.

As **Table 20.3** shows, ITA is proportionately divided over the phases for subjects that are taught over different semesters. For subjects that include other allied subjects (e.g., Medicine includes Dermatology, Psychiatry, etc.), a proportion of ITA is to be allocated to allied subjects based on the teaching time allotted. Students would need to secure passing marks (>50%) in theory and practical separately for allied subjects also.

TABLE 20.1: Example of Division of Marks for Internal Assessment in one subject*

Theory (Maximum marks: 100)		Practical/clinical (Maximum marks: 100)	
Knowledge tests: using multiple tools as explained above, (including one question from AETCOM per professional year)	80	Practical and clinical skills (including communication skills, bedside manners): using multiple tools as explained in text	60
Assignment preparation, participation in class – group discussion, role play, attendance* **(Logbook record)**	10	Professionalism, preparation for case presentation, presentation	10
Other academic activities: quiz, seminar, poster making, etc. **(Logbook record)**	10	ICMR projects, Other research projects, community work	10
		Log book record including: attendance*, skill certification	20

*Marks for attendance over and above minimum cutoff eligibility criteria of 75% in theory and 80% in practical respectively.

---

* This table has been modified in line with the 2019 MCI guidelines in its Module on Competency Based Assessment for Undergraduate Medical Education

TABLE 20.2: Example for PHYSIOLOGY - 'Quarter Model' as applied to Internal Assessment of Theory*

Maximum marks 100; Suggested 4 ITAs over entire course of Phase I MBBS *(The regulations suggest a minimum of 3)*

IA no.	Knowledge tests (Maximum marks: 80)#					Other skills (Maximum marks: 10) - Logbook		Other academic activity Logbook
	Essay/ MEQ	SAQ	MCQ	AETCOM SAQ	ECE/Rea- soning	Participation (discussion, group work, role play)	Attendance	
Maximum marks	20	20	20	10	10	5	5	10
1	10	5			5			Participation in quiz: 5
2		5	10	5		5	76–80%: 1 / 81–90%: 3 / >90%: 5	
3 (Pre-university)	10	10	10	5	5			Seminar: 5

\# The distribution of 80 marks can be altered as per requirements; No single assessment event will contribute to over 25% of the marks; No single assessment tool will contribute to over 25% of the marks
Depending on seats and faculty availability, this scheme may be modified suitably. No single faculty will contribute over 25% of the total marks.

* This table has been modified in line with the 2019 MCI guidelines in its Module on Competency Based Assessment for Undergraduate Medical Education

All results should be declared within 2 weeks of the assessment. Students should sign on the result sheet in token of having seen the results. The results should also be uploaded on the college website within 2 weeks of being put up on the notice board. Students who do not pass in any of the assessments should have the opportunity to appear for it again—however, any repeat assessment should not be conducted earlier than 2 weeks of the last to allow students to meaningfully make good their deficiencies. Only one additional assessment may be provided to make good the deficiency. If a student is unable to score passing marks even after an additional assessment, he should repeat the course/posting and appear for the university examinations 6 months later.

Teachers should provide feedback to students regarding their performance. A group feedback session should be organized within a week after declaration of results. However, for persistently low-achieving students, one-to-one feedback sessions may be organized.

To use the power of assessment meaningfully for better learning and to ensure stability in assessments, all colleges should appoint a Coordinator for ITA. All the teaching departments should also appoint

TABLE 20.3: Example for PEDIATRICS - 'Quarter Model' as applied to Internal Assessment of Theory*

Maximum Marks (MM) 100; Suggested minimum 7 ITAs over entire course including End of Posting (EOP) Theory assessment and the Pre-University examination]

MBBS phase	Clinical posting (weeks)	Tests	Theory (Maximum marks: 80)#					Logbooks (20)	
			Essay/MEQ	SAQ	MCQ	AETCOM	Clinical reasoning	Group work, role play, ICMR project, quiz	Attendance
Maximum Marks			20	20	20	10	10	15	5
Phase II	2	EOP-Th-1		5					
Phase III-Pt-1	4	EOP-Th-2			10			15 (distributed over various phases and different activities)	76–80%: 1 81–90%: 3 >90%: 5
		Th-1		5		2	3		
		Th-2	10	3		2			
Phase III-Pt-2	4	EOP-Th-3			10				
		Th-3		3			2		
		Th-4 (Pre-Univ)	10	4		6	5		

The distribution of 80 marks can be altered as per requirements; No single assessment event will contribute to over 25% of the marks; No single assessment tool will contribute to over 25% of the marks No single faculty will contribute over 25% of the total marks. Depending on seats and faculty availability, this scheme may be modified suitably.

*This table has been modified in line with the 2019 MCI guidelines in its Module on Competency Based Assessment for Undergraduate Medical Education

a teacher as a coordinator to plan and organize ITA. Departments should coordinate among themselves and with the Chief Coordinator to ensure that students do not have assessment in more than one subject during the same week. As far as possible, all ITAs should be scheduled on Monday mornings so that students get the weekend to prepare and do not miss classes. For clinical subjects, the practical component of the ITAs should be scheduled at the end of clinical postings. The minimum number of ITAs for each subject should be specified in the beginning of the term. The plan and tentative dates of assessment should be put up on the notice board within the first month of starting that phase of training. The ITA plan of each department should be developed as a standard operating procedure (SOP) document, approved by the Curriculum/Assessment committee of the college and reviewed (and revised if required) annually. This document should be made available to the students at the beginning of each phase.

Record-keeping: It is important to maintain a good record of performance in ITA to ensure credibility. Students should have access to this record and should sign it every 3 months. A sample format for record-keeping has previously been published (Singh et al., 2009).

Faculty development: Unless both the assessors and students understand the purpose of this exercise, this powerful tool will continue to be trivialized and acceptance will remain suboptimal. Success of this model will require training the faculty in use of multiple assessment tools. Currently, faculty development is carried out through the basic course workshops on medical education; this needs to be scaled up for capacity building of medical teachers. It is also imperative that the students be sensitized to the ITA program for MBBS during the proposed foundation course (the first 2 months before Phase I of MBBS).*

Utility of the Model

The quarter model addresses several commonly leveled criticisms against IA. The strength of ITA is expected to be realistic in its continuous nature and in the fact that it is based on longitudinal observations in authentic settings. Provision of feedback not only allows for mid-course correction of the learner's trajectory (Burdick, 2012) but also reinforces their strong points.

Medical competence is an integrated whole and not the sum of separate entities. No single instrument will ever be able to provide all the information for a comprehensive evaluation of competence (Dijkstra et al., 2010). Single assessments, howsoever well planned, are flawed (Vleuten et al., 2012). By including assessment in various settings and by use of multiple tools in this model, the intention is to increase the sampling and to make more well-informed and defensible judgments of students' abilities. Use of multiple examiners is expected to help reduce the examiner biases involved in the process of assessment, and also minimize misuse of power.

Understandably, this model may demand more effort and work from the faculty members. However, we feel that the added benefits of this model would be a better distribution of student assessment tasks within the department and an opportunity for the tutors/senior residents to be trained in assessment methods under supervision. It must be reiterated here that assessment requires as much preparation, planning, patience and effort that research or teaching does. Assessment has been taken rather casually for far too long and at least semi-prescriptive models of ITA based on educational principles are a need of the day. Ignoring educational principles while

---

* The article was written prior to the introduction of revised Basic Course Workshop, and the Curriculum Implementation Support Program (CISP) by the MCI/Board of Governors in supersession of the MCI

assessing students, merely because it results in more work, seriously compromises the utility and sanctity of assessment.

Black & Wiliam (1998) state that any strategy to improve learning through formative assessment should include: clear goals, design of appropriate learning and assessment tasks, communication of assessment criteria, and provision of good quality feedback. Students must be able to assess their progress toward their learning goals (Burdick, 2012). The Quarter model largely considers all these elements. Our model gives a broad overview of what is and what is not being measured. It also balances the content and counteracts the tendency to measure only those elements which are easy to measure. By involving students early in the process, informing them of the criteria by which they will be judged, the assessment schedules and most importantly, giving them feedback on their learning, the model is expected to provide them an opportunity to improve performance. The display of ITA grades alongside the ETA marks is expected to demonstrate the consistency of student performance and prevent manipulation of marks.

This model has been conceptualized using accepted theories of learning and assessment. *Multiple* tests on *multiple* content areas by *multiple* examiners using *multiple* tools in *multiple* settings in the Quarter model will improve the reliability and validity of IA, and thereby improve its acceptability among all stakeholders.

REFERENCES

Black, P., & Wiliam, D. (1998). Assessment and classroom learning. *Assessment in Education, 5(1)*, 7–74.

Burdick, W.P. (2012). Foreword. In: Singh, T. and Anshu (Eds). *Principles of assessment in medical education*, (1st ed). New Delhi, India: Jaypee Brothers Medical Publishers (P) Ltd.

Dijkstra, J., van der Vleuten, C.P.M., & Schuwirth, L.W. (2010). A new framework for designing programmes of assessment. *Advances in Health Sciences Education: Theory and Practice, 15(3)*, 379–93.

Feldt, L.S., & Brennan, R.L. (1989). Reliability. In: Linn, R.L. (Ed). *Educational measurement*, 3rd ed. New York: Macmillan. pp. 105–46.

Gitanjali, B. (2004). Academic dishonesty in Indian medical colleges. *Journal of Postgraduate Medicine, 50(4)*, 281–4.

Government of India. (2019). The Gazette of India, Extraordinary, Part III-Section 4. Board of Governors in super-session of the Medical Council of India - Regulations on Graduate Medical Education (Amendment) 2019, published 6 November 2019. Available from: https://mciindia.org/ActivitiWebClient/open/getDocument?path=/Documents/Public/Portal/Gazette/GME-06.11.2019.pdf [Last accessed 28 August 2020]

Hattie, J.A. (1987). Identifying the salient facets of a model of student learning: a synthesis of meta-analyses. *International Journal of Educational Research, 11(2)*, 187–212.

Medical Council of India. (2012). *Regulations on graduate medical education, 2012*. [online] Available from http://www.mciindia.org/tools/announcement/Revised_ GME_2012.pdf. [Last accessed August, 2020].

Medical Council of India. (1997). *Regulations on graduate medical education, 1997*. [online] Available from http://www.mciindia.org/RulesandRegulations/GraduateMedicalEducationRegulations1997.aspx. [Last accessed August, 2020].

Medical Council of India. (2019). Competency Based Assessment Module for Undergraduate Medical Education Training program, https://www.nmc.org.in/wp-content/uploads/2020/08/Module_Competence_based_02.09.2019.pdf (Last accessed March 2021).

National Accreditation and Assessment Council (2002). *Best practice series-6: curricular aspects*. [online] Available from http://naac.gov.in/sites/naac.gov.in/files/Best%20Practises%20in%20Curricular%20Aspects.pdf [Last accessed August, 2020].

RGUHS does it again, alters MBBS marks. [online] Available from http://articles.timesofindia.indiatimes.com/2006-04-25/bangalore/27804396_1_internal-assessmentrguhs-medical-colleges. [Last accessed August, 2020].

Rushton, A. (2005). Formative assessment: a key to deep learning? *Medical Teacher*, *27(6)*, 509–13.

Singh, T., & Anshu. (2009). Internal assessment revisited. *National Medical Journal of India*, *22(2)*, 82–4.

Singh, T., Gupta, P., & Singh, D. (2009). Continuous internal assessment. In: *Principles of medical education*, 3rd ed. New Delhi, India: Jaypee Brothers Medical Publishers (P) Ltd. pp. 107–12.

Singh, T., & Natu, M.V. (1997). Examination reforms at the grassroots: teacher as the change agent. *Indian Pediatrics*, *34(11)*, 1015–9.

University Grants Commission (2012). *Action plan for academic and administrative reforms*. New Delhi. [online] Available from http://ugc.ac.in/policy/cmlette2302r09.pdf [Last accessed August, 2020].

van der Vleuten, C.P.M., Norman. G.R., & De Graaff, E. (1991). Pitfalls in the pursuit of objectivity: Issues of reliability. *Medical Education*, *25(2)*, 110–8.

van der Vleuten, C.P.M., Scherpbier, A.J., Dolmans, D.H., Schuwirth, L.W., Verwijnen, G.M., & Wolfhagen, H.A. (2000). Clerkship assessment assessed. *Medical Teacher*, *22(6)*, 592–600.

van der Vleuten, C.P.M., Schuwirth, L.W., Driessen, E.W., Dijkstra, J., Tigelaar, D., Baartman, L.K., et al. (2012). A model for programmatic assessment fit for purpose. *Medical Teacher*, *34(3)*, 205–14.

van der Vleuten, C.P.M., & Schuwirth, L.W. (2005). Assessing professional competence: from methods to programmes. *Medical Education*, *39(3)*, 309–17.

Chapter 21

Assessment in Online Settings

Anshu

KEY POINTS

- The principles underlying good assessment remain the same for traditional classroom -and online settings
- Online platforms offer the opportunity not just to test what students have learnt, but also to design assessment as rich learning experiences (assessment as learning).
- Technology is not a substitute for the teacher. It merely provides a way to implement good assessment practices.

The need to provide newer strategies for online learning and assessment is clearly visible in the wake of the coronavirus disease 2019 (COVID-19) pandemic. However, even otherwise, new educational environments with changed requirements of students demand the use of blended learning, where e-learning complements classroom or clinical teaching (James, et al., 2002).

Teacher-centered approaches do not work when transferred from the classroom to the online platforms. A shift to the student-centered approach is essential in both settings. Secondly, the system we follow is heavily based on testing, and encourages a strong culture of examination-oriented learning. Course design, teaching strategies, and assessment procedures heavily influence whether students will adopt surface or deep approaches to learning (Gibbs, 1992). The pandemic has perhaps ushered in an opportunity to bring about major upheavals in the way we teach and assess our students (Fuller et al., 2020).

Online assessment allows us to rethink how assessment can be delivered in health professions settings. It is time we captured the potential of online learning to conduct assessment in a more meaningful manner. In this chapter, we will review some of the concepts that underlie design and implementation of online assessment.

Designing Online Assessment

The following principles help in designing good assessment in online settings:

Assessment as Learning

Traditionally, assessment has been used to test what students have learnt. However, it is time to rethink and review this concept. Assessment can work as a surrogate for providing learning experiences. Online settings provide several opportunities to innovate and experiment with newer assessment designs. Assessment can be creatively designed offline or online to provide students with rich learning experiences. For instance, students can be asked to visit a pharmacy or a blood bank and submit a report online about how things are organized and functioning. Here, while the report tests their understanding, it also makes them learn in an authentic environment. In this manner, assessment can be fully integrated with the teaching–learning processes. Assessment can thus actually contribute to student learning.

Aligning Assessment with Learning Outcomes and Teaching Methods

The 'whys' of assessment must not be forgotten. The purpose of assessment in each educational situation must be kept in mind. Is assessment being carried out for ranking, selection, or provision of formative feedback? Further, the type and level of learners who are being assessed are factors which determine the framework of assessment. Assessment must be aligned to the learning outcomes, and tasks must be designed to ensure that these outcomes are being attained (Norcini et al., 2018). As mentioned earlier, assessment should be integrated with the teaching–learning processes. It is always pertinent to ask how a particular assessment task will add to the learning experience being offered to students.

Learning *with* Technology, Rather than *from* Technology

There is this peculiar tendency to be excited about every new application or technological advance that comes our way. But it is important to remember that technology cannot substitute a teacher. The design of each assessment needs to be weighed in terms of its educational impact. Technology can be of assistance in achieving that design. However, one needs to go sequentially from intended educational outcome to assessment task, and then ask how technology can help simplify the conduct of the assessment; and not start vice versa just because a new-fangled application (app) is available.

One of the problems with telling students to learn *from* technology is that we are encouraging students to merely become knowledge users. The correct approach will be to make them construct their own knowledge *with* technology (Hallas, 2008). This again will require innovative thinking to design authentic assessment tasks which will require them to create original work.

Let's think of a clinical or community setting, which students are asked to explore. Suppose the task at the end of that learning exercise is that they are asked to develop a checklist or an algorithm or a management protocol which works specific to that setting. Here, they will have to understand the setting, explore existing literature using technology, and then adapt it to their specific setting. Merely cutting and pasting from the internet will not suffice. Such tasks can become more meaningful if learners are asked to collaborate with their fellow students, or with peers from other allied health professions. With one integrated task, we can teach them several elements, such as analysis, synthesis of new knowledge, team work, professionalism, and communication skills. It is important to stimulate higher-order thinking and be aware of the educational impact of assessment at all times.

Reducing Faculty Workload and Providing Feedback by use of Automation

Technology has the potential to reduce workload of the faculty by using automation. Submission of assignments, scoring, provision of immediate feedback, and preparation of results can easily be automated in several settings. It is also important to have multiple assessments using the principles of programmatic assessment. Technology makes this task simpler.

Online settings allow individualized feedback to be given to learners. It is possible to design self-assessments at the end of each module which help learners assess their learning themselves. Self-assessment modules offer learners the flexibility of learning at their own pace and place. Technology makes it possible to build in feedback depending on the response of the learner. While designing this takes time at the first instance, a good number of items in the question bank can enable one to reuse these questions for subsequent batches of students.

When dealing with large numbers, online assessment can enable monitoring of start and stop times, quicker declaration of results, and reduction in costs. However, simply because automation makes things easier, one must be careful not to succumb to encouraging lower-order thinking, by giving linear assessment tasks. The gains acquired in terms of efficiency and reduced cost must not be lost by encouraging poor learning habits.

Using Alternative Formats in Online Assessment

It is often perceived that online assessments are restricted to objective assessment formats. This is because e-assessments first began with formats, such as multiple choice questions, true-false questions, and extended matching questions, which were adapted from classrooms for online use (Dennick, et al., 2010). However, there are several more interesting avenues to explore, which can improve the validity of assessment. Visual and audio triggers can be used as simulations. Use of technology makes it possible to design assessment tasks which involve complex scenarios and interactivity.

The advantage of using e-assessment is that a whole range of question formats are possible. Some of them are tabulated below (**Table 21.1**):

TABLE 21.1: Question formats that can be used in online assessment

Text formats	❖ Multiple choice questions (with feedback) ❖ True/false questions ❖ Extended matching questions ❖ Assertion-reason type questions ❖ Online polls ❖ Short answer questions ❖ Structured long answer questions ❖ Scavenger hunt (students are asked to search for credible references from online resources on a topic or theme) ❖ Calibrated peer review
Audiovisual formats using multimedia	❖ Picture-based questions (using clinical photos, X-rays, microscopic images, investigation reports, and graphs) ❖ Sound-based questions (auscultation sounds, etc.) ❖ Video- or animation-based questions (showing clinical signs, patient interviews, procedures, animated mechanisms, processes, flowcharts)
Simulations and gaming formats	❖ Electronic patient management problems ❖ Simple and complex simulations such as virtual patients ❖ Virtual trainers and simulators (e.g., laparoscopy trainer) ❖ Dosage simulations with graphs ❖ Gaming style quizzes
Live interactive formats	❖ Assessment using standardized patients ❖ Virtual objective structured clinical examination (OSCE) ❖ Objective structured video examination (OSVE) ❖ Assessment of communication skills or history-taking skills by trainer
Activity-based	❖ Project-based assessment ❖ Assessment of reflective writing after an authentic experience ❖ Assessment-based on group activity and report ❖ Electronic logbooks ❖ Electronic portfolios

Once faculty have got used to the standard formats, their hesitation will reduce and they will begin to explore higher forms of assessment, which can be an exciting process.

Asking Higher Order Questions

Instead of restricting ourselves to the lower levels of Bloom's taxonomy, we need to ask questions from the higher levels. **Table 21.2** below lists the different verbs and the assessment methods which can be used to do this easily.

TABLE 21.2: Verbs and assessment methods to test different levels

Levels of Bloom taxonomy	Verbs	Assessment methods
Knowledge	❖ Define ❖ List ❖ Recall ❖ State ❖ Name ❖ Arrange ❖ Order ❖ Describe ❖ Label ❖ Recognize ❖ Tabulate ❖ Arrange	❖ Multiple choice questions ❖ Short answer questions ❖ Scavenger hunt ❖ Basic questions-based on illustrations and photographs
Comprehension	❖ Compare ❖ Classify ❖ Differentiate ❖ Distinguish ❖ Summarize ❖ Contrast ❖ Estimate ❖ Explain ❖ Interpret ❖ Identify ❖ Review	❖ Multiple choice questions ❖ Short answer questions ❖ Match the following ❖ Interpretation of investigation report, video, and diagram ❖ Written report preparation ❖ Summary
Application	❖ Apply ❖ Calculate ❖ Demonstrate ❖ Predict ❖ Solve ❖ Prepare ❖ Classify ❖ Interpret ❖ Examine ❖ Use ❖ Create	❖ Scenario-based questions ❖ Project ❖ Demonstration ❖ Simulation ❖ Role play ❖ Draw flowchart or concept map ❖ Propose solution to a problem ❖ Create educational material ❖ Interpretation of graph or data

Contd...

Contd...

Analysis	❖ Appraise ❖ Critique ❖ Contrast ❖ Infer ❖ Compare ❖ Examine ❖ Analyze	❖ Problem-solving exercises ❖ Case studies ❖ Discussion ❖ Critical incident analysis ❖ Analysis of data from a survey or questionnaire
Synthesis	❖ Construct ❖ Create ❖ Plan ❖ Prepare ❖ Organize ❖ Arrange ❖ Integrate ❖ Explain ❖ Invent ❖ Design ❖ Manage	❖ Projects ❖ Case studies ❖ Develop plans ❖ Design a model ❖ Organize an event
Evaluation	❖ Estimate ❖ Evaluate ❖ Critique ❖ Justify ❖ Discriminate ❖ Prove ❖ Support ❖ Interpret ❖ Defend ❖ Assess ❖ Appraise ❖ Argue ❖ Convince ❖ Conclude	❖ Projects ❖ Simulations ❖ Case studies ❖ Appraisal ❖ Survey

The use of open-book examinations and take-home examinations (discussed later in this chapter) must be explored to test higher-order thinking, synthesis and application of knowledge, and problem-solving skills. When designed well with creativity, these open-ended exercises engage the student better than closed-ended questions which propagate examination-oriented rote learning.

Exploring Patient Management Problems as Clinical Learning Exercises

No assessment task can achieve its full potential unless it also serves as a learning exercise. Technology offers means to convert traditional patient management problems (PMPs) into clinical exercises which can serve as assessment tasks. Electronic PMPs can be a wonderful method to explore various facets of clinical competence, and evaluate the *process* of providing healthcare which is often ignored in traditional teaching.

In a PMP, the learner is given a hypothetical scenario which is as close to real life as possible, with details of available resources. The examinee is then asked to choose from a series of alternatives, some of which are appropriate, while other might be contraindicated or simply not feasible. If he chooses a particular investigation, the results of that investigation might pop up on the screen (Vaughan, 1979).

The choices made by the student are not just scored on the basis of their correctness, but they are also shown the consequences of their decisions. The ease at which technology can provide feedback to students here, must be exploited during this process. For example, if a student chose a costly drug, he might be told why this could not be economically feasible for the patient to buy, or why it might have cross-reactions with his existing medication, or why it might lead to terrible side-effects. There might also be opportunities to take corrective action if a particular clinical decision is wrongly taken. PMPs can be linear or branching. The branching ones are more complex. When validated by experts, these problems have the potential of presenting several decision points, which can teach students how to make clinical judgments or even to prioritize the actions in the management plan.

Let's look at one example of how this can be done in **Figure 21.1**. In the above example, students can be scored for the decisions they take. Scores may even be negative if critical decisions are wrong. The computer inbuilt program can give them specific feedback on their decisions and propel learning. In a pen and paper-based PMP, the final outcome can be exposed, which enables a student to go backward and decipher the answers. However, technology allows us the benefit of not allowing students to backtrack. It makes them commit to a decision, and then face the consequences of their actions. The impact then is much better in terms of learning.

Assessment in Clinical Settings

It will be worthwhile to explore use of online assessment in clinical situations. Advances in artificial intelligence have now enabled more such devices such as virtual patients who are visually more appealing, and can give feedback on history-taking and train students in communication skills as well. When based on real cases, with videos and sounds, they augment the learning experience by providing authenticity. An added advantage is that all students get exposed to a necessary set of clinical cases, even if real patients are not available during a certain clinical posting.

There have been efforts during the pandemic to conduct objective structured clinical examinations online using the break-out rooms feature of web platforms. This requires a great deal of coordination, collaboration, and planning between the academic and technical teams. Except for palpation, elements of history-taking, inspection, percussion, and auscultation can be assessed in online settings. Say, e.g. students can be shown a video of a patient with stridor and be asked to count

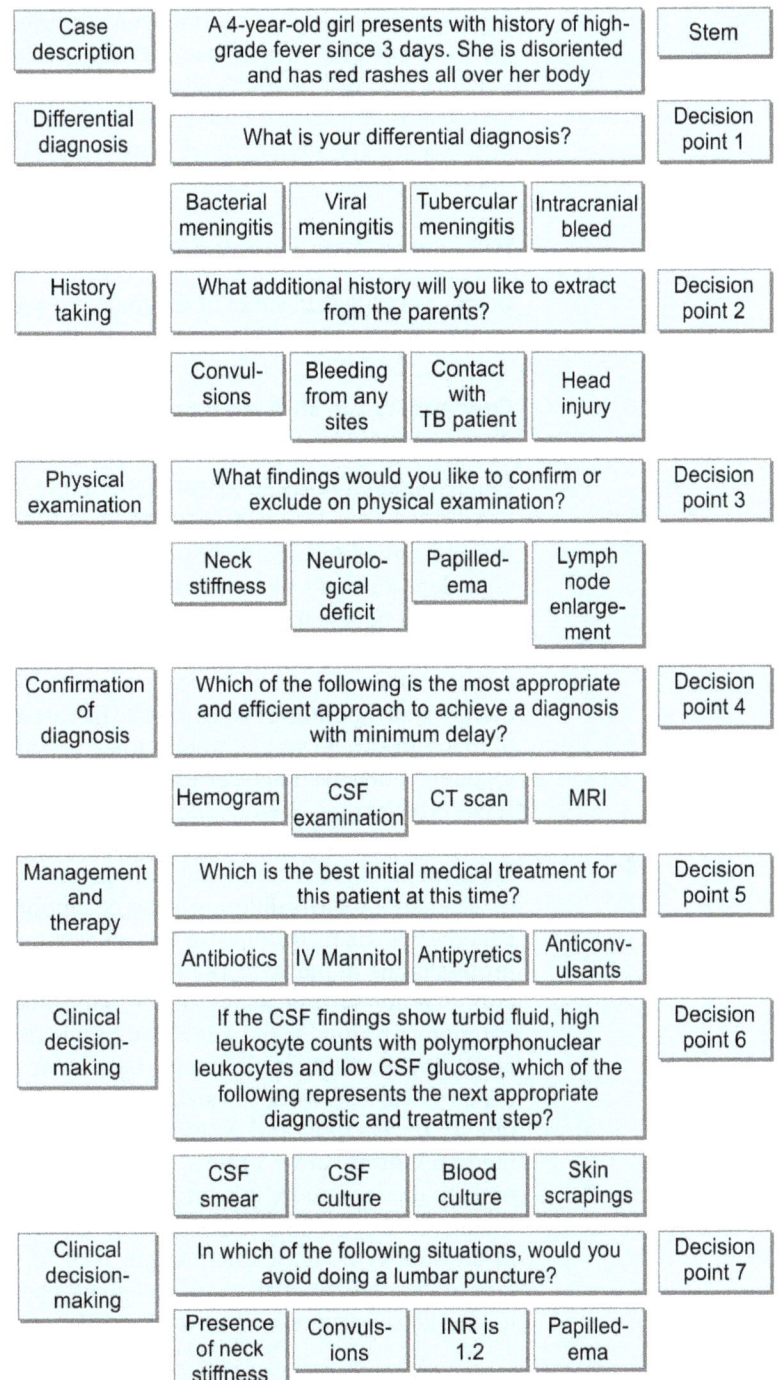

Fig. 21.1: Example of a patient management problem (PMP) which can be converted into an electronic PMP to teach clinical approach to a case of meningitis.

the respiratory rate. Heart sounds can be played as audio files and learnt much better than on real patients. It is possible to use standardized patients who will interact with students online and test their history-taking and communication skills. While nothing beats the clinical touch, in times of adversity, we need to resort to whatever we can do within our constraints.

Implementing Online Assessment

Below, you will find some of the major concerns which surround the implementation of online assessment:

Concerns While Shifting from Traditional Offline to Online Assessment

When transitioning from traditional to online assessment, some factors need to be kept in mind. Initially, the shift will require significant investment in terms of infrastructure and training. An important consideration in developing countries will be to ensure that all students have good access to internet connectivity and that their devices are installed with the latest technology. Keep in mind that some students might not have individual devices and might be sharing them with other members of the family (Pynos, 2016). The cost of printing large quantities of material can be great. Overall, some groups of students should not be put at a disadvantage because of the shift to online mode. It makes sense to have some sessions on study skills and technology support at the beginning of a course for every new batch of learners so that technology skills, metacognition, and time management can be emphasized.

The other issue is differing levels of comfort with use of technology. Faculty will need training in use of technology and support of IT professionals along with the students. Issues of passwords, access, connectivity during heavy traffic, etc., need to be handled by a competent trained team. There will be a learning curve, and patience is the key. Faculty development must be accompanied by a team of experts who will work toward maintaining standards and achieving quality in teaching and assessment. It is important to take student feedback about how online sessions are being perceived. When making the transition, it is important to start small, and focus on the quality of assessment rather than immediately shifting completely to an online mode. It might augur well to use assessment first for formative assessment, use web-based self-paced modules, and provide feedback to learners, and then try out summative assessment online.

Need for Regular and Good Communication

There might be significant challenges when dealing with large classes. There has to be smooth coordination between faculty within the department and across different departments. This will ensure that the students are not overburdened with assessment tasks from several departments at one time. There might be disparate understanding of why a particular assessment has been given or about the scoring pattern. A consensus has to be reached so that there is reasonable consistency of marking across different scorers. Newer faculty will need to be mentored in these areas. Teachers might be overwhelmed with the task of providing individualized feedback, and technology must be explored to make this task more efficient. It is always better to assess early in the semester so that there is enough time for teachers to provide feedback, and for learners to make improvements. Students must be aware of the criteria on which they are being assessed. Rubrics and templates must be shared with them. Examples of good quality assignments can be made available. The assessment policies must be transparent and public.

Plagiarism and Cheating in Online Examinations

One of the important concerns by of teachers about the difficulty of implementing online assessment is the ease with which students can cheat. Randomizing questions in electronic formats is one way of reducing cheating. Having separate examination centers where students can come and appear is not always feasible. There are a multitude of proctoring applications which are now available which monitor the examinee's presence through webcams or eye movements, but they are rather expensive.

Students need to be educated about what constitutes plagiarism. There is a tendency to pass off another students' work as their own. Further easy access to resource material online makes students resort to 'cut and paste' from other sources. Strict guidelines must be conveyed about non-tolerance to plagiarism and how students will be penalized for doing so. Students must be taught how to paraphrase, critically analyze, and summarize information. Appropriate instructions must be given about how to acknowledge their sources of information using citations and referencing software.

Open-book examinations and take-home examinations can be the way forward to reduce the incidents of cheating or plagiarism. In these examinations, there is no emphasis on time constraint, and the questions are more open-ended. These are questions which cannot be easily answered using a search engine. They test higher-order thinking and problem-solving skills. It is best to avoid assignments that require students to gather and present information that is available in a direct form (Carroll, 2000). Another way of ensuring that the references are genuine, are by asking students to supply copies of any references that have been used (Culwin & Lancaster, 2001). It is possible to use meta-assignments, such as asking students to answer questions like 'What problems did you encounter while doing this assignment?' or 'What did you learn from this assignment' after they complete the task at hand (Evans, 2000). A review of take-home examinations showed that they allowed time for reflection, were more aligned with constructivist theories, and succeeded in turning assessment into learning activities (Bengtsson, 2019).

The other way of countering cheating is to give group assignments rather than individual assignments. This will build in team spirit and collaboration, and also cut down the tendency to be hypercompetitive.

Sharing Resources: Skills Labs and Consortia

Resource-limited settings call for more collaborative efforts on the part of administrators. Just as expensive skills laboratories are not available at most centers, availability of simulators or electronic PMPs can be shared between different colleges of a university or region based on mutual reciprocation.

Electronic question banks can be created using the concept of consortia. In the past, we have seen efforts at collating questions between different institutes. Participating institutes share the administrative expenses to maintain these question banks. They are bound to submit a certain number of questions each year, which are included after proper validation procedures. Only then are they allowed to retrieve a certain percentage of questions for their assessments. If the number of questions is very large, a section of these question banks can be opened for students for self-assessment purposes.

The Concept of Triage in Medical Education During a Crisis

Unexpected crises such as that we have experienced during the COVID-19 pandemic require strategic decision-making. Medical education is not just about curriculum delivery, but also about harnessing our workforce efficiently and prioritizing at all levels of implementation. It will be imperative to triage all resources and take decisions about what activities can be continued, what needs to be stopped, what can be postponed, what modifications are required and what needs to be added. There are practical problems such as learner safety, faculty involvement in clinical care, and shortage of faculty due to quarantine and self-isolation. Such negotiations will not be easy, but one will have to be pragmatic about feasibility issues (Tolsgaard et al., 2020). During the pandemic, clinical teaching has been disrupted. We will have to rethink about what aspects can be delivered online, and do the best we can. Additionally we will have to envision the impact of what the students are missing out on. Can remediation measures be implemented during internship when the situation normalizes? Will this cohort need extra supervision when they come back to work in the clinics? Such questions need to be dealt with and the focus needs to be on what is essential and possible.

Online assessment has the potential of taking assessment into hitherto unexplored territories. As a faculty member, one can no longer be reluctant and avoid jumping in to experiment with radically newer formats. Since this is a rapidly developing area, newer strategies are emerging at break-neck speed. Keeping up with these can be overwhelming. We have tried to provide you a list of web resources at the end of this book which can be useful in implementing online learning and assessment.

When we published the first edition of this book, Dr William Burdick wrote in the foreword: '*Assessment is an approximation of the truth. The science of assessment is really a science of probability. It is important to retain this humility about assessment.*' Let us not presume that online assessment will work miracles and achieve the impossible. However, it can be a good genie to befriend and make tasks simpler!

REFERENCES

Bengtsson, L. (2019). Take-home exams in higher education: A systematic review. *Educ Sci 9(4)*, 267.

Carroll, J. (2000). *What kind of solutions can we find for plagiarism?* The Higher Education Academy. URL: https://www.gla.ac.uk/media/Media_13513_smxx.pdf [Last Accessed September, 2020].

Culwin, F., & Lancaster, T. (2001). *Plagiarism, prevention, deterrence and detection.* Institute for Learning and Teaching in Higher Education.London, UK: South Bank University.

Dennick, R., Wilkinson, S., & Purcell, N. (2010). *Online e-Assessment.* AMEE Guide 39. Dundee, UK: Association for Medical Education in Europe.

Evans, J. (2000). The new plagiarism in higher education: From selection to reflection. Warwick Interactions Journal. 11 (2) URL: https://warwick.ac.uk/fac/cross_fac/academic-development/resource-copy/interactions/issues/issue11/evans [Last accessed September, 2020]

Fuller, R., Joynes, V., Cooper, J., Boursicot, K., & Roberts, T. (2020) Could COVID-19 be our 'There is no alternative' (TINA) opportunity to enhance assessment? *Medical Teacher.* 42(7), 781–6.

Gibbs, G. (1992). *Improving the quality of student learning.* Bristol: Technical and Education Services Ltd.

Hallas, J. (2008). Rethinking teaching and assessment strategies for flexible learning environments. In *Hello! Where are you in the landscape of educational technology? Proceeding sascilite Melbourne 2008.* URL: http://www.ascilite.org.au/conferences/melbourne08/procs/hallas.pdf. [Last Accessed September, 2020].

James, R., McInnis, C., & Devlin, M. (2002). *Assessing learning in Australian Universities.* Centre for the study of Higher Education. Victoria, Australia: The University of Melbourne.

Norcini, J., Anderson, M.B., Bollela, V., Burch, V., Costa, M.J., Duvivier, R., et al. (2018). 2018 Consensus framework for good assessment. *Medical Teacher.* 40(11), 1102–9.

Pynos, R. (2016). Student engagement and its relationship to mobile device ownership and the role of technology in student learning [Doctoral dissertation]. Pittsburgh (PA): Duquesne University.

Tolsgaard, M.G., Cleland, J., Wilkinson, T., & Ellaway, R.H. (2020). How we make choices and sacrifices in medical education during the COVID-19 pandemic. *Medical Teacher.* 42(7), 741–3.

Vaughan VC III. (1979). Patient management problem as an evaluative instrument. *Pediatrics in Review.*1, 67–76.

Chapter 22

Item Analysis and Question Banking

Ciraj AM

KEY POINTS
- Item analysis is a useful tool to improve the quality of multiple choice questions (MCQs).
- Items need to be analyzed to find their level of difficulty and ability to differentiate good from average students.
- Question banking requires such data about the items.

Very often as an examiner or paper setter, there are two questions that keep haunting you after the test. How do I ensure that the items designed for the test were not too difficult or not too easy? Will the test administered differentiate effectively between students who do well on the overall test (higher group) and those who do not (lower group)? Item analysis and test analysis are valuable, yet relatively easy, procedures that can answer both your questions.

What is Item Analysis?

Item analysis is an important step in the development of any assessment strategy (Ebel & Frisbie, 1991). It is the phase that helps us identify an item that is either too easy, or too difficult for the examinee. This process also helps in detecting items that fail to discriminate between skilled and unskilled examinees.

Item Statistics

Assuming that the overall quality of the test is dependent on the quality of items used, item statistics are used to assess the performance of individual test items. Statistical methods are used for these purposes. The common methods adopted in an item analysis are the facility value

(FV; item difficulty), discrimination index (DI; item discrimination), and distractor efficiency (Thorndike, 1967).

Facility value is a measure of the proportion of examinees who responded to an item correctly. A measure of how well the item discriminates between examinees who are knowledgeable in the content area and those who are not is called **discrimination index** or item discrimination. The **distractor efficiency** provides a measure of how well each of the incorrect options contributes to the quality of a multiple choice item. Once the item analysis information is available, an item review is often conducted.

Process

Item analysis may be performed using the following steps:
- The answer sheets (papers) are evaluated. As mentioned in Chapter 5, most of them rely on computer software for the assessment of MCQs.
- A list is generated with the marks of the student scoring highest marks at the top followed by other scores arranged in a descending order.
- The whole list is then divided into two equal groups: the group of high achievers (Higher Ability Group, HAG) and low achievers (Lower Ability Group, LAG).
- If your student group is a bigger one (with more than 100 students), the first 30% of students (high achievers) and the last 30% of them (low achievers) can be your two groups.

Look at the following example: In a test conducted for a group of 100 students, for an item selected (e.g., item no. 5), the number of students answering to the options a, b, c, and d are arranged as given here.

Item No. 5

	a*	b	c	d
HAG (n = 50)	40	02	0	08
LAG (n = 50)	10	26	12	02

(*a is the key or correct answer)

After having performed this, we re-examine the terms related to item analysis.

Facility Value

This is the number of students in the group answering a question correctly. If 75% of your students have answered your item correctly then Facility Value (FV) will be 75.
It can be calculated using the formula:

$$FV = \frac{HAG + LAG}{N} \times 100$$

where,

HAG: the number of students in the higher ability group who chose the right answer

LAG: the number of students in the lower ability group who chose the right answer; and

N: the total number of students who appeared in the test

If you apply this formula to the example provided above (on item no. 5), you will see that the FV will be: $\frac{40+10}{100} \times 100 = 50\%$.

Facility value or item difficulty index ranges from 0 to 100; a lower FV indicates that the question was difficult for many students who appeared. In other words, the higher the FV, easier the question was. When an alternative is worth other than a single point, or when there is more than one correct alternative per question, the item difficulty is the average score on that item divided by the highest number of points for any one alternative. To maximize item discrimination, desirable difficulty levels are slightly higher than midway between chance and perfect scores for the item. For example, the chance score for five-option questions is 0.20, because one-fifth of the students responding to the question could be expected to choose the correct option by guessing. Many arbitrarily classify item difficulty as 'easy' if the index is 85% or above; 'moderate' if it is between 51 and 84%; and 'difficult' if it is 50% or below.

Significance of Facility Value

* Facility value is relevant for determining whether students have learnt the concept being tested. It helps to understand about the learning that happened in your classroom (Haladyna, 1999).
* It also plays an important role in the ability of an item to discriminate between students who know the tested material and those who do not. The item will have low FV, if it is so difficult that almost everyone gets it wrong or guesses, or so easy that almost everyone gets it right.
* Knowledge of FV helps in better design of the paper.
* It is recommended that the test begins with items with high FV. If the more difficult items (items with low FV) occur at the start of the test, students can become upset early during an examination which is likely to adversely affect the student's overall performance in that particular examination.

Discrimination Index

Calculating Discrimination Index (DI) helps in detecting the ability of items to discriminate between skilled and unskilled examinees. In other words, it helps to differentiate between students who are knowledgeable in the content area from those who are not.

The formula employed is DI = $\frac{2 \times (HAG - LAG)}{Total\ number}$

Let us apply this formula to the previous example, $\frac{2 \times (40 - 10)}{100} = \frac{60}{100} = 0.6$

The maximum value for DI an item can have is 1.0. An item with DI = 1 indicates that the item perfectly discriminates between high achievers and low achievers.

This would be the right context, to consider another term— 'negative discrimination'. If a greater number of students from lower group are answering an item right when compared to the higher group, we call it negative discrimination. The reasons are often due to an ambiguous question or an answer key that was wrongly marked.

For selection purposes, items with high DI are preferred. It is difficult to attain a DI with 1.0. Therefore, a DI of 0.35 is considered good and items with DI less than 0.2 are considered unacceptable, items with an intermediate value (above 0.2 and below 0.35) are generally accepted based on type of the test and what it intends to measure (Pyrczak, 1973).

Significance of Discrimination Index

- Flaws in the item may be identified.
- Assessing DI provides with improvement options.
- Learning can be improved.
- Misconceptions in learning can be identified.

Distractor Efficiency

In Chapter 5, we had mentioned that distractors used as options need to be plausible. Any distractor that is not picked up by at least 5% of students fails to qualify as a good distractor. If you look at our previous example, distractor "c" may be considered a good one as no HAG student has been attracted toward it. However, if you consider the option "d" a greater number of students from HAG have been attracted to it compared to LAG. We will discuss this a little later.

At the end of the Item analysis report, test items are listed according their degrees of difficulty (easy, medium, and difficult) and discrimination (good, fair, and poor). These distributions provide a quick overview of the test and can be used to identify items which are not performing well, and which can perhaps be improved or discarded.

Point-Biserial Correlation

Point-biserial correlation (PBS) is yet another important parameter which gives information about the 'fit' of an item with the remaining test. Let us look at an example. A group of fresh MBBS students have been taught and given a test for their understanding of physiology of the heart. However, by chance, one question on physiology of the brain has also crept in the test. Presuming that students have learnt the subject well, they will score high on the test, except in the item which does not fit the test, i.e., the item related to brain physiology. In general, PBS helps us to identify items which are not testing the same domain/construct as rest of the test, and thereby helps to improve the validity and reliability of the test.

Point biserial coefficient measures the correlation between a student's performance on a single item and her performance in the examination as a whole. Let us look at this table which shows the response of ten students to a 10-item MCQ test.

Student number	Item 1	Item 2	Item 3	Item 4	Item 5	Item 6	Item 7	Item 8	Item 9	Item 10	Total score
A	1	1	1	1	1	1	1	0	1	1	9
B	1	0	1	1	1	1	1	0	1	1	8
C	1	0	0	1	1	0	1	1	1	1	7
D	1	1	0	1	1	0	1	0	1	1	7
E	1	0	1	1	1	0	0	0	1	1	6
F	0	0	1	1	1	1	0	0	1	0	5
G	0	0	1	1	0	1	0	0	1	1	5
H	1	0	0	1	0	1	0	0	1	0	4
I	0	0	1	1	0	0	0	0	1	1	4
J	0	0	0	1	0	0	0	0	1	0	2
Item Total	6	2	6	10	6	5	4	1	10	7	

Here the score of a student on a single item is scored dichotomously, i.e., it is scored as 0 if the response is incorrect, and 1 if correct. The score of the student on the entire test is a continuous variable ranging from 1 to 10 if (each item has a score of one mark). Thus, PBS is a correlation between a dichotomous variable and a continuous variable.

PBS is calculated as a correlation between the score on that item with the total score on the test minus that item. The calculation of 'total score on the test minus that item' for PBS for item 1 will be 6-1=5; for item 2 it will be 1, for item 3 it will be 5, for item 4 it will be 9, and so forth. We do not intend to go into the mechanics of calculating PBS, for which many free software are available.

PBS values can range from −1.0 to +1.0. A large PBS value indicates that students with high scores on the test are also getting that item correct (which is anyway expected). A low PBS value either indicates that the students who got the item correct have done poorly on the total test, or that students have who answered the item wrong have done well on rest of the test. Both of these are anomalies which we do not want. This could be because of some error in framing of the item. Such faulty questions should be removed. Values of PBS between 0.15 and 0.35 are considered acceptable. Similarly, a consistently high value will indicate that same concept is being tested repeatedly and some items need to be changed. A zero value means that all students got the item correct or incorrect.

Another quick and reliable use of PBS is to detect wrongly entered keys in MCQ tests. After a test is conducted, items which have a PBS of 0.10 and less must be examined. Quite often, this occurs because the key has inadvertently been wrongly fed into the system (Varma, 2008)

So, in short, an item analysis helps in:
- Assessing the quality of items used in a test and of the test as a whole.
- Improving items which may be used again in the later tests.
- Eliminating ambiguous or misleading items.
- Enhancing instructors' skills in the construction of flawless items.
- Identifying specific areas of course content which need greater emphasis or clarity.

Test Analysis

It is logical to say that assessing the quality of items used in a test can assess the test as a whole. However, there are two other statistical expressions that help to evaluate the performance of the test as a whole: the reliability coefficient and the Standard Error of Measurement (SEM).

Reliability Coefficient

The reliability of a test refers to the extent to which the test is likely to produce consistent scores over time. For results of assessment to be defensible, they must be consistent and reproducible. In the absence of adequate reliability, assessment data cannot be interpreted properly as they have a component of random error (Downing, 2004). Even when the exactly same test is administered more than once to the same student, the student may not get the exactly same score due to this error. The degree to which test scores are unaffected by these errors is an indication of the reliability of the test.

Reliability coefficients (written as 'r') provide an estimate of random error in assessment data. They are expressed as an absolute number between 0 and 1. Here r=0 indicates complete lack of reliability, while r=1 indicates perfect reliability. Reliability coefficients above 0.8 are considered good. The larger r is the more reliable test scores are.

The reliability coefficient reflects three characteristics of the test:
1. *The inter-correlations among the items:* The reliability of a test will be high if the relative numbers of positive relationships are high, and the stronger those relationships are.
2. *The length of the test:* Any test with more items will have a higher reliability.
3. *The content of the test:* Reliability of a test is brought down if the subject matter tested is diverse.

Methods of Estimating Reliability

The acceptable level of reliability will depend on the type of test and the reliability estimate used. There are three strategies generally used for estimating reliability (Downing, 2004):
1. **Test-retest reliability:** Here, a reliability estimate is calculated by administering a test on two occasions and calculating the correlation between the two sets of scores. This reliability estimate will reflect the stability of the construct being measured. For example, tests which measure a student's ability to read and comprehend a paragraph might be more stable over time and have a higher test-retest reliability. On the other hand, a test which measures anxiety levels will not have high reliability coefficient values. The time interval between the administrations of the two tests is important. The longer the time gap, the greater is the chance that the two scores may change due to random error, and the lower will be the test-retest reliability.
2. **Equivalent (or parallel) forms reliability:** Each test can have more than one version. For example, if four sets of the same exam are prepared with different items. These different forms of a test are called parallel forms. These sets are supposed to measure the same construct and have similar measurement characteristics. But a student might do better in one version than on another as the items are not exactly the same. Here, the reliability estimate is calculated by administering two forms of a test within a short period of time, and the estimating correlation between the two sets of scores. In other words, we are trying to know if tests scores remain the same when two different instruments are used.
3. **Internal consistency reliability:** This indicates the extent to which items on a test measure the same thing, or in other words, how well test components contribute to measuring the construct. The reliability estimate is calculated based on a single form of a test, administered on a single occasion using one of the many available internal consistency equations. If a test has a high internal consistency, it indicates that the items on the test are homogeneous, i.e. they are very similar to each other. If a test is very long, the reliability coefficient can be falsely elevated. If a test measures

different characteristics, then the internal consistency reliability coefficient for each component is reported separately. Estimating the internal consistency is the easiest strategy because it does not require administering the test twice and eliminates the need of having two forms of the test.

However, one should remember that regardless of the strategy used to obtain it, reliability is not a characteristic inherent in the test itself, but it is rather an estimate of the consistency of a set of items when they are administered to a particular group of students at a specific time under particular conditions for a specific purpose.

The most familiar methods for estimating internal consistency reliability are (Maberly, 1967):
- Split-half method
- Kuder–Richardson formulas 20 and 21 (also known as KR-20 and KR-21)
- Cronbach's alpha

Split-half method: Here the test is split into two halves. This could be done randomly, for example, all even-numbered questions versus odd-numbered questions. Students are given both parts of the test together to solve. The scores from both parts of the test are correlated. If reliability coefficient values are high, it will indicate that a student has performed equally well (or equally poorly) on both halves of the test. This method works only for tests which have a large number of items all of which measure the same construct.

Split-half method is different from parallel forms reliability. In parallel forms reliability, the two sets are given to students at different times rather than simultaneously. Secondly, in parallel forms reliability, the two tests are equivalent and independent of each other. In split-half reliability, the two sets do not have to be equivalent or 'parallel'.

The most frequently reported internal consistency estimates are the KR-20 and Cronbach's alpha. The KR-20 formula is based on the split halves, while Cronbach's alpha is based on analysis of variance.

Kuder–Richardson formulas: These formulas are used to measure reliability of a test with dichotomous or binary variables (i.e. right or wrong). It can be used on for tests which have only one correct answer. The KR-20 formula is used for items that have varying difficulty. The KR-21 formula is used if all the items are equally challenging. The higher the KR-20 score (range from 0 to 1), the stronger is the relationship between test items. A score of at least 70 is considered good reliability. The KR-20 may be affected by difficulty of the test, the spread in scores and the length of the examination.

Cronbach's alpha: Cronbach's alpha is a measure of internal consistency that tells us how closely related a set of items are as a group. It has the advantage over KR20 of being applicable even when items are weighted (Bland & Altman, 1997). This formula can be used for items which have more than one correct answer. This is often used to see if multiple question surveys using Likert scales are reliable. These scales can be used to measure variables which are difficult to measure in real life like: anxiety, conscientiousness, or quality of life.

Cronbach's alpha is used to estimate the proportion of variance that is consistent in a set of test scores. Cronbach's alpha can be written as a function of the number of test items and the average intercorrelation among the items.

Here, for conceptual purposes, we show the formula for the standardized Cronbach's alpha:

$$\alpha = \frac{N \cdot \bar{c}}{\bar{v} + (N-1) \cdot \bar{c}}$$

Here, N is equal to the number of items, $\bar{c}$ is the average inter-item covariance among the items and $\bar{v}$ equals the average variance. One can see from this formula that the value of alpha is sensitive to the number of items in the test. If you increase the number of relevant items, you increase Cronbach's alpha. Additionally, if the average inter-item correlation is low, alpha will be low. As the average inter-item correlation increases, Cronbach's alpha increases as well.

Cronbach's alpha can range from 0 (if no variance is consistent) to 1 (if all variance is consistent) with all values between 0 and 1 also being possible. If the Cronbach's alpha for a set of scores turns out to be 0.80, you can interpret that as meaning that the test is 80% reliable, and by extension that it is 20% unreliable (100% − 80% = 20%).

However, the following points are worth considering while interpreting Cronbach's alpha:
- Cronbach's alpha will be higher for tests with a greater number of items than for shorter tests. Low alpha values might mean that there are not enough questions in the test. It is important to note that if you increase the number of redundant items which ask the same thing also, alpha will increase. Hence alpha must be carefully interpreted considering the particular test length involved.
- Cronbach's alpha is appropriately applied to norm-referenced tests and norm-referenced decisions (e.g., admissions and placement decisions), but not to criterion-referenced tests and criterion-referenced decisions (e.g., diagnostic and achievement decisions).
- Cronbach's alpha must be interpreted in the light of a distribution involved. Tests that have normally distributed scores are more likely to have high Cronbach's alpha reliability estimates than tests with positively or negatively skewed distributions.

Standard Error of Measurement (SEM)

The standard error of measurement (SEM) is an additional reliability statistic calculated from the reliability estimate. It is directly related to the reliability of the test. It is an index of the amount of variability in an individual student's performance due to random measurement error.

If it were possible to administer an infinite number of parallel tests, a student's scores would be expected to change from one administration to the next due to several factors. For each student, the scores would form a 'normal' (bell-shaped) distribution. The mean of the distribution is assumed to be the student's 'true score', and reflects what she 'really' knows about the subject.

While the reliability of a test always varies between 0 and 1, the SEM is expressed in the same scale as the test scores (Kehoe, 1995). The SEM may prove more useful than the reliability estimate itself when you are making actual decisions with test scores. As you are aware, the standard deviation helps you estimate the dispersion in a given distribution, and the standard error of the mean helps you to estimate the dispersion of sampling errors when you are trying to estimate the population mean from a sample mean. However, the SEM helps you estimate the dispersion of the measurement errors when you are making decisions about students' scores at a certain cut-point. It is conceptually related to test reliability in that it provides an indication of the dispersion of the sampling errors when you are trying to estimate students' true scores from their observed test scores.

Let us try to simplify this concept by explaining the terms that were used. The observed test scores are scores that the students got on whatever test is being considered. However, students' true scores are different. If you were to administer the test an infinite number of times to a group of students and you could average the students' scores over the infinite number of administrations, the average of each person's scores would probably be the best estimate of that person's true knowledge in whatever is being tested, or in other words it is that student's true score. The standard deviation of all those scores averaged across persons and test administrations is the SEM. It is impossible to administer a test an infinite number of times in real practice. So, we assume that each student's test score is our best estimate of the true score, but we recognize that there are sampling errors in that estimate. Those sampling errors are normally distributed and have a standard deviation called the SEM. Thus the SEM represents the degree of confidence that one has in stating that a student's 'true' score lies within a particular range of scores. For example, a SEM of 4 indicates that a student's true score probably lies within 4 points in either direction of the score she has obtained on the test. This means that if a student obtains 80 on the test, there is a good chance that the student's true score lies somewhere between 76 and 84. The smaller the SEM, the more accurate are the measurements.

An estimate of the SEM can be calculated from the test score standard deviation and reliability estimate using the following formula:

$$SEM = S\sqrt{1-r_{xx}}$$

Where,
SEM: standard error of measurement; S: standard deviation of the test; and rxx: reliability of the test.

If you have a test with a standard deviation of 4.89, and a Cronbach's alpha reliability estimate (rxx) of 0.91, the SEM would be calculated as follows:

$$SEM = S\sqrt{1-r_{xx}} = 4.89\sqrt{1-.91} = 4.89\sqrt{.09}$$
$$4.89(.3) = 1.467 \approx 1.47$$

The SEMs provide an estimate of how much variability in the actual test score points one can expect around a particular cut-point due to unreliable variance (with 68% probability if one SEM plus or minus is used, or with 95% if two SEMs plus or minus are used, or 98% if three are used). For instance, if the test in question had a cut-point for failing of 30, you should recognize that, if you want to be 68% sure of your decision, the SEM indicates that the students within one (SEM) of the cut point (i.e., 30 ± 1.47, or 28.53 to 31.47) might fluctuate randomly to the other side of the cut-point if they were to take the test again. So, it might force you to gather additional information (e.g., other test scores, homework grades or whatever is appropriate) in deciding whether they should pass the test or not. If you want to be 95% sure of your decision, the SEM indicates that the students within two (SEMs) of the cut point (i.e., 30 ± 2.94, or 27.06 to 32.94) might randomly fluctuate to the other side of the cut-point, (Driscoll et al., 2000).

Question Banking

A question bank besides having a large pool of questions will also provide a set of information pertaining to that question. The primary goal of question banking is ability to deposit, discover, and retrieve questions. In order to support discovery and retrieval of questions, each question needs to be described with certain information.

This information includes:
- The content area
- Learning outcome being measured using that particular item
- Time allotted to answer the question
- Marks allocated
- Facility value of the item

- Discrimination index
- Source of the question.

Process of Question Banking

The following steps are followed in the construction of a question bank (Singh et al., 2013):

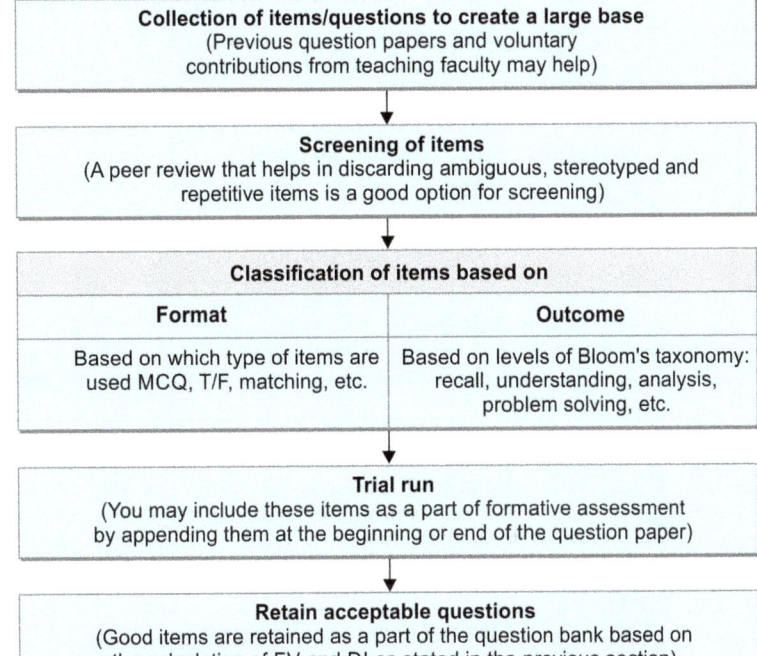

Sorting the Questions

Sorting is achieved by following the library catalog pattern. Questions are typed on cards (8" × 6") like the ones used in library cataloging. The obverse side (Side A) has information pertaining to the subject matter, the objective being assessed, item, key and reference. The reverse side (Side B) contains information related to the use of the item including its FV and DI for that examination. The data is updated every time the question is used. By making these cards, the blueprint of the weightage attached to different subject areas and intended learning objectives can easily be adhered on to. In other words, with this information available it is very easy to pull out items of desired objectives with known FV and DI values. You may then arrange the items accordingly to make the question paper that suits your examination. A model illustrating the details is provided here:

Side A

Content Area: Clinical Bacteriology
Chapter: 17 (Gram positive rods of medical importance)

Item

Stem:
Five hours after eating fried rice at a restaurant, 25-year-old man developed nausea, vomiting, and diarrhea. Which one of the following organisms is the **MOST** likely to be involved?

Responses:
a. *Clostridium perfringens*
b. Enterotoxigenic *Escherichia coli*
c. *Bacillus cereus*
d. *Salmonella typhi*

Key: c

Reference: Review of Medical Microbiology and Immunology, Warren Levinson. 10th edition.

Side B

Year	Class	No.	Options				Facility value	Discrimination index
			a	b	c	d		
2016	4th Semester	125	21	18	61	25	49	0.35
2017	4th Semester	112	11	16	72	13	64	0.29
2018	4th Semester	132	28	21	69	14	52	0.31
2019	4th Semester	126	25	15	78	08	62	0.25

Uses of Question Banking

The facilities provided by question banking as mentioned here should emphasize its importance in education:

- It provides a well-arranged collection of questions which are usually organized into topics.
- It provides easy access to questions based on search parameters. Search parameters include: topic, keywords, or attributes of a question, such as FV and DI.
- It minimizes the time and energy required to construct a test.
- It helps you choose the right kind of questions for the right kind of examination; like generalized to test the ability of students, peeked tests to select students with ability above a predetermined cutoff, entrance examinations, etc. in a very short time.
- It facilitates monitoring the performance of questions across varying testing criteria.
- It can be used to support the quality assurance of questions. Reuse of a question in different types of test, allows us to analyze the students' responses and comments about the difficulty level, usefulness, etc. of the question.

- It enhances skills of item writing and reviewing.
- Student access to the question bank may be permitted if the bank has large number of questions. In this way, it helps to facilitate student learning.
- It provides transparency to the evaluation process which helps in building faith in the examination systems.
- It helps in setting uniform standards of teaching and assessment.

REFERENCES

Bland, J.M., & Altman, D.G. (1997). Statistics notes: Cronbach's alpha. *British Medical Journal, 314(7080)*, 572.

Downing, S.M. (2004). Reliability: on the reproducibility of assessment data. *Medical Education, 38(9)*, 1006–12.

Driscoll, P., Lecky, F., & Crosby, M. (2000). An introduction to everyday statistics—2. *Journal of Accident and Emergency Medicine, 17(4)*, 274–81.

Ebel, R.L. & Frisbie, D.A. (1991). *Essentials of educational measurement*, 5th ed. Englewood Cliffs, NJ: Prentice-Hall.

Pyrczak, F. (1973). Validity of the discrimination index as a measure of item quality. *Journal of Educational Measurement, 10(3)*, 227–31.

Haladyna, T.M. (1999). *Developing and validating multiple-choice test items*, 2nd ed. Mahwah, New Jersey: Lawrence Erlbaum Associates.

Kehoe, J. (1995). *Basic item analysis for multiple-choice tests. ERIC/AE digest.* [online] Available from http://www.ericfacility.net/ericdigests/ed398237.html [Last accessed August, 2020].

Maberly, N.C. (1967). Characteristics of internal consistency estimates within restricted score ranges. *Journal of Educational Measurement, 4(1)*, 15–9.

Singh, T., Gupta, P., & Singh, D. (2013). *Principles of medical education*, 4th ed. New Delhi, India: Jaypee Brothers Medical Publishers (P) Ltd.

Thorndike, R.L. (1967). The analysis and selection of test items. In: Messick, S. and Jackson, D. (Eds). *Problems in human assessment*. New York: McGraw-Hill.

FURTHER READING

Burton, R.F. (2005). Multiple-choice and true/false tests: myths and misapprehensions. *Assessment and Evaluation in Higher Education, 30(1)*, 65–72.

Downing, S.M. (2005). The effects of violating standard item writing principles on tests and students: the consequences of using flawed test items on achievement examinations in medical education. *Advances in Health Sciences Education: Theory and Practice, 10(2)*, 133–43.

McCoubrie, P. (2004). Improving the fairness of multiple-choice questions: a literature review. *Medical Teacher, 26(8)*, 709–12.

Tarrant, M., & Ware, J. (2008). Impact of item-writing flaws in multiple-choice questions on student achievement in high-stakes nursing assessments. *Medical Education, 42(2)*, 198–206.

Chapter 23

Standard Setting

Tejinder Singh, Ara Tekian

KEY POINTS
- Standard setting is crucial to ensure validity/reliability and maintain quality in assessment.
- Standards can be relative or absolute.
- Efforts should be made to set defensible standards rather than taking 50% as cutoff.

Deciding which student is competent enough to be certified and practice medicine is one of the major purposes of assessment. The process through which decisions are made to decide the cut-off score for passing or failing a student is called standard setting. We discussed in Chapter 1 that assessment could be norm-referenced (relative) or criterion-referenced (absolute). While norm-referenced assessment looks at performance of students in relation to one another, criterion-referenced assessment compares the performance of students against a preset, agreed upon criteria. We also discussed that these criteria have to be determined *before* the examination is administered for criterion-referenced approach and *after* the examination for norm-referenced approach.

The Need

In most examinations in medicine in India, we use the cut-off criteria of 50% to classify students as pass or fail. This criteria is applied to all examinations, irrespective of the type and purpose of examination. Thus, a student who gets 50% marks in an essay type test is considered at par with another who may have scored 50% in a Multiple Choice Question (MCQ)-based test. The same is true of various tests used for the assessment of practical skills. Moreover, this cut-off applies in absolute terms to different universities and different cohorts of students. Although using 50% as a cut-off is simple, it is neither defensible nor fair. Further, it creates problems as all test content is chosen with these criteria in mind and may lose much of its validity (Tekian & Norcini, 2015).

Unless we set defensible standards for ourselves, the validity of assessment is threatened. Improperly set standards can act as double-edged swords. If they are not defensible, i.e., based on scientifically acceptable approaches, then they will allow the poor students to pass; on the other hand, some competent students may be classified as fail if the standards have been set unrealistically high. For certifying examinations, standard setting comprises of identifying a cut-off score based on criteria agreed upon by several judges. Consequently, only those who are above the cut-off score pass the examination. Standard setting is also important to ensure that test content is appropriately selected and to be as fair to students and other test users as possible.

There are various, well-established methods which can be used for standard setting (Ben-David, 2000). This chapter will provide you a select number of standard setting procedures which are commonly used to determine the cut-off scores. The intention is to provide a broad overview of standard setting procedures and encourage you to incorporate one of these methods in your future examinations. A list of additional readings and references is provided for those who are interested in reading more about this topic.

Absolute or Relative?

Viewpoints differ on whether the standards should be criterion-referenced (absolute) or norm-referenced (relative). Each method has its strengths and limitations, and therefore, it is important to upfront identify the purpose of the test to be administered upfront. It can be argued that criterion-referenced standards would be more useful as they allow comparison of performance against a level or mastery which is required of competent physicians. A standard is defined as absolute if a certain level of mastery or competence is required and this is not dependent on the performance of other students within the same cohort or group. An absolute standard stays the same over multiple administrations of the same test for the same or similar cohorts. This helps to separate the competent from the non-competent students/physicians and allows to decide on the degree of competence independent of the performance of other students in the group. However, it may be difficult to define a criterion, which is universally applicable without taking the content and context into consideration.

Relative standards, on the other hand, tell us how students performed in relation to one another—but it does not tell us about their competence or mastery level. Theoretically, it is possible to have a distribution where even the top student may have only 20% marks, and it is also possible to have the student at the lowest rank with 90% marks. Despite this shortcoming, people believe that norm referencing can provide useful information and that it is a practical way to motivate students. Most of the examining bodies still resort to norm-referencing in reporting scores (Barman, 2008). Relative standard or norm-referenced grading is commonly known as 'grading on the curve'. Although the students are rank ordered in such a system, yet the range of distribution of marks is another important consideration.

Relative standards are expressed in terms of proportion of students. An example would be to identify the top 2% of a cohort who could be considered for the award of a scholarship, or the bottom 10%, who are identified for remedial teaching. Absolute standards are expressed as proportion of test items that are correctly answered. Passing all those who answer more than 70% of the items in an examination might be an example. Absolute standards are more often used for final or certifying/high-stakes examinations. In practice, though, both methods may be used. In our settings, for example, we classify all those scoring more than 50% as pass and then rank order them.

Compensatory or Non-compensatory?

Another terminology which is also used in context of standard setting is compensatory or conjunctive standards. In compensatory standards, the standard relates to the total test and the examinees can compensate for low performance on some parts/components of the test by a good performance on other parts. In our setting, a student can compensate for their fewer marks in theory by getting more marks in viva voce examination. Conjunctive standards, on the other hand, are set on individual components of the examination and the examinees cannot compensate for their poor performance on one part of the test. A student failing in internal assessment, for example, cannot compensate for it by getting more marks in the final examination. This method has, however, the advantage of providing remedial tutoring as each part is separately marked. The adoption of compensatory or conjunctive standards is a policy decision. In general, if there is a high correlation between marks on various items, compensatory standards may be acceptable.

Effect on Learning

Standard setting has been reported to promote deep learning and develop a sense of professional identity (Norcini & Guille, 2002). It could also have a positive effect on intrinsic motivation. It can be argued that setting acceptable and defensible standards would help the students to be assessed against explicit criteria. This becomes especially important in the context of competency-based curricula. Setting absolute standards takes away the underlying competition, but has no effect on the proficiency demonstrated by students.

A standard could be considered an expression of professional values in the context of a test's purpose and content, the ability of the examinees, and the wider educational and social settings (Norcini, 2003). Following this perspective, standard setting seems more than a method—it is a technique for gathering value judgments, getting consensus and expressing that consensus as a single score on the test. An extrapolation of this thought is that standards will be more credible and defensible if they are aligned with the context and purpose of the test.

Methods of Standard Setting

Several standard setting methods have been described in literature (Yudkowsky et al., 2019) and it would be beyond the scope of this chapter to review and provide the details of each of those methods. Several good readings/references have been included in the references for the interested readers who wish to learn more about them. However, a broad overview of these methods will be quite useful. In general, standard setting methods can be classified as relative methods, test/item-based absolute methods, individual examinee performance-based absolute methods, and composite or mixed methods.

The basic steps involved in all the methods include deciding the purpose of the examination and the nature of standards, identifying content expert judges and training them, collecting ratings or judgments, deciding on the cut-off points and providing results and validity evidence to decision makers (Yudkowsky et al., 2019). Since almost all the methods are based on the expert opinion of the judges, the number and expertise of the judges are extremely important and could influence the quality of standards heavily.

Standard Setting for Knowledge Tests

Let us now discuss some of the commonly used (Ben-David, 2000; Downing et al., 2006) standard setting methods.

a. **Relative method:** This is probably the simplest of all methods. The judges make an estimate of the percentage of examinees that are qualified to pass the examination. They discuss their views and are open to change their ratings if required. This method is easy to use and is applicable to a variety of test types and situations. Its limitation, however, is looking at the relative performance of the examinees, rather than at the content of a test or the competence of the student. Standards arrived using this method will naturally vary with each cohort of examinees, and therefore, it makes it difficult to compare performances across institutions and over a period. It may be a useful method though in situations where there is a need to identify a certain percentage of examinees or rank order them, *e.g.,* for a selection or placement.

b. **Angoff method:** It is an absolute method where the judgment is based on the test items and this process could be carried out before the examination (Angoff, 1971). Let us illustrate the method in the context of a MCQ test **(Table 23.1)**. The judges are asked to think about a group of borderline students, i.e., those who are neither clearly pass nor clearly fail. The judges discuss the characteristics of these examinees and come to a consensus. The judges then discuss the difficulty of each item on the test and make an estimate regarding the proportion of borderline students, who will be able to answer this item correctly. This process is repeated for each item. The estimates are then averaged to get a cut-off point for passing students. Whenever the estimates between the different judges exceed 20% or more, the judges that gave a high and low estimate might hold a discussion to explore the reasons for such a wide spread. After such discussions, the judges are free to modify their ratings. An example of such a widespread is item number four where the lowest rating is 0.40 and the highest 0.75.
(*Note*: Judges usually think of round numbers/percentages, such as 70 or 80% instead of 69 or 81%. Therefore, these numbers are rounded as much as possible to be realistic.)

TABLE 23.1: Angoff method

Question	Judge 1	Judge 2	Judge 3	Judge 4	Judge 5	Average
1	0.75	0.80	0.70	0.75	0.80	0.76
2	0.90	0.75	0.65	0.70	0.80	0.76
3	0.80	0.75	0.70	0.75	0.80	0.76
4	0.50	0.45	0.65	0.75	0.40	0.55
5	0.75	0.70	0.70	0.80	0.85	0.76
6	0.65	0.80	0.70	0.75	0.80	0.74
7	0.90	0.75	0.65	0.70	0.80	0.76
8	0.80	0.75	0.70	0.60	0.65	0.70
9	0.80	0.70	0.70	0.75	0.80	0.75
10	0.60	0.60	0.70	0.65	0.75	0.66
Cut-off point						0.72
Passing score						72%

In the above example, anyone who score 72% and above passes the examination, and the ones who score 71% and below fail. Angoff method has been used very widely for standard setting in education. It produces absolute standards and is therefore useful for certifying examinations.

c. **Contrasting groups method:** This method uses the entire examination rather than an individual item (Livingston & Zieky, 1982). A random sample of examinees is chosen. The judges then consider the responses of each examinee on the entire test and then by discussion and consensus decide on pass or fail. After a decision has been made for all the examinees, the scores of all those who are considered as pass and those who are considered as fail are plotted on a graph. The point at which the scores cross is taken as the cut-off point.

This method has the advantages of producing absolute standards based on the actual performance—rather than a subjective opinion of the judges—of the examinees. It also has the added advantage of sliding the cut-off marks to either side/direction to suit the purpose of the test. For a competency-based test, for example, the scores can be moved to right, making sure that no incompetent student is certified as competent.

d. **Hofstee method:** This is a composite/compromise method, which combines features from both absolute and relative standard setting methods (Hofstee, 1983). Like absolute methods, it seeks judges' opinion about maximum and minimum cut-off scores and like relative methods, it also seeks minimum and maximum acceptable fail rates. The judges should be content experts and quite familiar with both the students and the performance examinations. The cut-off score is determined by the intersection/midpoint of the frequency curve which is usually a rectangle with a diagonal like intersecting the curve.

Most of these standard setting methods were developed for written examinations, mainly MCQs. Also, different standard setting methods will produce different passing scores. For setting standards of clinical assessments, a somewhat different approach may be required. It should be possible to use relative and composite methods without any major modifications. For absolute methods, particularly Angoff, there may be problems if judges were to use each item on the checklist as unit. To obviate this problem, each station is considered a unit. Judges give their estimates of the proportion of examinees that would pass that station and these scores are then averaged as described above.

Standard Setting for Practical/Clinical Skills

Standard setting methods have also been proposed for practical/clinical skills. For basic clinical skills, a patient safety approach has been described. It basically involves criteria for identifying essential items. Judges apply criteria to each checklist item to decide if it is essential or non-essential and determine separate passing scores for both categories. Learners must attain x% of essential and y% of non-essential items. Non-essential items cannot compensate for essential ones (Yudkowsky et al., 2014). Similarly, procedures for setting passing scores of objective structured clinical examination (OSCE) have also been described (Bouriscot et al., 2006).

One final consideration is the selection of the judges. Who can be a judge in a standard setting exercise? The most important characteristic of a judge would be his/her content expertise. Judges should also be aware of the examinee characteristics. Certain interventions can make the method more useful and realistic. The first is the sensitization of the judges to the level of examination. Often judges tend to set too high expectations from examinees. It has been suggested that asking the judges to take the test themselves before the meeting can help. Yet another method is to provide them with actual examination data so that they can calibrate their responses accordingly. Therefore, the selection and training of content expert judges is an important consideration.

REFERENCES

Angoff, W.H. (1971). Scales, norms, and equivalent scores. In: Thorndike, R.L. (Ed.) *Educational measurement*, 2nd ed. Washington, DC: American Council on Education. pp. 508–600.

Barman, A. (2008). Standard setting in student assessment: is a defensible method yet to come? *Annals of the Academy of Medicine, Singapore*, 37(11), 957–63.

Bouriscot, K., Roberts, T., & Pell, G. (2006). Standard setting for clinical competence at graduation from medical school: a comparison of passing scores across five medical schools. *Advances in Health Sciences Education: Theory and Practice*, 11(2), 173–83.

Ben-David, M.F. (2000). AMEE guide no. 18: standard setting in student assessment. *Medical Teacher*, 22(2), 120–30.

Downing, S.M., Tekian, A., & Yudkowsky, R. (2006). Procedures for establishing defensible absolute passing scores on performance examinations in health professions education. *Teaching and Learning in Medicine*, 18(1), 50–7.

Hofstee, W.K. (1983). The case for compromise in educational selection and grading. In: Anderson, S.B. & Helmick, J.S. (Eds). *On educational testing*. San Francisco: Jossey-Bass. pp. S107–27.

Livingston, S.A., & Zieky, M.J. (1982). *Passing scores: a manual for setting standards of performance on educational and occupational tests*. Princeton, NJ: Educational Testing Service.

Norcini, J.J. (2003). Setting standards on educational tests. *Medical Education*, 37(5), 464–9.

Norcini, J.J., & Guille, R. (2002). Combining tests and setting standards. In: Norman, G.R., van der Vleuten, C.P. and Newble, D.I. (Eds.). *International handbook of research in medical education*. London: Kluwer Academic. pp. 811–34.

Tekian, A., & Norcini, J.J. (2015). Overcome the 60% passing score and improve the quality of assessment. *GMS Zeitschrift für Medizinische Ausbildung*, 32(4), Doc43.

Yudkowsky, R., Downing, SM., & Tekian, A. (2019). Standard setting. In: Downing, S.M. and Yudkowsky, R. (Eds). *Assessment in health professions education*. New York, NY: Routledge, Taylor and Francis Group.

Yudkowsky, R., Tumuluru, S., Casey, P., Herlich, N., & Ledonne, C. (2014). A patient safety approach to setting pass/fail standards for basic procedural skills checklists. *Simulation in Healthcare*, 9(5), 277–82.

Chapter 24

Educational Feedback to Students

Rajiv Mahajan

KEY POINTS

☞ Educational feedback is the single most powerful factor which can enhance students' learning.
☞ Educational feedback should be based upon observable behavior of the learners.
☞ Educational feedback is not a one-time activity, rather it is a process.
☞ Ample opportunities for educational feedback to students must be incorporated in the curriculum.

Ludwig W Eichna, who took a second turn at being a medical student before stepping down as the Chairman of the Department of Medicine, State University of New York, Downstate Medical Center, Brooklyn has written in her seminal paper of the 1980s, "We are training future physicians who have never been observed" (Eichna, 1980). Is the situation not the same even now? Medical students are not observed, seldom guided and hardly any educational feedback is provided to them for course correction.

It is well documented that regular test-based assessment can enhance the whole spectrum of learning in medical students, ranging from diagnostic skills to clinical application of knowledge as well as retention (Roediger & Karpicke, 2006; Baghdady et al., 2014). While this regular test-based improvement in learning usually happens without feedback, the addition of feedback helps in correcting errors and reinforcing correct responses (Watling & Ginsburg, 2019).

What is Feedback?

In medical education settings, educational feedback refers to the information given by the instructor/facilitator to students, describing their performance in each task with an intention to guide their future performance in that same task or in a related activity. Dinham (2008) has defined feedback as "any form of response by a teacher to a student's performance, attitude or behavior, at least where attitude or behavior impinges upon performance, with a realization that feedback in not only an outcome of student performance but an essential part of the learning process". van de Ridder et al., (2008) in an effort to propose an operational definition of feedback defined feedback in clinical education as "specific information about the comparison between a trainee's observed performance and a standard, given with the intent to improve the trainee's performance". Ramaprasad (1983) defined feedback as "information about the gap between the actual level and the reference level of a system parameter which is used to alter the gap in some way".

In all these definitions, the crux about educational feedback is—identifying gaps between student's observed performance and standard reference, giving back this information to the student, identifying strategies to plug these gaps and continuous monitoring to check if these gaps have been plugged.

Feedback Loop: Corollary with the Human Body

You must be familiar with the feedback loops in the human body, where endocrinal functions are kept under control through feedback from outcomes, making a feedback loop. The same is true for feedback in any other system, including medical education.

A similar corollary of educational feedback loops can also be drawn to 'short-loop' and 'long-loop' feedback systems of the human body. Have a look at **Figure 24.1**, which depicts the educational feedback loop. The student is at the center of the loop. The other important person involved in this feedback cycle is the teacher (or may be peers also). The feedback provided by teachers or peers forms the long-loop feedback system. With longitudinal development, ultimately students come to hold the concept of quality roughly similar to that held by the teacher, and this promotes self-monitoring. Thus the short feedback loop involves self-monitoring and reflection by the student. This requires metacognitive skills. This concept has been proposed based upon the work of Sadler (1989).

If the information which proceeds backward from the performance is able to change the general method and pattern of a learner's performance, the process is called learning. The information thus proceeding backward from such a performance is referred to as feedback. In simple words, a task leads to outcomes, the outcomes are analyzed and information is given back to the performer (feedback), the feedback is processed leading to change in behavior, thus leading to learning and completing the educational feedback cycle. In a way, this educational feedback cycle is closely related to Kolb's learning cycle (Kolb, 1984). As can be seen in **Figure 24.2**, 'task' corresponds to 'concrete experience'; 'outcome analysis' corresponds to 'reflective observation'; 'feedback' corresponds to 'abstract conceptualization'; and 'processing corresponds to 'active experimentation'.

Chapter 24: Educational Feedback to Students

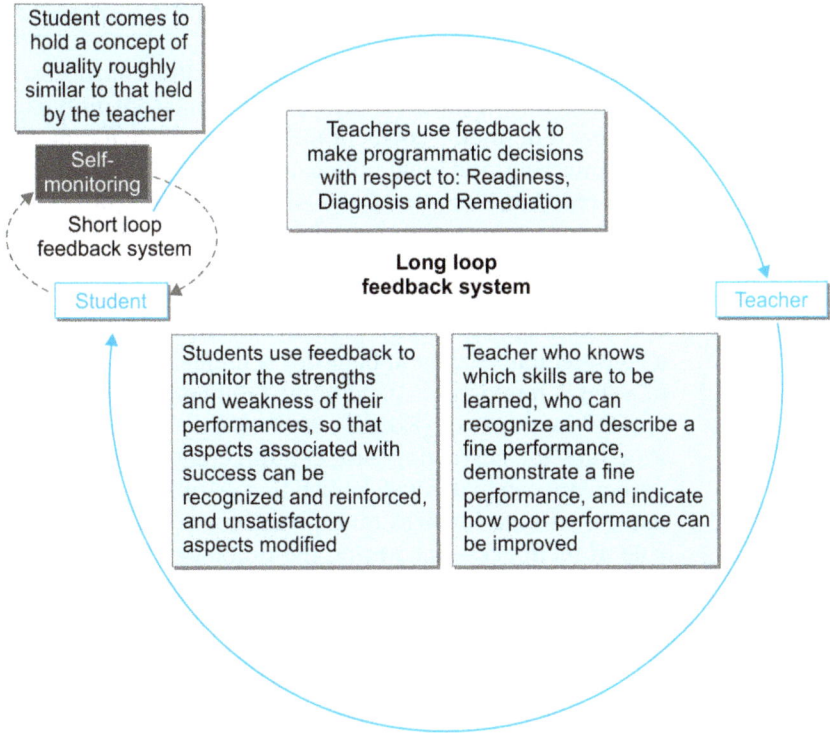

Fig. 24.1: Educational feedback loop: Short-loop and long-loop feedback systems.

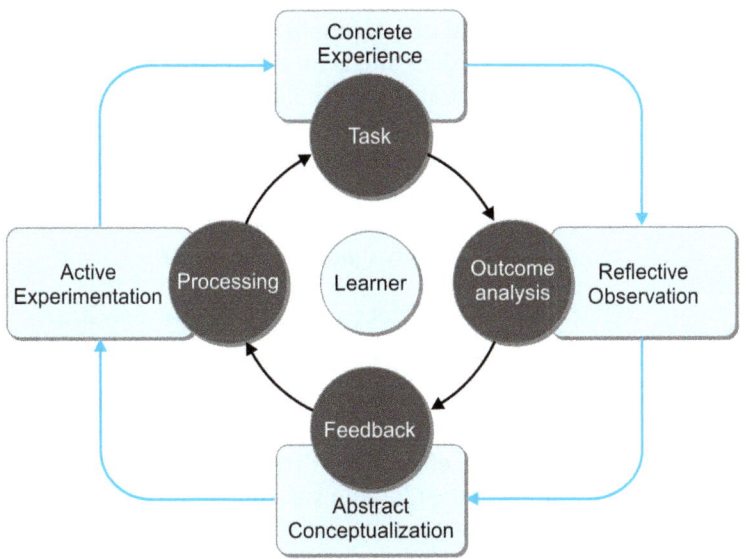

Fig. 24.2: Proximity of educational feedback cycle and learning cycle.

Hierarchy of Role-categorization of Educational Feedback

Educational feedback has been used for multiple purposes. Five broad role-categories of educational feedback, though not mutually exclusive, have been defined—correction, reinforcement, forensic diagnosis, benchmarking, and longitudinal development (Price et al., 2010).

Correction, the central role of feedback is to put things right by taking a corrective action with a focus on error treatment and achieving accuracy, most often restricted to the cognitive domain (Zohrabi & Ehsani, 2014). The role of **reinforcement** through educational feedback is to encourage the student to strengthen an existing behavior. Though a considerable change in behavior is frequently evident as the result of a single reinforcement, continued reinforcements are pertinent to sustain the behavior (Skinner, 2003). Utility of educational feedback as a tool for correction and reinforcements seems very limited, particularly when it is well known that learning is multi-dimensional, and assessment involves multiple criteria. Here comes the **forensic role of feedback**—diagnosing the problem with performance. This is connected with the **benchmarking** role of feedback—determining the gap between present performance and the standard of expected performance. For educational feedback to be effective, it must possess a concept of the standard being aimed for; compare the actual level of performance with the standard, and engage the learner in appropriate action which leads to some closure of the gap.

Educational feedback must explicitly address the future activity of learners by a concept called 'feed-forward' (Molloy, 2010). This concept emphasizes that the feedback opportunities should focus on **longitudinal development** of the learner through development of metacognitive skills and learning processes. These five role-categories of feedback act as a closely nested ladder—every category building on the information provided by the previous category; nevertheless major time and efforts in giving feedback to students are invested in 'correction' and 'reinforcement' aspects of feedback. The longitudinal development of learner, the most relevant aspect of feedback often remains substantially ignored **(Fig. 24.3)**.

Attributes of Effective Educational Feedback

Educational feedback has been widely cited as an important facilitator of learning and performance. Though feedback has been marked as the most powerful single factor that enhances learners' achievement with an overall effect size of 1.13 (Hattie, 1999), many meta-analyses have shown considerable variability, indicating that some types of feedback are more powerful and effective than others. The highest effect sizes involved students receiving information feedback about a task and how to do it more effectively, while lower effect sizes relate to praise, rewards, and punishment (Hattie & Timperley, 2007). This makes a case to identify the attributes of effective educational feedback:

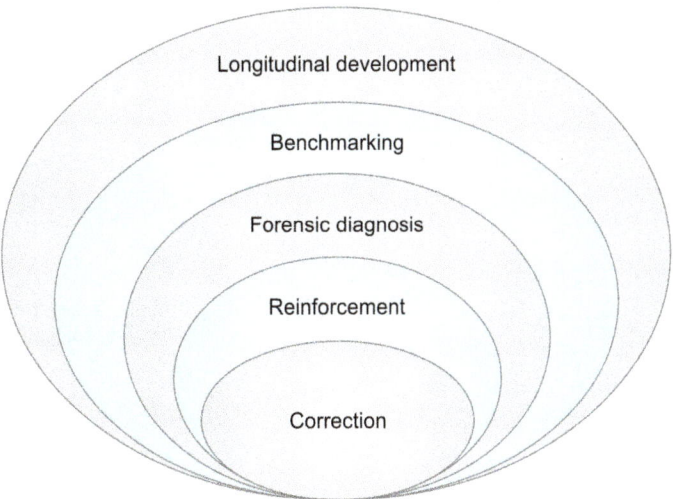

Fig. 24.3: Hierarchy of role-categories of educational feedback—every category building upon the information provided by the previous category.

Based upon observations: Educational feedback to students must be based upon their observable behaviors and performance; and not on the personality of the students. Feedback should never turn into personal criticism of the student. Feedback based upon observation has been the highest rated feedback technique (Hewson & Little, 1998).

Respectful, friendly teaching environment: The effectiveness of feedback is directly linked to instituting a respectful and friendly teaching environment, where students do not feel threatened while receiving feedback.

Non-judgmental: Feedback is not synonymous with evaluation. The purpose of feedback should not be to judge students but to suggest mid-course corrective measures.

Specific: Specificity of feedback means the amount and level of information offered by the feedback. Specific feedback tends to be more directive than facilitative. Directive feedback tells the student what needs to be fixed, while facilitative feedback only provides comments and suggestions to help guide students in their own revision and conceptualization. Feedback is significantly more effective when it offers details of the ways to improve the work, rather than when it just indicates the correctness of students' work. Feedback deficient in specificity may be regarded as useless and/or frustrating by students.

Right amount of feedback: While more specific feedback is generally regarded as better than less-specific feedback, a related attribute to consider is length or complexity of the feedback—many students will not pay attention to too long or too complicated feedback rendering it useless (Shute, 2007). Same can be the case with too less information. More feedback does not always mean more learning.

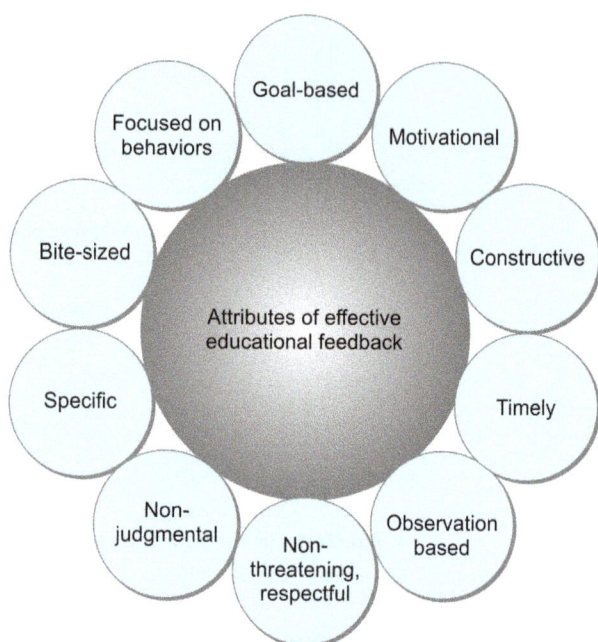

Fig. 24.4: Attributes of effective educational feedback to the students.

Some of the other attributes of effective educational feedback are—it should be goal-based, should elicit students' feelings and emotions, should be timely, and should be motivational and constructive for students. None of these attributes are standalone features; all are interwoven. In short, an effective feedback is the one which is delivered in an appropriate setting, focusing on the performance (and not on the individual), which is clear, specific and based on direct observation, is delivered using neutral, non-judgmental language emphasizing the positive aspects, and is descriptive (rather than evaluative) **(Fig. 24.4)**. The same has been explained as 'ABCDEFG IS' a mnemonic—**A:** amount of information, **B:** benefit to the trainees, **C:** change behavior, **D:** descriptive language, **E:** environment, **F:** focused, **G:** group check, **I:** interpretation check, **S:** sharing information (Bhattarai, 2007).

Types of Educational Feedback

Feedback has been categorized as oral and written feedback, evaluative and descriptive feedback, informal and formal feedback, and peer and self-feedback. Oral feedback usually occurs during a task, while written feedback is given usually at the end of a task. Evaluative feedback can make good students feel better, but generally tend to make less able students feel worse. Descriptive feedback on the other hand is designed to answer four important questions:
1. Where am I going?
2. How am I going?

3. What do I need to do to improve? and
4. How do I do that?

Descriptive feedback is always regarded as specific feedback. Formal feedback can be planned for specific goals, and can be structured to address the individual needs of a student.

Peer feedback has already been regarded as 'long-loop feedback', with an added advantage that students get to see other students' work which can also deepen understanding of the learning goals. Self-feedback should be the ultimate goal of any feedback system and has already been termed as 'short-loop feedback' system. Feedback has also been classified as one-to-one feedback and generic feedback.

Notwithstanding the types, the basic purpose feedback tends to serve is the same—identifying gaps in learning and promoting strategies to bridge that gap.

Models for Giving Educational Feedback to Students

Not only is the type of feedback important, but the chronological order in which statements are made is also important. It has been reported that the sequence of feedback statements and their timing influence performance (Henley & Reed, 2015). Thus, it is pertinent to discuss an outline of some of the prevalent models in use for providing educational feedback to the students.

Feedback sandwich: In its most basic form, a feedback sandwich consists of one specific criticism 'sandwiched' between two specific praises, also known as PCP (praise-criticism-praise or positive-corrective-positive) model. This technique of giving educational feedback is fast, efficient and suited to the time constraints of physician practice (Dohrenwend, 2002). However, feedback sandwich has been criticized on the grounds that information presented before the corrective statement makes the feedback less efficacious. An experimental design has shown that for post-session feedback, CPP (corrective-positive-positive) sequence is more efficacious and ending feedback with a corrective statement results in a decrease in the performance of the students (Henley & Reed, 2015).

Pendleton model: Pendleton model is an adaptation of the feedback sandwich in which the learner's observations precede teacher's comments. It basically consists of four steps: (1) The learner states what was good about her performance; (2) The teacher states areas of agreement and elaborates on good performance; (3) The learner states what was poor or could have been improved; (4) The teacher states what she could have improved. This model provides opportunity for more detailed review of the performance of the student and encourages her to become better equipped at recognizing her performance and the learning gaps (Pendleton et al., 2003).

Some of the other prevalent models have been outlined in **Box 24.1**.

Hewson & Little (1998) have proposed a six-step model for providing educational feedback which includes: orientation and

> **BOX 24.1:** Some other models of giving educational feedback
>
> **Stop-Start-Continue model:** More involvement of student; model works around three basic assumptions answered by the students concerned—what they feel they should: stop doing; start doing; and continue doing (Hoon et al., 2015).
>
> **SET-GO model:** For an agenda-led, problem-based analysis for descriptive educational feedback; based upon mutual goal seeking interaction of the learner and the facilitator. Basic five steps in this model include: What I **S**aw?; What **E**lse did you see?; What do you **T**hink?; Can we clarify what **G**oal we would like to achieve?; Any **O**ffers of how we should get there? (Silverman et al., 1997).
>
> **STAR model:** First teacher understands the situation or task (**ST**) which lead her to give feedback to the student for improvement; then she accesses the action (**A**); at last the result (**R**) produced, meaning the feedback-effect is monitored (UNM Human Resources, 2010).
>
> **Reflective model:** More emphasis on student's own ability to recognize performance deficit and planning strategies for improvement, thus encouraging students to reflect more on their actions and to motivate subsequent improvement in performance (Cantillon & Sargeant, 2008).

climate; elicitation; diagnosis and feedback; Improvement plan; application; and review. This emphasizes the role of monitoring the effect of the feedback. A 'stage of change model' has been proposed by Milan et al. (2006). It is pertinent to reemphasize here that irrespective of the model and method used, the three basic questions which need to be answered from a student's point of view are the same: Where am I going?, How am I going?, and Where to next? (Hattie & Timperley, 2007). Based upon the above discussion, a simple, feasible model to be incorporated in undergraduate medical training, largely based on Pendleton model is being proposed **(Box 24.2)**.

> **BOX 24.2:** A model of educational feedback for undergraduate training
>
> Step 1: Student asked to reflect about what they did well in their performance
> Step 2: Teacher elaborates on areas of good performance.
> Step 3: Student identifies the areas which can be improved.
> Step 4: Student seeks teacher's opinion about the areas which can be improved and how to improve them.
> Step 5: Teacher explains the areas which need to be worked upon and the strategy to improve those areas, giving specific information—what should be stopped?, what should be started?, and what should be continued?
> Step 6: Both student and teacher reach an agreement and discuss the ways to monitor progress.

Feedback Opportunities during Undergraduate Training

As already stated, feedback can be formal or informal; though in an educational setting, formal feedback carries much more impact. During undergraduate medical training, ample opportunities are available to the teachers to provide educational feedback to the students, and these opportunities can be incorporated in day-to-day activities as well as for special feedback purposes.

Written assignments: Even today, the 'red pen' by far is the most used instrument by the teacher for conveying their message across to learners. Written comments on written assignments can provide a good feedback strategy, if the basic rules of providing feedback are followed. Firstly, written feedback should not contain vague or general comments. Secondly, tutors should provide specific assessment criteria on how marks have been computed. When written assessment criteria is provided beforehand and used subsequently for marking, it benefits both teachers and students (Weaver, 2006).

Care should be taken while writing comments for providing feedback. Feedback such as 'concentrate more', 'get help with your spelling', 'improving', 'poor punctuation', 'some good ideas', 'did you write this?', and 'satisfactory' provides little reassurance or guidance. The criteria used for assessing student work need to be clear, understood by the student and used to frame personalized feedback (Dinham, 2008). Explaining the grades remains the best strategy to provide effective feedback.

Oral feedback: Tutorials, seminars and class viva are some of the opportunities for providing timely oral or verbal feedback. One-to-one verbal feedback may be better than written feedback in improving the performance of undergraduate medical students, and it may prove to be even more helpful in eliciting the learning gaps and motivating more accurate self-analysis by weaker students (Aggarwal et al., 2016).

Clinical encounters: Clinical case presentations, OSCE, mini-CEX and WBPA provide opportunities for giving educational feedback to the students in clinical skill areas. Such clinical encounters coupled with judicious use of feedback from standardized patients, peer feedback, and video recording followed by self-evaluation can enhance the effect of teacher-led feedback. Care should be taken that in such scenarios feedback should not be given in front of patients, lest it may discourage students.

Immediate feedback assessment technique: Immediate feedback assessment technique (IFAT) is commercially available answer form for feedback on MCQs. In contrast to other forms used for MCQ testing, IFAT, widely used in many colleges abroad, gives an opportunity to students to try second and subsequent choices if their first choice is wrong. IFAT provides immediate, corrective feedback for every item attempted by the student (DiBattista et al., 2004).

Self-monitoring: To make students lifelong learners, students need to transit from being recipients of feedback to learning metacognitive skills of self-efficacy, self-monitoring, self-reflection, and self-assessment. In fact, learners move across the learning horizon from being self-directed learners, to acquiring self-monitoring skills and reflective behavior to becoming metacognitive learners (Mahajan et al., 2016). Students are the best judge of their work, provided they have reached a level where they hold the concept of quality as held by the teachers. For this to happen, students have to possess a concept of the goal being aimed for, identify the gap between the current level and the standard, and engage in action to close that gap. Self-assessment has been marked by undergraduate students to be helpful in increasing their knowledge and interest in the subject and motivating them to develop self-directed learning skills (Sharma et al., 2016).

Issues with Giving Educational Feedback to Students

Students need feedback on their performance in cognitive aspects, clinical skills, communication with patients, and other aspects of clinical practice for improvement. However, there are many student-related, teacher-related and process/educational environment-related issues, which render educational feedback ineffective, thus making the whole exercise futile.

Student-related issues: Many times, students feel uncomfortable about interacting with faculty and seeking feedback. Feedback can be effective only if a student has the inetention to improve. Without a willing student, even most specific feedback would not be useful. Even if willing, students often view feedback as a statement about their personal potential. Students may apparently want information about their performance but only insofar as it confirms their self-concept ultimately converting feedback into feeding (Hyman, 1980). Quite often, students are not able to interpret feedback properly, the problem being more common with written feedback where technical jargon has been used. Moreover, students' reflective behavior is often underdeveloped, and they are not aware about the questions to be asked (Brukner et al., 1999).

Teacher-related issues: The most critical teacher-related issue is lack of understanding about the process of giving educational feedback, lack of formal training and lack of experience in giving feedback to the students. As such, teachers lack confidence in their observations and feel uncomfortable giving specific feedback (Brukner et al., 1999). Teachers often start using feedback as opportunities for evaluation. It must be remembered that the purpose of feedback is only presenting formative information, and not making judgments. Evaluation is expressed as normative statements, whereas feedback is neutral (Hyman, 1980). This 'tagging of feedback' is often repulsive to the students.

A major issue which can take place while providing feedback even with well-trained and experienced teachers is invocation of expectation effect—referring to teacher's expectation of the students' achievements—self-fulfilling prophecy and self-sustaining expectation, to be more specific (Good, 1987). Self-fulfilling prophecy is good if the expectation is positive, but if the teacher's expectation is negative it can severely harm the student's progress. Similarly, sustaining expectations prevent change through a lack of acceptance in the teacher towards a student who is showing positive changes and improvement.

Process/educational environment-related issues: One process-related issue is that despite receiving the most honest and specific educational feedback, students are not aware of how to use it. It is a failure of the process, as students take-up the literal meaning of feedback and start looking back at the assignment they have already completed, rather than using this feedback for feed-forward and continued professional development (Burke, 2009). Another issue is lack of a supportive learning environment. For the feedback process to thrive, a conducive educational environment is needed.

Strategies for Enhancing Value of Educational Feedback

A comprehensive approach, targeting all stakeholders, and the educational environment can certainly improve the value of educational feedback given to students. Some of the target areas can be:

Sensitizing students: Students need to be sensitized about the importance of feedback in learning and professional development, so that it does not come as a surprise to them. They should not feel threatened by the prospect of receiving feedback and should be open to receiving it.

Faculty training: Giving educational feedback to the students is a skill which can be learnt over a period of time. Target-specific faculty development in the form of workshops and longitudinal programmes can be undertaken for capacity building.

Building a supportive environment: Educational feedback as a standalone process will never survive; it must be supported by instituting a supportive educational environment. Moving over to programmatic assessment with ample opportunities for formative assessment can be one example.

Follow rules: Providing feedback to students should not be treated as a casual affair. Though informal feedback too is important, but more often than not, the feedback process should follow certain ground rules. Many rules have been cited in literature and an attempt has been made here to specify them as SMARTER rule (**Box 24.3**).

BOX 24.3: SMARTER rule for providing educational feedback to the students

S: Specific—Feedback should be about specific performance, and should be non-judgmental
M: Measurable—Feedback should be based upon measurable and observed behavior of students
A: Acting as allies—Teacher and student should work together as allies
R: Remediable behaviors—Feedback should be limited only to the remediable behaviors
T: Timely—Feedback should be provided well with-in time to have its maximum effect
E: Expected—Students should be expecting feedback and it should not come as a surprise to them
R: Relaxed environment—Educational feedback should be provided in a relaxed, non-threatening environment

Feedback is an integral part of students' learning and professional development. For optimal growth of students, ample feedback opportunities should be interwoven into the educational curriculum by introducing a system of programmatic assessment. When given by following a set of rules after sensitizing the students and after proper faculty training, the educational impact of feedback can be optimally tapped.

REFERENCES

Aggarwal, M., Singh, S., Sharma, A., Singh, P., & Bansal, P. (2016). Impact of structured verbal feedback module in medical education: a questionnaire- and test score-based analysis. *International Journal of Applied and Basic Medical Research, 6(3)*, 220–5.

Baghdady, M., Carnahan, H., Lam, E.W., & Woods, N.N. (2014). Test-enhanced learning and its effect on comprehension and diagnostic accuracy. *Medical Education, 48(2)*, 181–8.

Bhattarai, M. (2007). ABCDEFG IS—the principle of constructive feedback. *Journal of Nepal Medical Association, 46(167)*, 151–6.

Brukner, H., Altkorn, D.L., Cook, S., Quinn, M.T., & McNabb, W.L. (1999). Giving effective feedback to medical students: a workshop for faculty and house staff. *Medical Teacher, 21(2)*, 161–5.

Burke, D. (2009). Strategies for using feedback students bring to higher education. *Assessment and Evaluation in Higher Education, 34(1)*, 41–50.

Cantillon, P., & Sargeant, J. (2008). Giving feedback in clinical settings. *British Medical Journal, 337*, a1961.

DiBattista, D., Mitterer, J.O., & Gosse, L. (2004). Acceptability by undergraduates of the immediate feedback assessment technique for multiple-choice testing. *Teaching in Higher Education, 9(1)*, 17–28.

Dinham S. (2008). Feedback on feedback. *Teacher, 191*, 20–3.

Dohrenwend, A. (2002). Serving up the feedback sandwich. *Family Practice Management, 9(10)*, 43–6.

Eichna, L.W. (1980). Medical-school education, 1975-1979: a student's perspective. *New England Journal of Medicine, 303(13)*, 727–34.

Good, T.L. (1987). Two decades of research on teacher expectations: findings and future directions. *Journal of Teacher Education, 38*, 32–47.

Hattie, J. (1999). *Influences on student learning*. Inaugural Lecture, University of Auckland, New Zealand. [online] Available from https://cdn.auckland.ac.nz/assets/education/hattie/docs/influences-on-student-learning.pdf [Last accessed August, 2020].

Hattie, J., & Timperley, H. (2007). The power of feedback. *Review of Educational Research, 77(1)*, 81–112.

Henley, A.J., & Reed, F.D. (2015). Should you order the feedback sandwich? Efficacy of feedback sequence and timing. *Journal of Organizational Behavior Management, 35(3–4)*, 321–35.

Hewson, M.G., & Little, M.L. (1998). Giving feedback in medical education: verification of recommended techniques. *Journal of General Internal Medicine, 13(2)*, 111–6.

Hoon, A., Oliver, E.J., Szpakowska, K., & Newton, P. (2015). Use of the 'stop, start, continue' method is associated with the production of constructive qualitative feedback by students in higher education. *Assessment and Evaluation in Higher Education, 40(5)*, 755–67.

Hyman, R.T. (1980). *Improving discussion leadership*. New York: Teachers College Press.

Kolb, D. A. (1984). Experiential learning: Experience as the source of learning and development (Vol. 1). Englewood Cliffs, NJ: Prentice-Hall.

Mahajan, R., Badyal, D.K., Gupta, P., & Singh, T. (2016). Cultivating lifelong learning skills during graduate medical training. *Indian Pediatrics, 53(9)*, 797–804.

Milan, F.B., Parish, S.J., & Reichgott, M.J. (2006). A model for educational feedback based on clinical communication skills strategies: beyond the 'feedback sandwich'. *Teaching and Learning in Medicine, 18(1)*, 42–7.

Molloy, E.K. (2010). The feedforward mechanism: a way forward in clinical learning? *Medical Education, 44(12)*, 1157–8.

Pendleton, D., Schofield, T., Tate, P., & Havelock, P. (2003). *The consultation: an approach to learning and teaching*. Oxford: Oxford University Press.

Price, M., Handley, K., Millar, J., & O'Donovan, B. (2010). Feedback: all the effort, but what is the effect? *Assessment and Evaluation in Higher Education*, 35(3), 277–89.

Ramaprasad, A. (1983). On the definition of feedback. *Behavioral Science, 28(1)*, 4–13.

Roediger, H.L., & Karpicke, J.D. (2006). Test-enhanced learning: taking memory tests improves long-term retention. *Psychological Science, 17(3)*, 249–55.

Sadler, D.R. (1989). Formative assessment and the design of instructional systems. *Instructional Science, 18*, 119–44.

Sharma, R., Jain, A., Gupta, N., Garg, S., Batta, M., & Dhir, S.K. (2016). Impact of self-assessment by students on their learning. *International Journal of Applied and Basic Medical Research, 6(3)*, 226–9.

Shute, V.J. (2007). *Focus on formative feedback*. Princeton, NJ: Educational Testing Services. p. 6.

Silverman, J., Draper, J., Kurtz, S.M., & Silverman, J. (1997). The Calgary-Cambridge approach to communication skills teaching II: the SET-GO method of descriptive feedback. *Education for General Practice, 8*, 16–23.

Skinner, B.F. (2003). The science of learning and the art of teaching. In: Vargas, J.S. (Ed). The *technology of teaching*, e-book. [online] Available from www.bfskinner.org/wp-content/uploads/2016/04/ToT.pdf [Last accessed August, 2020].

UNM Human Resources. (2010). *The star feedback model*. [online] Available from https://hr.unm.edu/docs/eod/the-star-feedback-model.pdf [Last accessed August, 2020].

van de Ridder, J.M., Stokking, K.M., McGaghie, W.C., & ten Cate, O.T. (2008). What is feedback in clinical education? *Medical Education, 42(2)*, 189–97.

Watling, C.J., & Ginsburg, S. (2019). Assessment, feedback and the alchemy of learning. *Medical Education, 53(1)*, 76–85.

Weaver, M.R. (2006). Do students value feedback? Student perceptions of tutors' written responses. *Assessment and Evaluation in Higher Education, 31(3)*, 379–94.

Zohrabi, K., & Ehsani, F. (2014). The role of implicit and explicit corrective feedback in Persian-speaking EFL learners' awareness of and accuracy in English grammar. *Procedia - Social and Behavioral Sciences, 98*, 2018–24.

Chapter 25

Student Ratings of Teaching Effectiveness

Anshu, Tejinder Singh

KEY POINTS

- ☞ Student ratings of teaching can be used to improve the quality of teaching, for decision making (renewals, promotions, awards, etc.) and for course evaluation.
- ☞ The purpose of these ratings must be established in advance. Tools to obtain such feedback should be carefully designed keeping the purpose in mind.
- ☞ The focus should be on specific teaching behaviors. Students should not be asked about what they cannot answer (e.g., knowledge or expertise of the teacher).
- ☞ Student ratings must be used in combination with multiple sources of information to make a balanced judgment about all of the components of teaching.

Gathering feedback from students about the effectiveness of teaching and the relevance of curriculum is universally accepted to be a useful method in improving the quality of courses. Student ratings are used for formative purposes, for decision making (renewals, promotions, awards, etc.), and for summative purposes (course evaluation) (Marsh, 1987; Theall & Franklin, 1991). In India, however, student feedback is not consistently used in educational institutions for curricular revision or faculty appraisal. Student evaluation of teaching is viewed with skepticism and faculty members are apprehensive about student ratings.

Student Ratings of Teaching: Misconceptions and Misuses

This negative opinion about the value of student ratings of teaching stems from misconceptions about the validity and reliability of this tool in improving quality of teaching. Issues around validity and reliability also arise when interpreting student feedback. 'Is student feedback valid?' 'Are the results obtained from student feedback reliable?' These questions continue to be asked by teachers the world over. Some of the common problems and prejudices against student feedback are outlined in **Box 25.1**.

> **BOX 25.1:** Common conceptions about student ratings of teaching.
> - Student feedback cannot be used to improve teaching effectiveness
> - Students are not competent to make consistent judgments
> - Students ratings are just popularity contests
> - Student feedback is not valid or reliable
> - Student feedback can be manipulated
> - Teachers will mark students more leniently to get better ratings

A good number of faculty and administrators lack knowledge about student feedback, and this ignorance about research correlates significantly with negative opinion about value of student feedback. These misconceptions also arise from personal biases, fear, as well as general hostility toward being evaluated (Theall & Franklin, 2001). However, credible research of more than 50 years in this area negates these misconceptions. Many of these can be addressed by judicious use of this tool.

Process of Collecting and Interpreting Student Ratings

Student ratings are viewed with skepticism because the process of collecting and interpreting feedback is wrought with flaws. Certain principles must be followed before using student feedback for formative purposes (Cashin, 1999). The purpose and uses of ratings should be established in advance (Theall & Franklin, 2001). Evaluation, improvement or advisements are all legitimate uses of such data. A prior discussion can help to alleviate the concerns of various parties involved. Some of the factors which have been shown to result in poor acceptance of the method include—absence of clear policy, use of poor instruments, misuse and misinterpretation of data, and arbitrary decision-making (Theall, 1996). The system for collection, analysis, and interpretation of feedback must be decided in advance and conveyed to the faculty. Involving all stakeholders is highly recommended (Miller, 1987) and not following this is a serious error (Centra, 1979).

Flaws in Design of Instrument

What we ask is more important and it is expected that we ask only what the students can answer. Students can tell us whether teachers helped them learn, or how well teachers taught, but they are not the best judges of the content, adequacy or depth of teaching. Some of the most common mistakes are to ask students whether the teacher is knowledgeable, or to ask whether the teacher used appropriate assessment tools. The focus should be on specific teaching behaviors.

Consensus exists in literature that students are unable to judge the currency of course content, clarity and realism of objectives, validity of assessment procedures and similar vital matters. Cashin (1989) lists 26 considerations relevant to instructional effectiveness, of which 11 cannot be validly commented upon by the students. It is therefore imperative that self-ratings, colleague ratings, ratings on indirect contributions to teaching, and department chair ratings should complement student ratings. The use of student feedback should focus attention on improving teaching and learning outcomes, rather than simply improving perceptions of the instructor.

Student feedback forms are multi-dimensional and reflect several different aspects of teaching. This is because no single item is useful for all purposes. Student rating forms have to be flexible enough to include items useful for all courses and teachers, yet be comprehensive to provide information on all dimensions of teaching. Studies recommend use of low-inference (individual behaviors) and high-inference global measure (enthusiasm, clarity, or overall effectiveness) items that align with purpose (Seldin, 1993). Low-inference (specific individual behaviors) items are important because a single score or measure of overall course cannot represent the multi-dimensionality of teaching. Specific behavior items can be clear to students and offer easy interpretation for instructors. High-inference (overall global measures) measures are also essential as low-inference ratings may be more affected by the systemic distortion hypothesis, i.e., traits can be judged to be correlated, when in reality they have little or no correlation.

Some studies have found a good correlation between ratings given by students and open-ended written comments provided by them (Ory, et al., 1980; Burdsal & Harrison, 2008), and that these can be used to make personnel decisions. Faculty find written comments from students useful for self-improvement, but these are not credible data to use for promotion decisions (Braskamp et al., 1981).

Seldin (1993) is of the opinion that for diagnostic purposes, 20-30 questions should provide sufficient information, provided the questions relate to specific teaching behaviors. In fact, for personal decisions, he suggests only 4-6 global questions. Grouping items by factors (e.g., organization, clarity of communication, etc.) may be the best method of providing meaningful feedback to instructors. Some of the items reflected on most forms are—course organization and planning, clarity of teaching, communication skills of instructor, student-teacher interaction, rapport developed, workload, difficulty of course, grading, examinations, and student learning (Centra, 1993; Braskamp & Ory, 1994).

Issues in the Logistics of Collecting Feedback

The questionnaires are often not administered at the appropriate time, have too many items and are answered by too few students. All these factors pose threat to the valid interpretation of data generated from their use.

To be meaningful, the questionnaires should be filled by not less than 10 raters or 75% of the class, whichever is more (Seldin, 1993).

For formative purposes, the scales should be administered about one-third of the way into a semester to give teachers a chance to adjust their teaching. Administrative guidelines ought to be clear and consistent. It is preferable if a neutral person (other than the faculty member) administers the evaluation. The administration should strive for quick processing and return of forms.

Teachers are often not convinced that students will give honest feedback. It is important to create an atmosphere of trust. Sadly, the teacher-student relation in India is still guided by the colonial culture, where the teacher is supreme, can decide the fate of the student and can spoil their career. Students, therefore, often find it much more sensible to keep their opinions to themselves than to risk their careers. The problem also lies with teachers who are not prepared to accept criticism. Students need to be convinced that their feedback is valued and must be assured of anonymity. Creating a climate of openness and transparency must precede the process of collecting feedback.

When students are given a questionnaire and asked for their comments, they are likely to be thinking 'Should I answer this? What should I say? Will they listen and take my comments seriously? What is the evidence that what I write will make any difference?', etc. Students then are having a conversation in their own way with the questionnaire and the teachers who give it to them. Their past experiences in the class and with questionnaires will guide their responses. Their answers are a reflection of their trust in the teachers and their school to listen to them. In this way, the design of the questions and the response of the students are not as simple as we might think. Honest feedback will not be received in a hostile climate where a student fears a backlash for criticism.

Problems with Interpretation of Data

Interpretation of the data also needs to be done with caution. Feedback is meant for improvement, not for comparisons. Data which are not meaningfully interpreted are seen as a threat to teachers, the meanings of ratings are not clear (e.g., how low is low?), and there is too much dependence on student ratings alone.

Data from student ratings should not be used to grade teachers as being good or bad. As Cashin (1999) points out, improvement in teaching effectiveness should not be viewed as improving from 3rd to 50th centile—rather, it should be seen as providing an opportunity for improvement at all levels; a change from 98th to 99th centile also signifies improvement. Further, since there are no absolute figures available, it is better to provide comparative data for teachers to make meaningful interpretations. It should also be clear that while low ratings may indicate dissatisfaction, they do not mean that the teacher is not doing an adequate job (Boice, 1992). We should also be careful to over interpret the significance of small differences in the scores (Seldin, 1993)—a teacher scoring 3.70 is not to be considered a better teacher than someone scoring 3.68. Personnel committees should use broad categories (e.g., promote/do not promote, deserves merit increase/deserves average increase) rather than 'attempting to interpret decimal-point differences' in making evaluations (McKeachie, 1997).

Cashin (1995) suggested that the teachers should view the whole exercise as a rating, rather than as evaluation. The term 'rating' implies data which is to be interpreted—while evaluation suggests a terminal connotation and the finality of the answer. There is yet another important benefit out of this paradigm—like any other assessment, use of multisource data becomes an inherent part of the process.

Are Student Ratings Valid and Reliable?

Faculty is often skeptical about the validity, reliability, and generalizability of student feedback. This prevents them from making any meaningful use of the data in addition to generating a lot of frustration. Persisting negative opinion takes its toll.

Machell (1989) coined the term 'professional melancholia' to denote increasing hostility, arrogance, alienation and even verbal and grade abuse toward students. Students spend a full course term observing the behavior of the teacher, and are therefore in a unique position to comment on teaching behaviors and rate the teachers. Cashin (1995) in his meta-analysis of research stated that 'In general, student ratings tend to be statistically reliable, valid and relatively free from bias or need for control; probably more so than any other data used for evaluation'.

There are a number of factors which come into play in student ratings. In the context of student ratings validity means: 'To what extent do student rating items measure some aspect of teaching effectiveness?' Unfortunately, not everyone agrees to the same definition of 'effective teaching'. Since teaching is a multidimensional activity, it is difficult to define the 'content' of good teaching. For this reason, most workers seek construct-related evidence to find out the validity of the process (Kulik, 2001). In essence, this means that ratings should correlate satisfactorily to other partial and/or imperfect measures of effectiveness. Cohen (1981), in his meta-analysis, found a significant relationship between student ratings and student learning. Ory et al., (1980) found a strong relation between student ratings and ratings of a class derived from written and interview comments. Feldman (1989) reported average correlation of 0.50 between student and observer ratings. These reports suggest a good evidence related to construct and concurrent validity. Here, it is important to caution that validity is not a characteristic inherent in a student questionnaire. Validity is determined by how the ratings are used, how they are interpreted, and what actions follow from those interpretations. Messick (1989) called this the consequential basis of validity.

A mention must be made here of the 'Dr Fox' effect. The study by Naftulin et al., (1973) created an impression that it is possible to get good ratings by judicious use of showmanship. However, as later publications (Frey, 1979) demonstrated, this study was full of methodological flaws and does not negate the validity of student ratings. Similarly, other variables like populist tendencies of the teachers, giving lenient grades, etc., have been shown to have an effect size of +0.22, suggesting that there may be some small influence of non-academic factors, but the magnitude is too small to negate the validity of student ratings (Abrami, 2001). There are reviews on the factors which are thought to have a bearing on student ratings (Cashin, 1995) and the published evidence showing that ratings maintain their validity despite these variables.

Like any other assessment, the importance of getting evidence from other sources cannot be overemphasized. As Benton and Cashin (2012) emphasize, no single source of information, including student ratings, provides enough information to make a valid judgment about overall teaching effectiveness. Instead of depending on student feedback alone, data ought to be complemented by self-ratings, peer feedback, and administrative feedback as well. Getting feedback from more than one source will improve both the validity as well as the reliability.

Reliability provides important evidence related to validity. The feedback itself is not reliable or unreliable—it is the inferences that we draw from the results which are. In respect to student ratings, reliability refers to the *consistency*, *stability*, and *generalizability* of data. In this context, reliability refers most to consistency or inter-rater agreement (Cashin, 1995). Reliability, in addition to other factors, is a function of the number of raters. Sixbury and Cashin (1995) reported a reliability of 0.69 for 10 raters, going up to 0.91, when the number of raters goes up to 40. To ensure reliability, feedback must be collected from at least 75% of the class. As a general rule, data obtained from multiple classes provide more reliable information than that obtained from a single class. Stability is concerned with agreement between raters over time (Benton & Cashin, 2012). Ratings of the same teacher across semesters tend to be similar.

Generalizability refers to how accurately the data reflect a teacher's overall teaching effectiveness, not just how effective he or she was in teaching a particular course in a particular semester. Marsh (1984) studied the differential effects of the teacher and the course. He found that the instructor, and not the course, is the primary determinant of students' ratings. Generalizability is especially relevant when making personnel decisions about a teacher's general teaching effectiveness. Benton & Cashin (2012) recommend that for most teachers, ratings from a variety of courses are necessary. They recommend data from preferably two or more courses from every term, for at least 2 years, totaling six to eight courses to use for this purpose.

Anonymity, timing of administration, culture of the institution, and use of the data all have an influence on reliability.

Purposes of Student Ratings of Teaching

Table 25.1 outlines what student ratings can be used for and should not be used for.

TABLE 25.1: Uses and misuse of student ratings	
Student ratings can be used for	**Student ratings should not be used for**
❖ Improvement of faculty teaching effectiveness ❖ Making administrative decisions about promotions, awards, renewal of job tenure ❖ Review and evaluation of course ❖ Helping students decide which course to choose	❖ Deciding course content ❖ Deciding subject expertise of teacher ❖ Making administrative decisions based on fine discriminations and comparisons between faculty scores ❖ Modifying administrative procedures

It has been found that the overall ratings given by students strongly correlate with several dimensions of teaching such as how clearly and concisely the course content is explained, whether the teacher finds ways for students to answer their own questions, the personal interest that teachers display in students and their learning, whether they demonstrate the relevance of the subject matter, and how they introduce stimulating ideas about the subject (Hoyt & Lee, 2002; 2002 b). Teachers who wish to improve their global ratings must focus on good teaching behaviors such as stimulating student interest, establishing rapport with students, encouraging student involvement, and fostering student collaboration.

Prospects of Using Student Ratings in India

Student feedback is only one mechanism of collecting feedback for improving teaching programs. It is essential that it be combined with other sources of feedback from teachers, peers, administrators, etc., to improve the validity and reliability of this data.

Institutions must decide in advance the purposes for which the data will be used. Teachers need to be made aware of literature on student feedback to improve acceptance of this method and to be able to use it effectively. Issues which make teachers averse to student feedback need to be talked about openly and all attempts must be made to address their apprehensions. They must be satisfied about the way this modality is used and must be aware of the utility, validity, and reliability of student feedback. It may be useful to have centralized guidance about using student feedback as a modality. Uniform questionnaires may make interpretations easier.

Given the initial resistance to student feedback from faculty, it may be essential to tread slowly. One way of approaching this issue is that results of their evaluation can be made available to individual teachers. They can see their own scores as well as the anonymous scores of their peers.

A mechanism to help the faculty who get poor ratings must be in place. Our own experience with student feedback showed that repeating the exercise after six months resulted in improvement in the scores. We had not provided any additional inputs—our hypothesis was that the better scores could be attributed to Hawthorne effect (Singh et al., 1991). An important issue is to provide some sort of development advice so that teachers can improve their specific behaviors. When rating information is coupled with knowledgeable assistance, improvement can result. It is imperative to provide an opportunity for teachers to discuss the scores with peers/administration in a nonthreatening atmosphere.

The student voice must be appropriately integrated with self-assessment of the instructor and peer/supervisor feedback. Integrating all three elements allows teachers to try out new teaching strategies and remain open to feedback that focuses on how they might improve. This feedback must not demoralize teachers, but be provided in an open environment that fosters challenge, support, and growth. The evaluation of teaching should become a rewarding process, and not a dreaded event (Benton & Young, 2018).

REFERENCES

Abrami, P.C. (2001). Improving judgements about teaching effectiveness using teacher rating forms. *New Directions for Institutional Research*, 109, 59–87.

Benton, S.L., & Cashin, W.E. (2012). *Student ratings of teaching: a summary of research and literature. IDEA paper no. 50*. Manhattan, Kansas: Kansas State University, Centre for Faculty Evaluation and Development.

Benton, S.L., & Young, S. (2018). *Best practices in the evaluation of teaching. IDEA paper no. 69*. Manhattan, Kansas: Kansas State University, Centre for Faculty Evaluation and Development.

Boice, R. (1992). *The new faculty member: supporting and fostering professional development*. San Francisco, CA: Jossey Bass.

Braskamp, L.A., & Ory, J.C. (1994). *Assessing faculty work: enhancing individual and institutional performance*. San Francisco, CA: Jossey-Bass.

Braskamp, L.A., Ory, J.C., & Pieper, D.M. (1981). Student written comments: dimensions of instructional quality. *Journal of Educational Psychology, 73(1)*, 65–70.

Burdsal, C.A., & Harrison, P.D. (2008). Further evidence supporting the validity of both a multidimensional profile and an overall evaluation of teaching effectiveness. *Assessment and Evaluation in Higher Education, 33(5)*, 567–76.

Cashin, W.E. (1989). *Defining and evaluating college teaching. IDEA paper no. 21*. Manhattan, Kansas: Kansas State University, Centre for Faculty Evaluation and Development.

Cashin, W.E. (1995). *Student ratings of teaching: the research revisited. IDEA paper no. 32*. Manhattan, Kansas: Kansas State University, Centre for Faculty Evaluation and Development.

Cashin, W.E. (1999). Student ratings of teaching: uses and misuses. In: Seldin, P. and Associates. *Changing practices in evaluating teaching: a practical guide* to improved faculty performance and promotion/tenure decisions. Bolton, MA: Anker Publishing. pp. 25–44.

Centra, J.A. (1979). *Determining faculty effectiveness: assessing teaching, research, and service for personnel decisions and improvement.* San Francisco, CA: Jossey-Bass.

Centra, J.A. (1993). *Reflective faculty evaluation: enhancing teaching and determining faculty effectiveness.* San Francisco, CA: Jossey-Bass.

Cohen, J. (1981). Student ratings of instruction and student achievement: a meta-analysis of multi-section validity studies. *Review of Educational Research, 51(3),* 281–309.

Feldman, K.A. (1989). Instructional effectiveness of college teachers as judged by teachers themselves, current and former students, colleagues, administrators, and external (neutral) observers. *Research in Higher Education, 30(2),* 137–94.

Frey, P.W. (1979). The Dr. Fox effect and its implications. *Instructional Evaluation, 3(2),* 1–5.

Hoyt, D.P., & Lee, E. (2002). *IDEA technical report no. 12: basic data for the revised IDEA system.* Manhattan, Kansas: Kansas State University, Centre for Faculty Evaluation and Development.

Hoyt, D.P., & Lee, E. (2002b). *IDEA technical report no. 13: disciplinary differences in student ratings.* Manhattan, Kansas: the IDEA Center.

Kulik, J.A. (2001). Student ratings: validity, utility and controversy. *New Directions for Institutional Research, 109,* 9–25.

Machell, D.F. (1989). A discourse on professional melancholia. *Community Review, 9(1–2),* 41–50.

Marsh, H.W. (1984). Students' evaluations of university teaching: dimensionality, reliability, validity, potential biases, and utility. *Journal of Educational Psychology, 76(5),* 707–54.

Marsh, H.W. (1987). Students' evaluations of university teaching: research findings, methodological issues, and directions for future research. *International Journal of Educational Research, 11(3),* 253–388.

McKeachie, W.J. (1997). Student ratings: the validity of use. *American Psychologist, 52(11),* 1218–25.

Messick, S. (1989). Validity. In: Linn, R.L. (Ed) *Educational measurement,* 3rd ed. New York: Macmillan.

Miller, R.I. (1987). *Evaluating faculty for promotion and tenure.* San Francisco, CA: Jossey-Bass.

Naftulin, D.H., Ware, J.E., & Donnelly, F.A. (1973). The Doctor Fox lecture—a paradigm of educational seduction. *Journal of Medical Education, 48(7),* 630–5.

Ory, J.C., Braskamp, L.A., & Pieper, D.M. (1980). Congruency of student evaluative information collected by three methods. *Journal of Educational Psychology, 72(2),* 181–5.

Seldin, P. (1993). The use and abuse of student ratings of professors. *Chronicle of Higher Education, 39,* 40–5.

Singh, T., Singh, D., Natu, M.V., & Zachariah, A. (1991). Hawthorne effect: a tool for improving the quality of medical education. *Indian Journal of Medical Education, 30,* 33–7.

Sixbury, G.R., & Cashin, W.E. (1995). *IDEA technical report no. 9: description of database for the IDEA diagnostic form.* Manhattan, Kansas: Kansas State University, Centre for Faculty Evaluation and Development.

Theall, M. & Franklin, J.L. (1991). Using student ratings for teaching improvements. In: Theall, M. and Franklin, J.L. (Eds). *Effective practices for improving teaching*. San Francisco, CA: Jossey-Bass.

Theall, M., & Franklin, J.L. (2001). Looking for bias in all the wrong places: a search for truth or a witch hunt in student ratings of instruction? *New Directions for Institutional Research, 109*, 45–56.

Theall, M. (1996). When meta-analysis isn't enough: a report of a symposium about student ratings, conflicting results, and issues that won't go away. *Instructional Evaluation and Faculty Development, 15*, 1–14.

FURTHER READING

Abrami, P.C., d'Apollonia, S. & Rosenfeld, S. (2007). The dimensionality of student rations of instruction: an update on what we know, do not know, and need to do. In: Perry, R.P. and Smart, J.C. (Eds). *The scholarship of teaching and learning in higher education: an evidence-based perspective*. Dordrecht, the Netherlands: Springer. pp. 385–445.

Abrami, P.C., Rosenfeld, S. & Dedic, H. (2007). Commentary: the dimensionality of student rations of instruction: what we know, and what we do not. In: Perry, R.P. and Smart, J.C. (Eds). *The scholarship of teaching and learning in higher education: an evidence-based perspective*. Dordrecht, the Netherlands: Springer. pp. 385–446.

Davis, B.G. (2009). *Tools for teaching*, 2nd ed. San Francisco, CA: Jossey-Bass.

Feldman, K.A. (2007). Identifying exemplary teachers and teaching: evidence from student ratings. In: Perry, R.P. and Smart, J.C. (Eds). *The scholarship of teaching and learning in higher education: an evidence-based perspective*. Dordrecht, the Netherlands: Springer. pp. 93–129.

Forsyth, D.R. (2003). *The Professor's guide to teaching: Psychological principles and practices*. Washington, DC: American Psychological Association.

Marsh, H.W. (2007). Students' evaluations of university teaching: dimensionality, reliability, validity, potential biases and usefulness. In: Perry, R.P. and Smart, J.C. (Eds). *The scholarship of teaching and learning in higher education: an evidence-based perspective*. Dordrecht, the Netherlands: Springer. pp. 319–83.

Murray, H.G. (2007). Low-inference teaching behaviors and college teaching effectiveness: recent developments and controversies. In: Perry, R.P. and Smart, J.C. (Eds). *The scholarship of teaching and learning in higher education: an evidence-based perspective*. Dordrecht, the Netherlands: Springer. pp. 145–200.

Theall, M. & Feldman, K.A. (2007). Commentary and update on Feldman's (1997). 'Identifying exemplary teachers and teaching: evidence from student ratings.' In: Perry, R.P. and Smart, J.C. (Eds). *The scholarship of teaching and learning in higher education: an evidence-based perspective*. Dordrecht, the Netherlands: Springer. pp. 130–43.

Svinicki, M. & McKeachie, W.J. (2011). *McKeachie's teaching tips: strategies, research, and theory for college and university teachers*, 13th ed. Belmont, CA: Wadsworth.

Wachtel, H.K. (1998). Student evaluation of college teaching effectiveness: a brief review. *Assessment and Evaluation in Higher Education, 23(2)*, 191–211.

Chapter 26

Is Objectivity Synonymous with Reliability?

Tejinder Singh, Anshu

KEY POINTS

- Objectivity is neither synonymous with, nor is it the *sine qua non* of reliability.
- Reliability is a necessary condition for validity. However it is not the only sufficient condition, as more evidences are needed, especially those that infer construct validity.
- Reliability of assessment improves by increasing testing time and wider sampling of content, rather than by standardization of assessment.
- Too much trivialization in the pursuit of objectivity takes its toll on validity.
- Subjective assessment by expert raters can provide very reliable information provided these are accompanied by prolonged and close observation, first-hand knowledge of the trainee, and training of raters in the use of scales
- There is a resurgence of expert subjective assessments in the context of competency-based medical education.

We have already learnt in Chapter 19, that internal assessment is a very useful tool, especially in view of its ability to assess areas which cannot be tested during a traditional term-end examination (Singh & Anshu, 2009). However internal assessment has hardly been implemented in India in the manner in which it was visualized. This is partly because of some reluctance on the part of teachers to accept the internal assessment guidelines in their entirety (Medical Council of India, 2019). The reason often advanced by teachers is that subjective measures are not reliable, and therefore only objective measures should be used for student assessment (Tongia, 2010).

Let us examine the notion—'all that is objective is inherently reliable, and all that is subjective is unreliable'—and see if this is true.

Objective assessments refer to assessments that are conducted within a restricted domain, using methods like multiple choice questions (MCQs), objective structured clinical examinations (OSCE), and patient management problems (PMPs), which are at a lower level of simulation. These methods have the advantage of sampling large domains of knowledge within a small time frame. Generally, objective assessments use a norm-referenced approach with no specified criteria (although some cut-off like 50% may be used).

Subjective assessment, on the other hand, could mean assessment where experts rate performance at a higher level of simulation, e.g., during an extended period of supervised practice. Here ratings are generally comparisons with a pre-determined set of criteria, and therefore this approach is criterion-referenced (Keynan et al., 1987).

To understand this issue better, it would be pertinent to recapitulate what we learnt in Chapter 1 about the contemporary concepts of validity and reliability.

Validity and Reliability: A Quick Recap

Validity refers to the appropriateness of the inferences that we draw from assessment scores. Validity is now considered a unitary concept which requires collection of evidences to infer its degree. These evidences can be in the form of content, criteria, educational impact of testing, construct, and reliability.

The most important step is determining the construct that we intend to measure. Cronbach and Meehl (1955) called this *construct formulation*. In assessment we are more interested in measuring the overall construct (e.g. clinical competence or problem solving) rather than testing for isolated bits of knowledge. Remember that when patients visit a doctor, they are looking for someone who can diagnose their problem, communicate properly, and treat them. They are not interested in fragmented skills such as whether their doctor can palpate the abdomen as per a protocol, or can rattle off a list of ten causes which can lead to their symptoms. The biggest threats to validity come from *construct underrepresentation* (CU) and *construct irrelevance variance* (CIV) (Messick, 1989). Not sampling all the domains adequately contributes to CU, while not sampling the actual construct leads to CIV. Asking trivial questions, asking too few questions, asking questions outside the syllabus, or asking only questions which require rote memorization and avoiding higher-order questions, all contribute to CU. Flawed question writing, test-wiseness, using unfair practices during a test, or teaching to the test are all sources of CIV that tend to erroneously alter test scores. We have already discussed these concepts in Chapter 1.

Construct is considered most important evidence related to validity (Downing, 2003). Construct validity refers to the sources of multiple evidences that we use to support or refute (a) our interpretation of assessment scores, (b) the inferences we draw from assessment, and (c) the decisions we make based on these tests. As the stakes get higher, our need to gather more sources of evidence increases. To do this, we will need to look in detail at the procedures of how a test is developed, what exactly is being measured, how the test is administered, scored and how the results are used in practice.

Kane (1992) talked about an argument-based approach to determine validity. He looked at the process of validation as an investigation where we present plausible arguments about how we interpret test scores, collect evidences to support our arguments, and evaluate existing evidences to justify our viewpoint. He identified the different dimensions on which our arguments can be based. These are:

❖ *observations*: how is the construct being measured, what kind of test is being used, what kind of items are used in the test, how is scoring being done, how is the test being administered, what are the qualifications, expertise and experience of the assessors, etc.;

❖ *extrapolation*: what kind of conclusions are being drawn from the scores, is there any actual relationship between test scores and predicted behaviour; and

❖ *generalizability*: will results obtained from this test conducted at a specific time and place be similar to results of the same test being conducted in other settings.

The last aspect on the list, i.e., generalizability, reinforces the importance of reliability. Kane (1992) calls 'construct' and 'reliability' the cornerstones of validity. It is important to note that reliability is a necessary condition for validity. However it is not the only sufficient condition as you see, that to determine validity, one needs more inferences than only reliability. To explain this better, let us take the familiar example of the single entrance examination scenario for post-graduate courses which are based exclusively on MCQs. While having a so-called objective examination has a high 'reliability', one will surely question if it really measures the intended construct. Do the scores obtained by students in the exam actually determine their clinical acumen and performance after they finish post-graduation?

Reliability needs to be discussed separately, although it is part of validity evidence, as there are several misgivings associated with it. Traditionally, reliability was defined as 'consistency of results' or 'obtaining the same results under same conditions'. While this definition of reliability is perfectly alright for a laboratory test, it is not appropriate for educational testing for several reasons. In the first place, doctors will encounter a wide variety of clinical contexts in real life, which are unlikely to be the same as those that they face as students in examination settings. One can hardly recreate real-life situations for each clinical case in an examination. You will see therefore, that educational testing always involves a certain degree of prediction. After all, we do not certify students as competent to handle a case of central nervous system (CNS) or a case of cardiovascular system (CVS), but we certify them as *competent to practice medicine.* Case specificity, thus, is one of the major threats to reliability and in addition, contributes to construct under-representation or construct irrelevance variance (Vleuten & Schuwirth, 1990).

Viewing reliability as 'consistency of results' also needs careful consideration. Linn and Miller (2005) point out that an estimate of reliability always refers to a particular type of consistency. We could be looking for consistency over a given task, consistency over time, or consistency across tasks. Each of these has its own uses. For example, if we are looking for how students will fare over a period of time, time consistency is more appropriate. But for certification purposes, consistency across tasks will be crucial. Thus, for different purposes, a different analysis of consistency is required, and treating reliability as a general characteristic can lead to erroneous interpretations.

Since the calculation of reliability looks at the variability of scores among students, this is useful only for norm-referenced tests—meaning thereby that if a test is reliable, a student will obtain the same rank as before (Gronlund & Waugh, 2009). It should be specifically noted that here, that the consistency is for the rank, and for not actual marks (Wass et al., 2007). Applying reliability calculations to criterion-referenced tests may lead to erroneous interpretations.

Viewing reliability only as a statistical concept has its own disadvantages. First, it is possible to mathematically manipulate reliability by interventions unrelated to the test itself. For example, by adding 20 students who do not know anything about that subject—or know everything—one can markedly improve the Cronbach alpha for that test. Secondly, it is difficult to reach the acceptable level of reliability due to logistic reasons. To give you an example, a reliable estimate of communication skills would need a minimum of 37 encounters or 6 hours of testing time. And thirdly, the generalization to other situations is poor. For instance, performing well in a CNS case is no guarantee that a student will do equally well in a case of malnutrition. As you can see, more than inter-rater variability, it is the content specificity which poses a major threat to reliability.

From these points of view, it is better to view reliability as *the degree of confidence that we can place in our results*—i.e., how confident are we that the student whom we are certifying as competent is *really* competent. This confidence will not stem from precisely measuring very limited knowledge (e.g., by using only one or two cases in the examination), but will come only from examining the student multiple *times* on multiple *cases* in multiple *situations* by multiple *assessors*. Similarly, if we strive for statistical reliability, it is more advisable to send four examiners on one case, hand each one of them a checklist, and highly structure the assessment. On the other hand, if we strive for confidence in our results, we will allot only one examiner per case, but will keep four cases for assessment. Inter-rater reliability may be high in first situation, but *inter-case reliability* will be higher in the second. In the second situation, although the marking on each case may be 'subjective', the inter-rater variability will be offset by the increased number of observations. Increasing the number of cases or test items is accepted as a useful method to increase reliability (Downing, 2004) and is considered better than minimizing inter-rater variability.

Testing time (in hours)	MCQ	Case-based essays	PMP	Oral exam	Long case	OSCE	Mini-CEX	Video assessment	Incognito SP
1	0.62	0.68	0.36	0.50	0.60	0.47	0.73	0.62	0.61
2	0.76	0.73	0.53	0.69	0.75	0.64	0.84	0.76	0.76
4	0.93	0.84	0.69	0.82	0.86	0.78	0.92	0.93	0.82
8	0.93	0.82	0.82	0.90	0.88	0.96	0.93	0.93	0.86

TABLE 26.1: Reliability as a function of testing time

(MCQ: multiple choice question; PP: patient management problem; OSCE: objective structured clinical examination; mini-CEX: mini-clinical evaluation exercise; SP: standardized patient
Source: Adapted from Vleuten (2006)

Countering Variability

Most of the times, an objective test is perceived as being more reliable. This belief has its flaws. While objectivity is an important attribute of an assessment tool, it is *not synonymous* with reliability.

Have a look a **Table 26.1** where the reported reliability of some of the assessment methods in literature have been summarized. A one-hour OSCE has a reported reliability of 0.47 compared to 0.60 of a one-hour long case. The reliability of both methods keeps increasing with increase in testing time. This implies that the reliability of OSCE is not related to either its objectivity or its structure—because if it was so, then even a one-hour OSCE would have been as reliable as an eight-hour one. Reliability therefore seems to be a function of testing time—indirectly implying that when more tasks are given to the student, it makes the test more reliable. Similarly, a mini-clinical evaluation exercise (mini-CEX), which would be regarded by many as highly subjective in comparison to an OSCE, has a much higher reliability of 0.73 even for an hour's testing time by virtue of its wider sampling of tasks, situations, and examiners. "More"—rather than precision—seems to be the keyword for reliability. **Table 26.1** also makes the point that no tool is inherently reliable (or unreliable), the degree of objectivity notwithstanding. In fact, it is possible to increase the reliability of any tool if adequate testing time is given, thereby increasing the sample of competencies to be tested.

Accuracy of measurement is always more important than its precision. Translated into educational parlance, it means concern for validity should always get priority over concern for reliability. In any case, most of the so-called objective tests like MCQs and OSCEs do not deliver the required reliability unless the testing time is stretched to 6–8 hours, something which is logistically impossible in most institutions (Cox, 1990). Unfortunately, in the process, it takes its toll on validity directly by trivializing the content (CIV), and indirectly by way of low reliability.

The Impact of 'Objectification' and the Value of 'Subjective' Expert Judgment

During the second half of the 20th century, 'subjectivity' became a bad word and began to be associated with unreliability (Eva & Hodges, 2012). Any sort of rating scale or assessment format which was viewed as 'subjective' fell out of favour. The world of assessment moved towards rigid standardization in an effort to reduce measurement error.

Norman et al., (1991) have argued that there is nothing totally objective in assessment. All assessment is ultimately subjective— there is no such thing as an 'objective test'. Even when there is a high degree of standardization, the judgment of what will be tested and what constitutes a criterion of satisfactory performance is in the hands of the assessor (Anonymous, 2010). If a test was purely objective then all teachers in all colleges would have come out with exactly similar test items for a given class. But that does not happen because a paper setter's thoughts, beliefs, and preferences play a large role in deciding which questions should make it to the test paper. What we actually do is, subjectively decide the test format/content and then try to measure it objectively. Vleuten et al., (1991) call it 'objectification'. Norman et al., (1991) have rightly pointed out that objective measures of clinical competence focused more on trivial and easily measured aspects at the cost of more important, critical but difficult to measure attributes. Eva & Hodges (2012) called it 'the atomization of medicine' saying that too much objectification seemed to have stretched the argument too far, to almost to the point of distorting it.

Variability is an inseparable part of the clinical process. The patient, the illness, the context, and the student—all contribute to variability (Cox, 1990). Standardization curbs variability. The better approach, would have been to gauge how a student responds to that variability. We do not issue grade sheets and degrees with the fine print saying "under standard test-taking conditions"—we certify our students as being competent in the real world. Over-reliance on objectification goes contrary to this premise.

A useful way to take care of the problem of variability, is to increase the breadth and size of the sample. In the educational context, it would mean that instead of limiting the assessment to precise but limited occasions, we need to have more testable opportunities. Increasing the number of observations in multiple settings and contexts, with multiple examiners over multiple periods of time is likely to give more valid and reliable results. Rigid examination structures are inappropriate for clinical tasks requiring eclectic responsive skills controlled by clinical judgment.

Checklists versus Global Rating Scales

The quest to undermine expert judgment and standardize assessment, has had its impact on performance assessment, more than on knowledge tests. The classic prototype is the use of checklists in OSCE. There have been reports to suggest that OSCEs marked with a checklist do not effectively measure knowledge, clinical skills or clinical reasoning—the three major components that go into making of clinical competence (Chumley, 2008).

The major problem with checklists is that they contain a combination of content-specific and content-non-specific items, which may not give an indication of competence. Extreme disagreements have been reported even among experts when designing OSCE checklists, which leads to inclusion of only those items which everyone agrees upon. These are usually general items (duration of symptoms, treatment history, etc.) where a student does not require content-specific knowledge to obtain credit. Consider an example of a history-taking station in neonatology. Typically, a checklist for this station would contain items related to date, time and place of birth, type of delivery, natal and immediate postnatal events, respiration, colour and need for resuscitation. A student who asks any of these questions would get appropriate credit on the checklist. However, what is interesting is that these very same points will be applicable to a neonate presenting with prematurity, birth asphyxia, neonatal jaundice or bleeding. You can see that these items on the checklist become non-content-specific. These items lower the reliability of the test by failing to distinguish between a student who asks them based on his prior knowledge of birth asphyxia, and a student who asks them mechanically. In the latter case, the exercise in history-taking becomes a test of memory, rather than being a test of clinical skills or reasoning, inducing CIV and therefore threatening validity. It has been demonstrated that while preparing for OSCEs, students pay less attention to practicing clinical skills as compared to memorizing checklists (van Luijk et al., 1990).

Checklists are appropriate for situations where several steps need to be completed in a particular sequence each time. Cardiopulmonary resuscitation provides a classic example. However in actual practice, no two students (or two consultants) ask the same questions or perform physical examination in the same sequence. Returning to the earlier example of neonatal history-taking, consider two students taking history in a neonate with suspected intrauterine infection. One student might enquire about a history of maternal lymphadenopathy because some feature in the history may indicate the possibility of toxoplasmosis; whereas, the other one may ask it regardless of the presentation. Both will get credit on the checklist, but both are operating at different levels. A trained observer will be able to see the first student applying relevant knowledge to the given situation, but a checklist will not discern this difference. Vleuten & Schuwirth (2005) feel that the validity of OSCE may be threatened by checklists.

Any test of clinical competence should be able to distinguish the level of expertise of the student. There is evidence to suggest that experts generally score low on OSCE checklists because they are able to make diagnostic and therapeutic decisions with fewer steps and do not need to go through all the steps. This creates a divergence between what experts do and what students should be taught to do at an OSCE. There are measurable differences between levels of expertise, which checklists fail to capture (Hodges et al., 1999). An expert observer passing global judgments over performance is likely to do it better than checklists, howsoever elaborate they may be.

Is Subjective Expert Judgment Reliable Then?

'Subjective' expert assessment of performance through global rating scales have been reported to have high reproducibility (Keynan et al., 1987). The reliability of a 5-point rating scale about communication skills has been reported to be higher than a 17-item checklist (Cohen et al., 1996). Another study reported acceptable reliability of 5-point global ratings compared to a 25-item checklist (Morgan et al., 2001). van Luijk & Vleuten (1992) compared the global ratings of physician raters in OSCEs, with checklist scores obtained by the same raters prior to assigning the global rating. The inter-rater reliability of the checklist was found to be higher than the global rating, but the *inter-case generalizability* of global ratings was higher than the checklists, resulting in similar test reliability.

Subjective expert assessment is considered superior for domains where art and science are interwoven (Eisner, 1979). Even untrained patients have been shown to provide reliable opinion about students' clinical skills (Wilkinson & Fontaine, 2002). Subjective evaluation has the advantage of being low cost, flexible and able to assess domains not amenable to measurement by objective methods (Neufeld & Norman, 1985). Leaving out these areas will create a serious setback to our efforts in producing competent physicians (Norman, 2010).

Certain factors postulated as being responsible for high reproducibility include—prolonged and close observation, first-hand knowledge of the trainee, and training of raters in the use of scales. In this context, it is interesting to take note of the concept of *valid* and *invalid* subjectivity (Cassidy, 2009). Valid subjectivity refers to situations where teachers have 'substantiated' opinions of students. This generally requires a long-term observation of the students in a climate of trust and commitment. Invalid subjectivity pre-supposes a deficit in the interaction and the 'unconfirmed' nature of opinion. Callaham et al., (1998) also demonstrated that the quality of subjective ratings correlated with expertise. Expertise of the raters is a crucial factor in ensuring validity and reliability. Together, these two arguments demand that the rater should not only be a subject expert, but also be well-versed with students' working over a period of time (Virk et al., 2020). The trustworthiness of subjective assessments is improved when there is a sense of mutual reciprocity between the teachers and students (Gillespe, 2005).

Implications for Educational Practice

What are the implications of this knowledge in clinical practice? For assessing isolated clinical skills, especially during early clinical years, checklists might be a better option as they are easy to mark and may not require expert examiners for marking. However, one needs to exercise caution against unintended educational effects of checklists like encouraging rote memorization without an understanding of the outcome of the skills, and subsequent CIV. When assessing clinical cases, rating scales appear to be better, as there is less emphasis on details of the procedure, and more on the effectiveness and proficiency of the student. For complex skills like communication or professionalism, checklists are difficult to be constructed without trivialization of the content. However, when standardized patients are used, rating scales may be better in order to avoid non-expert opinion.

Similarly, open-ended questions might be better for classroom tests when the number of students is less, but for large-scale entrance examinations, MCQs from a validated question bank may be more appropriate. Norman et al., (1991) rightly point out that

> *"... it is clear that the choice of a test format—written or performance—cannot be made on the basis of an unconditional appeal to objectivity. Objectivity, in an empirical sense, does not necessarily result from strategies of objectification, and the application of these strategies may have undesirable consequences. Decisions must be made as a result of careful consideration to other issues resulting from the purpose of the testing situation—practicality, educational impact, acceptability—rather than on the dogma that objective methods, like Orwell's four-legged animals, are inherently superior".*

Since the 1990s, there have been a number of developments in trying to find 'new' approaches to assessment. These have been variously been referred to as authentic assessment, alternate assessment, direct assessment or performance-based assessment (Linn & Miller, 2005). The connecting thread for all these new approaches has been to move away from merely recognizing or knowing the right answer, to actually performing a task or constructing a response. This is in line with the constructivist approach to learning.

Much of the misinterpretation prevailing around reliability can be avoided if we recognize the limited nature of information that assessment scores provide. This recognition is a critical component of proper use of results. In most educational decisions, tests provide just one type of information, which should always be supplemented by past records of achievement and other types of assessment data. Linn and

Miller (2005) are right in saying that no major educational decision should be taken on test scores alone.

As is evident, the notion "everything objective is reliable" is certainly not true. However the corollary that "subjective is more reliable" is also not unconditionally true. Subjective assessment requires an expert opinion and cannot be left to lay observers. We will also remind you of Cassidy's (2009) viewpoint again, that valid subjectivity comes only with 'substantiated' opinions of students requiring their long-term observation in a climate of trust and commitment.

With the introduction of competency-based medical education (CBME), medical education has entered a 'post-psychometric' phase of assessment, with very diverse domains of expertise. Most of us would agree that perhaps in our pursuit to standardize and objectify assessments, we may have moved too far in its criticism. Nevertheless, a renewed interest in the revival of subjective judgment in assessment (Rotthoff, 2018; Virk et al., 2020) puts forth some interesting questions about what judgment is and how to rationally aggregate multiple judgments without compromising on the abundant expert perspectives.

The Medical Council of India (MCI, 2019a) module on assessment for undergraduate medical education lays emphasis on use of ongoing developmental feedback, direct observation, multiple assessors, and use of multiple tools for students' assessment under its competency-based curriculum. Such a system can only be strengthened with the relevant use of expert subjective assessment. Having implemented CBME, the big challenge that now lies ahead is to understand how subjectivity in assessment can be reintroduced while retaining 'rigor' in assessment.

Hodges (2013) argues, and rightly so, that the clinical assessment of students can be compared to clinical judgment:

> "With experience, expert clinicians become more rapid and more accurate in their recognition of patterns. There is no reason to believe that this process does not operate in education."

We should not be depriving students of this all-important source of learning. There seems to be a resurgence of subjective assessments worldwide (ten Cate & Regehr, 2019; Hodges, 2013) and this looks like a welcome trend!

REFERENCES

Anonymous (2010). Assessment. [online] Available from http://www.learningandteaching.info/teaching/assessment.htm [Last accessed August, 2020].

Callaham, M.L., Baxt, W.G., Waekerley, J.F., & Wears, R.L. (1998). Reliability of editors' subjective quality ratings of peer review of manuscripts. *Journal of the American Medical Association, 280,* 229–31.

Cassidy, S. (2009). Subjectivity and the valid assessment of pre-registration student nurse clinical learning outcomes: implication for mentors. *Nurse Education Today, 29(1),* 33–9.

Chumley, H.S. (2008). What does an OSCE checklist measure? *Family Medicine, 40,* 589–91.

Cohen, D.S., Colliver, J.A., Marcy, M.S., Fried, E.D., & Schwartz, M.H. (1996). Psychometric properties of a checklist and rating scale form used to assess interpersonal and communication skills. *Academic Medicine, 71,* S87–9.

Cox, K. (1990). No OSCAR for OSCA. *Medical Education, 24,* 340–5.

Cronbach, L.J., & Meehl, P.E. (1955). Construct validity in psychological tests. *Psychological Bulletin, 52,* 281-302

Downing, S.M. (2003). Validity: on the meaningful interpretation of assessment data. *Medical Education, 37,* 830–7.

Downing, S.M. (2004). Reliability: on the reproducibility of assessment data. *Medical Education, 38,* 1006–12.

Eisner, E.W. (1979). *The educational imagination.* 2nd ed. New York McMillan Publishing Co Inc.

Eva, K.W., & Hodges, B.D. (2012). Scylla or Charybdis? Can we navigate between objectification and judgement in assessment? *Med Education, 46(9),* 914-9.

Gillespe, T.M. (2005). Student teacher connection: a place of possibility. *Journal of Advanced Nursing, 52,* 211–9.

Gronlund, N.E., & Waugh, C.K. (2009). *Assessment of student achievement,* 9th ed. New Jersey: Pearson.

Hodges, B., Regehr, G., McNaughton, N., Tiberius, R., & Hanson, M. (1999). OSCE checklists do not capture increasing level of expertise. *Academic Medicine, 74(10),* 1129–34.

Hodges, B. (2013). Assessment in the post psychometric era: learning to love the subjective and collective. *Medical Teacher, 35,* 564–8.

Kane, M. (1992). An argument-based approach to validation. *Psychological Bulletin, 112,* 527–35.

Keynan, A, Friedman, M., & Benbassat, J. (1987). Reliability of global rating scales in the assessment of competence in medical students. *Medical Education, 21(6),* 477–81.

Linn, R.L., & Miller, M.D. (2005). *Measurement and assessment in teaching,* 9th ed. New Jersey: Merrill Prentice Hall.

Medical Council of India. (2019). Graduate medical education regulations, 2019. [online] Available from https://mciindia.org/ActivitiWebClient/open/getDocument?path=/Documents/Public/Portal/Gazette/GME-06.11.2019.pdf [Last accessed August, 2020].

Medical Council of India. (2019a). Module on assessment for competency-based education. [online] Available from https://www.nmc.org.in/wp-content/uploads/2020/01/Module_Competence_based_02.09.2019.pdf [Last accessed November, 2020].

Messick, S. (1989). Validity. In: Linn, R.L. (Ed). *Educational measurement,* 3rd ed. New York: American Council on Education and Macmillan. pp. 13–104.

Morgan, P.J., Cleavehogg, D., & Guest, C.B. (2001). A comparison of global ratings and checklist scores from an undergraduate assessment using an anesthesia simulator. *Academic Medicine, 76,* 1053–5.

Neufeld, V.R., & Norman, G.R. (1985). *Assessing clinical competence.* New York: Springer.

Norman, G.R., van der Vleuten, C.P.M., & De Graaff, E. (1991). Pitfalls in the pursuit of objectivity: issues of validity, efficiency and acceptability. *Medical Education, 25(2),* 119–26.

Norman, G.R. (2010). Non-cognitive factors in health sciences education: from clinic floor to the cutting floor. *Advances in Health Sciences Education, 15,* 1–8.

Rotthoff, T. (2018). Standing up for subjectivity in the assessment of competencies. *GMS Journal for Medical Education, 35(3),* Doc29.

Singh T., & Anshu. (2009). Internal assessment revisited. *National Medical Journal of India, 22(2),* 82–4.

ten Cate, O., & Regehr, G. (2019). The power of subjectivity in the assessment of medical trainees. *Academic Medicine, 94(3),* 333–7.

Tongia, S.K. (2010). Medical Council of India internal assessment system in undergraduate medical education system. *National Medical Journal of India, 23,* 46.

van der Vleuten, C.P.M., Norman, G.R., & De Graaff, E. (1991). Pitfalls in the pursuit of objectivity: issues of reliability. *Medical Education, 25,* 110–8.

van der Vleuten, C.P.M., & Schuwirth, L. (2005). Assessing professional competence: from methods to programs. *Medical Education, 39,* 309–17.

van der Vleuten, C.P.M. (2006). Life beyond OSCE. [online] Available from http://www. fdg.unimaas.nl/educ/cees/wba [Last accessed August, 2020].

van Luijk, S.J., van der Vleuten, C.P.M., & van Schleven, S.M. (1990). Validity and generalizability of global ratings in an OSCE. Academic Medicine, 66, 545–8.

van Luijk, S.J., van der Vleuten, C.P.M., & van Schelven, S.M. (1990). The relationship between content and psychometric characteristics in performance-based testing. In: Bender, W., Hiemstra, R.J., Scherpbier, A.J. and Zwierstra, R.P. (Eds). (1990). *Teaching and assessing clinical competence.* Groningen: Boekwerk Publishers. pp. 202–7.

van Luijk, S.J., & van der Vleuten, C.P.M. (1992). A comparison of checklists and rating scales in performance-based testing. In: Hart, I.R., Harden, R., and Mulholland, H. (Eds). *Current developments in assessing clinical competence.* Montreal: Can-Heal Publications. pp. 357–82.

Virk, A., Joshi, A., Mahajan, R., & Singh, T. (2020). The power of subjectivity in competency-based assessment. *J Postgrad Med, 66,* 200-205

Wass, V., Bowden, R., & Jackson, N. (2007). The principles of assessment design. In: Jackson, N., Jamieson, A. and Khan A. (Eds). *Assessment in medical education and training: a practical guide,* 1st ed. New York: Radcliffe Publishing.

Wilkinson, T.J., & Fontaine, S. (2002). Patients' global ratings of student competence: unreliable contamination or gold standard? *Medical Education, 36(12),* 1117–21.

Chapter 27

Faculty Development for Better Assessment

Tejinder Singh

KEY POINTS

- Faculty development is crucial to build quality of assessment.
- Faculty development can be both, formal and informal.
- Training should promote application of skills and knowledge.
- Internal assessment provides a useful informal opportunity to train junior teachers in assessment.

We have discussed various means and ways to assess the learning of medical students in this book. One point which stands out very consistently is that validity and reliability are not inherent properties of any tool. Rather the way an assessment tool is used makes it valid or not. MCQs, for example, are very good tools for testing even higher domains of learning, but they are often used badly and are reduced to tests of simple recall. OSCEs, for example, can provide very useful inputs about attainment of practical skills, but end up being used as theory stations in the garb of tests of practical skills. Developing capabilities of teachers who are going to use newer and existing methods of assessment is crucial to ensure quality in assessment.

Faculty development (FD) is one such intervention, which can help us to develop the expertise of medical teachers. Although several definitions are available for FD, we prefer to see it as "a broad range of activities that institutions use to renew or assist faculty in their multiple roles" (Steinert, 2000). A perusal of this definition brings out some key points, i.e., it is a planned activity, it prepares teachers for various roles and that it aims to improve the knowledge and skills of teachers.

Literature is replete with reports describing various types of programs for FD (Centra, 1978). However, in this chapter, we shall restrict ourselves to FD for student assessment. To be able to use

various assessment tools in a meaningful way, the faculty needs to know about:
- Use of assessment in various settings
- Basic principles of assessment, including attributes (validity, reliability, educational impact) and utility of assessment tools
- Assessment for learning, formative assessment, internal assessment
- Taxonomy of learning, blueprinting, setting a question paper
- Miller's pyramid, authentic and integrated assessment
- Competency-based assessment
- Strengths and weaknesses of various tests and tools
- Writing quality MCQs and OSCE stations
- Standard setting (absolute and relative)
- Techniques of direct observation and providing meaningful feedback.
- Application of these concepts in designing tests to maximize learning

This is a long list, but since assessment has the most profound influence on learning, it is worth investing time and effort in this area. We would like to repeat here that in the event of any discrepancy between the written and taught curriculum, it is always the examinations which guide student learning. As an example, the new curriculum might stress integrated teaching, but if we continue to assess using conventional modalities, it is unlikely that students will learn in an integrated manner. We would also like to caution that the purpose of FD for better assessment is not to expect that most medical teachers will become competent to plan a high-stakes assessment (like for example pre-postgraduate examination, though *some* of them may do that). Rather, the purpose should be to ensure that *all* of them will be able to use the formative effect of locally developed assessment to enhance learning.

Of the two, formative assessment is considered more useful as an aid to learning than summative assessment (Rushton, 2005)—yet it is formative assessment which is also considered inferior to summative. Most of the times, assessment planning focuses on the summative function because of the stakes and the competitive nature attached to it—and hardly any guidelines are provided for formative assessment. Even where it is practiced in the garb of internal assessment, the purpose is still summative (Singh & Anshu, 2009).

Since there are generally no consequences attached to formative assessment, teachers see it as an extra effort and waste of time. Students on the other hand, do not take it seriously as it does not contribute to final grades. This is not to say that medical teachers in India do not value formative assessment. In one of our studies on the needs for FD in India (Singh et al., 2010), "formative versus summative assessment" and "providing feedback" emerged as important topics which made it to the list of top ten themes which teachers wanted to be included in assessment training. Many of these (mis)concepts may be related to lack of research in this area. Limited research available from India indicates a good predictive utility and construct validity of internal assessment (Badyal et al, 2017).

It is not that students do not like to receive feedback on how they performed—most of the times they shy away from feedback is because it becomes critical, judgmental and an exercise in fault finding. Honest feedback which is non-directive in nature is acceptable to most adult learners. In Chapter 24, we have emphasized the need for a culture of trust and understanding. Putting these two together, the skill of giving developmental feedback emerges as a key component for practice and acceptability of formative assessment.

Training alone however may not be the answer to the problem. In addition to providing training on various points listed above, FD also needs to include a component of attitudinal change and a component of student development. During some of the training sessions conducted by us on OSCE in colleges which had no exposure to it, students were shocked at the concept of someone standing there with a checklist and observing them! Such factors affect the acceptability of formative assessment and reduce its utility (Vlueten & Schuwirth, 2005).

The contemporary concept of authentic assessment means taking assessment to the setting where knowledge and skills are actually going to be used. Consequently, paradigms like WPBA (Norcini, 2010) are attracting more and more attention the world over compared to rigorously designed snapshot summative assessments. Almost all the tools used for WPBA like mini-CEX, DOPS and MSF rely a lot on direct observation and feedback. We have been using many of the concepts discussed above in the training programs that we conduct. In addition to theoretical inputs regarding attributes and utility of assessment tools using interactive training methodology, we have also started including two very important aspects in our training programs. One of them is the skill of providing feedback using an accepted framework (Pendleton et al., 1984). This is not restricted to any formal session but is liberally used during other sessions like microteaching also. Participants are encouraged to provide open-ended feedback to each other on various aspects.

The other important area is inclusion of tools using direct observation (e.g., mini-CEX). A live or a recorded demonstration of a clinical encounter which is followed by a detailed feedback on directly observed behavior is an integral part of this session. We also encourage our students and postgraduates/residents to be part of these sessions so that the participants can see the utility of immediate feedback. During exit interviews with participants, feedback emerges as the most important theme which they have been able to use back home.

Formal Approaches to Faculty Development

Workshops, seminars, and short-term trainings provide a good opportunity for FD. A 3-day program (12–15 hours) generally suffices to cover most issues related to assessment. We begin with a description of taxonomies of learning, emphasizing the need to include all domains of learning in the assessment plan. This is followed by interactive discussion on uses and attributes of good assessment. We also discuss about formative/summative assessment, and criterion/norm-referenced testing. Assessment of knowledge includes sessions on design of essay questions and their variants (structured essays, modified essays, short answers, etc.). A hands-on experience is provided for all sessions. Similarly, the session on MCQs includes critique of dummy MCQs, writing MCQs to test higher levels of learning and their variants (extended matching, key feature, etc.).

Assessment of practical skills is taught using OSCE, which includes a demonstration followed by practice in developing OSCE stations. For basic sciences, its variant objective structured practical examination (OSPE) is also included. Overcoming the limitations of a long case (lack of observation, content specificity, etc.) is discussed using role plays, as is mini-CEX. There are separate sessions on providing feedback.

Assessment of ethics, professionalism, and communication skills is also included. Internal assessment provides a very useful means for assessing these skills and participants are encouraged to design situations where these skills can be assessed. Taking feedback from students to improve teaching is used to encourage the concept of formative assessment. Acceptance of these sessions as indicated by participant reactions and change in perceptions about their utility using *retrospective pre-evaluations* are generally good (Pratt et al., 2000).

Informal Approaches to Faculty Development

In addition to formal training described above, we also make use of several informal approaches. The core faculty, for example, also conducts sensitization meetings in various departments to tide over the problem of collecting large number of teachers from busy areas. OSCE and mini-CEX have been the most common topics discussed and demonstrated in such on-site sessions. Developing peer mentoring is another useful approach, especially for younger faculty members. As already discussed, students are involved in many of these sessions.

Promoting Application: Transfer-oriented Training

Training programs—formal and informal—help to equip the participants with knowledge, skills and sometimes attitudes related to assessment. However, application of new knowledge and skills depends on several other factors. These include the culture within the organization/department, supervisor and peer support and regulatory issues. Since such rules are never specified by regulatory bodies, using assessment for learning is never a problem from that perspective. However, convincing students, colleagues, and superiors is generally a problem.

Convincing students becomes easy once they see the benefit of formative role of assessment. Several interventions have been tried to make formative assessment more acceptable. Some of these include use of "grade-less" assignments (Hattie, 1987), where only feedback is provided to the students. Students also seem to be more receptive to feedback in the absence of marks (Black & Wiliam, 1998). However, as already discussed, it is a challenge to sustain such assessment. The key to sustenance lies in making the feedback useful, developmental rather than critical, based on what is observed rather than on historical facts and making it immediately available. Feedback should be provided at a time when students still have time to improve their performance. Providing a nonthreatening culture is vital to success of a learning culture. We have already discussed these in Chapter 24.

Organizational support (in terms of support from Head of the department and Dean) is also important and needs to be systematically managed. Not only is this support required in terms of logistics, but also in terms of sustainability of efforts. Though it is still an alien concept in medical education, organizational development strategies have been very successfully used for designing and implementing many innovative programs in other areas (World Bank, 2010).

We will like to end this discussion by revisiting the doctrine of WYPIWYG *(what you put is what you get)*. Assessment can be a wonderful tool if appropriately used for better learning, but it could also be a potent destroyer of good learning if used inappropriately. FD can make all that difference between appropriate and inappropriate use of assessment.

Model Program for Training

This plan is being used for training on assessment. Suitable modifications in content and emphasis may be made **(Box 27.1)**. Throughout the program importance of feedback should be emphasized.

Chapter 27: Faculty Development for Better Assessment

BOX 27.1: Model training program

Day 1

9.00–9.45	Why assess	Discuss use of assessment as a learning tool
9.45–10.15	Types of assessment	Classifications based on purpose, timing or utility (formative/summative; criterion/norm-referenced) Differences and commonalities
10.30–11.30	Attributes of good assessment	Discuss validity, reliability, feasibility, acceptability, and educational impact
11.30–12.30	Domains of learning	Recap the three domains with appropriate examples Importance of each for a physician
12.30–13.00	What to assess	Miller pyramid
14.00–15.00	Assessment of knowledge: Essay questions	Strengths, weaknesses, how to improve, newer varieties Group work
15.30–17.00	Short answer questions	Supply type Strengths, weaknesses, how to improve, newer varieties Group work

Day 2

9.00–10.00	Multiple choice questions	Strengths, weaknesses, how to improve, newer varieties Critique of given MCQs Group work
10.00–11.00	Item analysis and question banking	Concept, uses, methods, interpretation of indices, role in improving assessment
11.30–13.00	Objective structured clinical examination (OSCE)	Concept, principles, demonstration, strengths, weakness, how to improve them
14.00–15.00	Designing OSCE stations	Group work to write stations
15.30–17.00	Educational feedback	Role in making learning better, how to give, framework for giving feedback, group work/ appreciative inquiry regarding best feedback experienced Group work

Contd...

Contd...

Day 3

9.00–10.00	Mini-clinical evaluation exercise (mini-CEX)	Rationale, process, advantages, demonstration
10.00–11.00	Oral examinations	Strengths, weaknesses, how to improve Group work
11.30–13.00	Assessment of soft learning areas	Ethics, communication, professionalism Direct observation, multisource feedback
14.00–15.00	Blueprinting and question paper design	Steps, advantages, sampling
15.30–16.15	Programmatic assessment	Concept, utility, logistics, application
16.15–17.00	Competency-based assessment	Peculiarities, tools, setting, reinforce the concept of feedback

REFERENCES

Badyal, D.K., Singh, S., & Singh, T. (2017). Construct validity and predictive utility of internal assessment in undergraduate medical education. *National Medical Journal of India, 30(3)*, 151–4.

Black, P., & Wiliam, D. (1998). Inside the black box: raising standards through classroom assessment. *Phi Delta Kappan, 80(2)*, 139–44.

Centra, J. (1978). Types of faculty development programs. *Journal of Higher Education, 49*, 151–62.

Hattie, J.A. (1987). Identifying the salient facets of a model of student learning: a synthesis of meta-analyses. *International Journal of Educational Research, 11(2)*, 187–212.

Norcini, J.J. (2010). Workplace-based assessment. In: Swanwick, T. (Ed) *Understanding medical education: evidence theory and practice*, 1st ed. West Sussex: Wiley-Blackwell.

Pendleton, D., Schofield, T., Tate, P., & Havelock, P. (1984). *The consultation: an approach to teaching and learning*. Oxford: Oxford University Press. pp. 68–72.

Pratt, C.C., McGuigan, W.M., & Katzev, A.R. (2000). Measuring program outcomes: using retrospective pretest methodology. *American Journal of Evaluation, 21(3)*, 330–2.

Rushton, A. (2005). Formative assessment: a key to deep learning? *Medical Teacher, 27(6)*, 509–13.

Singh, T., & Anshu. (2009). Internal assessment revisited. *National Medical Journal of India, 22*, 82–5.

Singh, T., Moust, J., & Wolfhagen, I. (2010). Needs and priorities for faculty development in India. *National Medical Journal of India, 23*, 297–302.

Steinert, Y. (2000). Faculty development in the new millennium: key challenges and future directions. *Medical Teacher, 22*, 44–50.

Van der Vleuten, C.P.M., & Schuwirth, L.W. (2005). Assessing professional competence: from methods to programmes. *Medical Education, 39(3)*, 309–17.

World Bank. (2010). *Organizational development as a framework for creating anti-poverty strategies and action*. [online] Available from http://info.worldbank.org/etools/docs/library/114925/eum/docs/eum/ethiopiaeum/Module2OrganizationalDevelopmentEth.pdf [Last accessed August, 2020].

Chapter 28

Online Resources for Assessment

Chinmay Shah, Anshu

KEY POINTS

☞ This is a list of resources available online which can be used to conduct online assessment.
☞ It is important to remember that the basic principles of assessment that are followed in classroom settings must be followed online as well. Technology is merely a medium to facilitate application of these principles in online settings.

Introduction

After the onset of the coronavirus disease (COVID) pandemic, academic institutions have been forced to explore online assessment. There are multiple tools available for online assessment. These range from assessment of multiple choice questions (MCQs), short answer questions and can go up to correcting traditional answer sheets using technology. Students can be provided instant feedback on their progress online. Teachers can more easily monitor learners' progress and achievement of milestones. The possibility of automated marking accelerates a once time-consuming burden for institutions (Cantillon et al., 2004; Dennick et al., 2009). Online lectures, video feedbacks and assessments, portfolio-based education and assessments, remote clinical response and virtual patients are going to be part of medical education in coming years (Sahi et al., 2020). However, it must be remembered that technology is merely a tool. The basic pedagogical aspects of delivering assessment must not be forgotten, and tools must be chosen depending on the needs of the teachers and students. Ultimately, the effectiveness of the assessment will be judged based on the content of the assessment and not on the technological format (Joshi et al., 2020).

Listed here are resources which can be useful in conducting online assessment. Each resource is accompanied by its Uniform Resource Locator (URL) (which is functional and verified as on 1st November 2020) and a short description of its use. Finally, at the end of the description is a mention of whether the application is freeware or a paid version in the parenthesis, as of 1st December 2020.

Learning Management Systems which Offer Resources for Integrated Learning and Assessment

1. **MOODLE:**
   URL: *https://moodle.org/*
   MOODLE (an acronym for Modular Object-Oriented Dynamic Learning Environment) is a free and open-source learning platform and course management system written in PHP and distributed under the GNU General Public License having full features of a virtual classroom including teaching and assessment. It is designed to provide educators, administrators, and learners with a single robust, secure, and integrated system to create personalized learning environments. (Free)

2. **G Suite for Education:**
   URL: *https://edu.google.com/products/gsuite-for-education/*
   G Suite for Education is a suite of free Google tools and services that are tailored for certain schools or higher non-profit educational institutions, accredited by an accepted accreditation body. It is available globally at a discounted price for all educational institutions. The tools include Google Meet, Google Classroom, 10,000 user licenses with Gmail accounts for faculty and students, Google Drive and other security features. (Free and paid versions available depending on institution)

3. **Blackboard:**
   URL: *https://blackboard.com/*
   Blackboard is an interactive learning management system (LMS) suitable for higher education institutions which offers integrated facilities for online, learning, collaboration, and assessment. The features include customized content authoring, virtual classroom facilities and calendars to warn learners of deadlines. (Paid)

4. **CANVAS:**
   URL: *https://www.instructure.com/canvas/*
   This is an LMS which helps in course organization, resource management, student guidance, and personalized learning. (Paid)

5. **Drupal:**
   URL: *https://drupal.org/*
   Drupal is an open-source content management system for creating digital experiences that will help to engage, enrol, and retain students, faculty, and alumni. (Paid)

6. **mCourse:**
   URL: *https://mcourse.co.in/*
   This is a Mobile LMS compatible with all mobiles having the following following features for competency-based education.
   For teachers: Option of creating and grading tests, assignments,

discussions, and certificate generation. This mobile app has features in test like review letter, autosubmission. Questions can be of an image, video or true/false format, etc. Other features include autograding with negative marking in MCQ tests, conduct of time-bound examination, generation of course completion certificate etc. *For students*: Access to all materials, assignments, discussions, tests in mobile. *For colleges*: Easy to use LMS. Can assign students to teacher, students to course, can post information to all students, user friendly app with option to upload teacher, student and test in bulk. (Free Trial + Paid versions)

Resources for Creating, Distributing and Grading Assessments

1. **Google Classroom:**
   URL: *https://classroom.google.com/*
   Google Classroom is a free web service, developed by Google for educational institutes, that aims to simplify creating, distributing, and grading assignments in a paperless way. The primary purpose of Google Classroom is to streamline the process of sharing files between teachers and students. (Free)
2. **Google Forms:**
   URL: *https://google.com/forms/about*
   Google Forms is a survey administration app that is included in the Google Drive Office Suite along with Google Docs, Google Sheets, and Google Slides. Google Forms features all the collaboration and sharing features found in Docs, Sheets, and Slides. It can be used to design assessments and quizzes. It has various question types like short answer text, paragraph text, multiple choice, checkboxes, dropdown select menus (lists), upload, linear scale, multiple choice grid, checkbox grid, etc. There is also the option of shuffling the questions. (Free)
3. **MyGradeBook:**
   URL: *https://www.mygradebook.com/*
   MyGradeBook allows teachers to grade assignments, print out reports, email learners automatically and let them access information, from wherever they have got an internet connection. (Free Trial version)

Interactive Tools for Formative Assessment and Enhanced Student Engagement in Online Sessions

1. **Pear Deck:**
   URL:*https://peardeck.com/*
   Pear Deck is a live slides presentation tool that works with Google Slides or PowerPoint presentations. It allows students to see the slides on their own devices. With Pear Deck, interactive slides can

be added to solicit feedback, do a quick formative check, or just see how your students are feeling today. Pear Deck helps in active learning and formative assessment during online as well as self-paced teaching. (Free + Paid versions)

2. **Mentimeter.com:**
URL: *https://www.mentimeter.com/*
Mentimeter can be used to create interactive presentations and get real-time input from online students with live polls, quizzes, word clouds, questions and answers (Q&As). Once the presentation is over, these results can be shared or exported for further analysis. (Free)

3. **AnswerGarden:**
URL: *https://www.answergarden.ch/*
AnswerGarden is an easy to use minimalistic feedback tool. This can be used to elicit real-time audience participation, online brainstorming, polling, and classroom feedback. Users can create, share, and answer questions without signing up for accounts. It can be used both in synchronous and asynchronous mode where responses appear like word clouds. (Free)

4. **QuizSlides:**
URL: *https://quizslides.co.uk/*
QuizSlides is a cloud-based quiz platform that enables easy creation of online quizzes from PowerPoint slides. It currently supports four different quiz formats—traditional, answer-until-correct (two types), subset selection, and elimination. These include novel multiple-choice test formats and marking schemes which have been designed to yield more reliable aggregate scores as compared with traditional multiple choice tests by reducing the occurrence of guesswork. (Free Trial version)

5. **GoSoapBox:**
URL: *https://www.gosoapbox.com/*
It is a web-based clicker tool to keep students engaged. A feature called Confusion Barometer can be used to gain real-time insight into student comprehension by anonymous responses. Besides this, there are features which enable polling, online discussions, Q&A, quizzes, and assignments. (Free for up to 30 students)

6. **Slido:**
URL: *https://www.sli.do/*
Slido makes it easy to engage online audience while running large video conferences, webinars or a small team meeting. It is compatible with video conferencing tools like Zoom, Skype, Webex or GoToMeeting. It allows online polls, discussions, and Q&A features. (Paid)

7. **Explain Everything:**
URL: *https://explaineverything.com/*
Explain Everything is a whiteboard app which provides teachers and students an opportunity to teach, present, sketch, and create

videos. This can be used in both synchronous and asynchronous settings to share thinking, reflect upon knowledge building, and assess both products and processes of learning. Explain Everything adds the opportunity to collaborate in real time. (Free)

8. **VideoNotes:**
   URL: *http://videonot.es/*
   VideoNotes enables one to take notes while watching videos. The right side of the screen plays the video, while the left side gives you a notepad to type on. This can be synchronized with Google Drive to share or save notes. Clicking on a note takes the viewer directly to the relevant video section. Teachers can easily see student feedback against the video. (Paid)

9. **Tozzl:**
   URL: *http://tozzl.com/*
   This is a digital pinboard that integrates media (such as YouTube videos, files, and images) and Twitter feeds. It is similar to other digital spaces for communication of student learning, ideas, and reflection. (Free)

10. **Blogger:**
    URL: *https://blogger.com/*
    This is a free Google tool which can be used to ask students to write reflections. (Free)

11. **Nearpod:**
    URL: *https://nearpod.com/*
    This tool helps in gathering evidence of student learning and works like an all-student response system but can also create differentiated lessons based on the data collected. The basic version (30 students or less) is free. (Free + Paid)

12. **Peergrade:**
    URL: *https://www.peergrade.io/*
    Peergrade is a platform that allows teachers to create assignments and upload rubrics. Students upload work and are anonymously assigned peer work to review according to the rubric. (Free + Paid versions)

13. **Plickers:**
    URL: *https://get.plickers.com/*
    Plickers allows teachers to collect real-time formative assessment data without the need for student devices. (Free)

14. **Backchannel Chat:**
    URL: *https://backchannelchat.com/*
    This site offers a teacher-moderated version of Twitter. It is an extension of the in-the-moment conversation that might be to capture the chat, create a tag cloud, and see what surfaces as a focus of the conversation. (Paid)

Resources to Create Customized Quizzes and Gamification Apps

1. **Kahoot!:**
   URL: *https://kahoot.it/*
   Kahoot is a game-based learning platform, used for creating learning games known as Kahoots. These are user-generated multiple-choice quizzes that can be accessed via a web browser or the Kahoot app. (Free Trial version)

2. **Socrative:**
   URL: *https://socrative.com/higher-ed/*
   Socrative is an all-in-one easy to use assessment tool which allows quizzes, surveys, and team activities to be created. These can be used to track learner understanding in real time during online sessions. (Trial version is free with restrictions on number of students)

3. **Hot Potatoes:**
   URL: *https://hotpot.uvic.ca/*
   The Hot Potatoes suite includes six applications, enabling you to create interactive multiple choice, short answer, jumbled-sentence, crossword, matching/ordering, and gap-fill exercises for the World Wide Web. Hot Potatoes is freeware, and can be used for any purpose or project. (Freeware)

4. **iSpring QuizMaker:**
   URL: *https://www.ispringsolutions.com/support/quizmaker*
   This is a quiz maker to build online assessments. With iSpring QuizMaker, one can create interactive tests and quizzes, set up custom scoring, and evaluate learner progress online. (Paid version)

5. **Quizizz.com:**
   URL: *https://quizizz.com/*
   This can be used to create and deliver quizzes in synchronous and asynchronous settings. Real-time input can be obtained from distant learners. (Free)

6. **Learnclick:**
   URL: *https://www.learnclick.com/*
   Learnclick is a very versatile quiz creator, which can be used by teachers to easily create creating online quizzes with formats like gap-filling exercises (also known as cloze tests), drag and drop questions, dropdown answers, MCQs, and more. (Paid version)

7. **QuizFaber:**
   URL: *https://quizfaber.com/index.php/en/*
   QuizFaber is a freeware software for Windows that enables you to create multimedia quizzes as HTML documents. This program simplifies quiz-making in HTML without any prior knowledge of HTML or JavaScript. The quiz is ready to be published on the internet, or on a local PC. It is possible to create and manage many types of questions: questions with multiple choices, true or false questions, questions with open answers, gap-filling exercises

and matching words. It can be fully customized for the choice of background images, colors, sounds, and font types. The quiz result can be saved on a web server, sent through e-mail, stored on Google cloud (Google Drive) or into internal server. The quiz can be exported into Moodle e-learning platform or imported from Moodle XML format. (Freeware)

8. **ViewletQuiz:**
URL: *https://www.qarbon.com/presentation-software/viewletquiz/*
ViewletQuiz allows one to create customizable interactive Flash-based quizzes and surveys without need for extensive training and development time. (Free Trial version)

9. **Helpteaching.com:**
URL: *https://www.helpteaching.com/*
This is mostly for elementary and high school students, but the test maker feature can be used to make your own multiple choice tests and quizzes in printable and online versions. (Free Trial version)

10. **Yacapaca.com:**
URL: *https://yacapaca.com/*
This tool allows creation of quizzes with six types of questions. Feedback on performance can be delivered to students online, and it allows monitoring of learner performance. (Free)

11. **Online quiz creator:**
URL: *https://www.onlinequizcreator.com/features/multiple-choice-test-maker/item10051*
This app can be used for creating online MCQs through online platform. (Free Trial + Paid)

12. **Triventy:**
URL: *http://www.triventy.com/*
Triventy is a free quiz game platform that allows teachers to create quizzes students and takes it in real time. These live quizzes provide teachers with real-time data on student understanding of classroom concepts. Students can respond to quiz questions with mobile devices and laptops. (Free)

Resources to Create Interactive Videos

1. **Edpuzzle:**
URL: *https://edpuzzle.com/*
Edpuzzle can easily create interactive video lessons for students and can be integrated into other LMSs. This app can reuse available videos from the internet, customize them with explanations and clarifications, as well as embed quizzes with the video. Students' understanding and progress can be tracked with these analytics. (Free + Paid versions)

2. **PlayPosit:**
URL: *https://go.playposit.com*
PlayPosit is an interactive web-based video platform that allows instructors and instructional designers to customize videos on

YouTube and other sites as much or as little as they would like. Educators can embed quiz type questions into videos, and this can be used for formative assessment inside and outside the classroom. Data can be analyzed to gain insights into educational trends in the classroom. (Paid version)

3. **H5p Content:**
   URL: *https://h5p.org/*
   H5P is a free and open-source content collaboration framework based on JavaScript. H5P is an abbreviation for HTML5 Package. It aims to make easy to create, share and reuse interactive content. The H5P plug in can be added to existing websites or virtual learning environments. Quizzes can be embedded into videos or slide presentations to make them interactive. Reasoning and simulation exercises can be created to assess diagnostic or clinical reasoning. (Free with LMS and its own server)

4. **Adobe Spark:**
   URL: *https://spark.adobe.com*
   Adobe Spark is a tool for creating visual content, to communicate effectively. It uses three options. Spark Post—for social media posts originally, has the capacity to simply add text and filters to images. Spark Page—can create web stories by turning images and text into magazine style communication tools. Spark Video—allows one to record voice, add images, icons, and soundtrack. (Paid)

5. **Voice Thread:**
   URL: *http://voicethread.com*
   Voice Thread app can be used to add voice to video or text. Learners can be invited to comment on content. (Paid)

Resources to Create Online Polls and Surveys

1. **Poll Everywhere:**
   URL: *http://polleverywhere.com/*
   Poll Everywhere provides a live safe platform for every student to ask questions, participate in group activities, and share thoughts and insights, right from their phone or computer during an online synchronous session. (Free + Paid versions)

2. **Survey Anyplace:**
   URL: *https://surveyanyplace.com/*
   This quiz generator software can be used to create fun, professional and interactive surveys and quizzes. (Paid version)

3. **Typeform:**
   URL: *https://www.typeform.com/*
   Typeform allows teachers to engage with learners using conversational forms and surveys and get access to data. (Free + Paid versions)

4. **SurveyMonkey:**
   URL: *https://www.surveymonkey.com*
   This can be used to create both surveys and online MCQ through online platforms. (Paid)

5. **FreeOnlineSurveys:**
   URL: *https://freeonlinesurveys.com/#/!/*
   This allows teachers to create surveys, quizzes, forms, and polls quickly and easily. (Free)
6. **Telegram:**
   URL: *https://telegram.org/*
   Polls can be added to your Telegram channel or group directly. Or just search @VOTE In Telegram search bar to create a simple poll. If some extra features are needed, @GroupAgreeBot can be used. (Free)

Resources for Online Collaboration

1. **Padlet:**
   URL: *https://padlet.com/*
   Padlet is the online equivalent to popping a Post-it Note on a wall. Padlet allows collaborative participation in a shared space. (Free)
2. **Lino:**
   URL: *http://en.linoit.com/*
   An alternative to Padlet, Lino is a free board for collaborative sharing of notes and images. It gives alternative presentation space for projects, posters, ideas. (Free)
3. **Wikis:**
   URL: Sites like MediaWiki or Confluence can be used to create wiki pages
   Wikis are collaborative web pages and online documents that can be edited by anyone with access to the page. The tool could be useful for collaborative writing.

E-portfolios

An electronic portfolio (e-portfolio) is a purposeful collection of sample student work, demonstrations, and artifacts that showcases a student's learning progression, achievement, and evidence of what students can do. The collection can include essays and papers (text-based), blog, multimedia (recordings of demonstrations, interviews, presentations, etc.), and graphic. Some LMSs have integrated options to create e-portfolios. Some free or low-cost tools are: Wix, Weebly, Wordpress, Google Sites, and Edublog.

1. **Evernote:**
   URL: *https://evernote.com/*
   This is an option for creating digital portfolios. Students record their thoughts using notes then enhance these notes using things such as photos, audio files, links, and attachments. Evernote provides various organizational features that enable users to effectively organize their work so it can be easily searched and accessed across different device. (Free)

2. **RCampus:**
   URL: *http://rcampus.com/*
   Students can build a lifelong e-Portfolios with RCampus. Learners can build e-Portfolios to reflect on learning activities, submit them for reviews, and communicate with teachers and peers. Educators can also build teaching e-Portfolios. (Free + Paid versions)
3. **Mahara:**
   URL: *https://mahara.org/*
   Mahara is an open source e-portfolio system with a flexible display framework. Mahara, meaning 'think', or 'thought' in Te Reo Māori, is a user-centered environment with a permissions framework that enables different views of an e-portfolio to be easily managed. Mahara also features a weblog, resume builder and social networking system, connecting users and creating online learner communities. (Free)
4. **PebblePad:**
   URL: *http://www.pebblepad.co.uk/*
   PebblePad is much more than an e-portfolio. It is a personal learning system being used in different learning contexts as diverse as educational institutes, colleges, universities, and professional bodies; by learners, teachers, and assessors. It has been used for personal development planning, continuing professional development, and learning, teaching, and assessment. PebblePad provides scaffolding to help users create records of learning, achievement and aspiration and has a reflective structure underpinning all its core elements. PebblePad provides a suite of tools to improve learning in institutional contexts. Conversation, communication, and collaboration are easy in PebblePad; items can be shared with trusted individuals, published to group pages or made public to the world-wide web. (Free 60-day trial and Paid version)

Resources to Conduct OSCEs and Simulation

1. **SimulationiQ:**
   URL: *https://www.simulationiq.com/*
   SimulationiQ has facilities to deliver video-based objective structured clinical examination (OSCE) encounters to remote locations. Standardized patient encounters can be provided in a fully virtual environment. The site provides standardized patient training services. There is a feature called DistanceSIM which utilize a combination of physical training rooms and teleconferencing connectivity to conduct live simulation and clinical observation scenarios online. (Paid)
2. **EOSCE:**
   URL: *https://eosce.ch/*
   EOSCE stands for electronic registration of objective structured clinical examination. It is a simple and efficient system which

enables OSCEs to be carried out without paper checklists. The iPad app enables examiners and observers to mark student performance on electronic checklists. There are provisions to schedule and time the stations. And also, analyze and store the examination data. (Paid)

3. **I-human:**
   URL: *https://www.i-human.com/*
   This software enables students to interact with virtual patients. The patient encounter from history to diagnosis to management helps in developing diagnostic reasoning skills. Students can be trained and assessed using this modality. (Paid)

4. **SkillGym:**
   URL: *https://www.skillgym.com/*
   This site provides AI-based technologies which can be used to create videos to train students in communication skills through role plays. The same technology can be used to train standardized patients for virtual OSCEs. (Paid)

5. **MedEd Portal OSCE resources:**
   URL: *https://www.mededportal.org/action/doSearch?AllField=OSCE*
   This link from MedEd Portal provides access to a series of OSCE modules and stations in different clinical contexts. (Free)

Resources to Create Rubrics

1. **Rubric-maker:**
   URL: *https://rubric-maker.com/*
   This software helps to make customized rubrics for learners using templates. (Free)

2. **ForAllRubrics:**
   URL: *https://www.forallrubrics.com/*
   This software is free for all teachers and allows to import, create, and score rubrics on your iPad, tablet, or smartphone. It can also collect data offline with no internet access, compute scores automatically, and print or save the rubrics as a PDF or spreadsheet. (Free for teachers)

Resources for High-stakes Examinations, Online Security and Proctor Devices

1. **Respondus LockDown Browser:**
   URL: *https://web.respondus.com/he/lockdownbrowser/*
   LockDown Browser prevents cheating during proctored online examinations. When the online examination is on, access to all other websites, messaging and screen-sharing, etc., is blocked. The assessments are displayed full screen and cannot be minimized. There are restrictions on browser and tool bar options. Printing, copy-pasting and screen capture functions are disabled. Assessments cannot be exited unless the students submit them

finally for grading. This device can be integrated with Blackboard Learn, Canvas, Brightspace, Moodle, and more. (Free Trial + Paid)

2. **Safe exam browser:**
   URL: *https://safeexambrowser.org/*
   Safe Exam Browser is a web browser environment to carry out e-assessments safely. The software turns any computer temporarily into a secure workstation. It controls access to resources like system functions, other websites and applications and prevents unauthorized resources being used during an examination. It can be integrated with some LMSs. The application is available for Windows, macOS, and iOS as freeware. (Free)

3. **ExamSoft:**
   URL: *https://examsoft.com/*
   ExamSoft is a portal which enables faculty and administrators to align assessment with objectives and teaching. It enables faster grading, collection of all assessment data in one place, analysis of examination results, and generation of reports to monitor student performance. This enables provision of detailed feedback to learners and targeted remediation. It also enables one to identify gaps in the curriculum and ensure that courses meet the accreditation standards. Reports are available on individual learners, departments or courses. (Paid)

4. **Timify.me:**
   URL: *http://timify.me/*
   This is an add-on with Google forms. Timify.me seamlessly injects a timer and behavior tracking tools in your Google form. The web camera is on for the whole test duration. (Paid)

5. **Surpass:**
   URL: *https://surpass.com/*
   Surpass is a professional end-to-end assessment platform used for the authoring, banking, administration, delivery, scoring, and reporting of computer and paper-based tests. It can be used to deliver secure and validate large-scale high-stakes paper examinations and computer-based assessment. (Free Trial version)

6. **Speedwell:**
   URL: *https://www.speedwellsoftware.com/exam-software/*
   This software enables online administration of examinations. It removes complexity from all online examinations including multiple choice, single correct answer, short written answer, and OSCEs. Being completely versatile, it accommodates all disciplines, and we can have as many candidates, stations and examiners as you need. All analytic reports are available. (Paid)

7. **Mettl:**
   URL: *https://mettl.com/*
   This can be used to create aptitude tests or psychometric tests. (Free Trial + Paid versions)

REFERENCES

Cantillon, P., Irish, B., & Sales D. (2004). Using computers for assessment in medicine. *British Medical Journal, 329(7466)*, 606–9.

Dennick, R., Wilkinson, S., & Purcell, N. (2009). Online eAssessment: AMEE guide no. 39. *Medical Teacher, 31(3)*, 192–206.

Fuller, R., Joynes, V., Cooper, J., Boursicot, K., & Roberts, T. (2020). Could COVID-19 be our 'There is no alternative' (TINA) opportunity to enhance assessment? *Medical Teacher, 42(7)*, 781–6.

Gikandi, J.W., Morrow, D., & Davisa, N.E. (2011). Online formative assessment in higher education: a review of literature. *Computers and Education, 57(4)*, 2333–51.

Joshi, A.,Virk, A., Saiyad,S.,Mahajan,R., & Singh T. (2020). Online assessment: concept and applications. *J Res Med Educ Ethics,10*, 79–89.

Perera-Diltz, D., & Moe, J. (2014). Formative and summative assessment in online education. *Journal of Research in Innovative Teaching, 7(1)*, 130–42.

Sahi, P.K., Mishra, D., & Singh T. (2020). Medical education amid the Covid-19 pandemic. *Indian Pediatrics, 57*, 652–6.

Index

360° Assessment (*see* Multisource feedback)

A

Admission procedures 248-251
   Medical College Aptitude Test (MCAT) 249-251
   multiple mini-interviews (MMI) 249, 251
   National Eligibility-cum-Entrance Test (NEET) 252-255, 257
   UK Clinical Aptitude Test (UKCAT) 249-250
AETCOM 69, 174-175, 290
Angoff method (*see* Standard setting)
Assessment tools
   acute care assessment tool (ACAT) 126, 194-195
   direct observation-based assessment of clinical skills 114-137
   directly observed procedural skills (DOPS) 125-126, 185-186, 189, 225
   ethics (*see* Ethics) 169-171
   long case (*see* long case) 83-90
   mini-clinical evaluation exercise (*see* Mini-clinical evaluation exercise) 117-125, 185-186, 188-189, 225
   mini-peer assessment tool (mini-PAT) 128-129, 185-186, 193
   multiple choice questions (*see* Multiple choice questions) 47-64
   multiple mini-interview (MMI) 111, 143-147, 249-251
   multisource feedback (360° assessment) 127-129, 170-171, 185-186, 192-193
   objective structured clinical examination (*see* Objective Structured Clinical Examination) 91-113
   objective structured long examination record (OSLER) 87, 129-130
   online assessment (*see* Online resources for assessment) 300-301, 371-383
   oral examination (*see* Oral examination) 138-148
   patient management problem 301-303
   portfolios (*see* Portfolios) 151-164
   professionalism (*see* Assessment of Professionalism) 169-171
   selection type questions (*See* Selection type questions) 39-46
   structured oral examination 142-143, 144-146
   team assessment of behavior (TAB) 129, 185-186, 193-194
   viva voce (*see also* Oral examination) 138-148
   workplace-based assessment (WPBA) (*see also* Workplace-based assessment tools) 184-196
   written assessment (*see* Written assessment) 32
Assessment
   assessment as learning 20, 26-28, 263
      assessment for learning (*see* Assessment for learning) 20, 25, 28, 233-246, 263, 266
   assessment of learning 20-25, 234, 263
   assessment versus evaluation 2
   attributes of good assessment 6
   basic concepts 1-17
   clinical competence 18-29, 84, 117, 120, 179, 275, 301, 353, 359
   community-based (*see* Community-based assessment) 221-232
   competency-based (*see* Competency-based assessment) 206-220
   COLE framework 16
   criterion-referenced versus norm-referenced 5
   difference between assessment of learning and assessment for learning 234
   end of training 288
   ethics 165-177
   expert judgment 28, 122, 262, 267, 357, 359
   for selection (*see* Admission procedures) 247-260
   formative (*see* Assessment for learning) 236
   in-training 288
   measurement versus assessment 2
   objective 352-353, 357
   objective versus subjective 359-361
   online (*see* Online assessment) 296-307
   professionalism (*see* Professionalism) 165-177
   programmatic (*see* Programmatic assessment) 243-244, 261-277
   purposes of 3
   reducing assessment stress 15
   subjective (*See* Subjective expert judgment) 353, 357
   summative assessment limitations 234-235, 279-280
   summative versus formative 3-6
   test versus tool 3
   triangulation of data 267

types 3
utility 15, 262
Vleuten's formula 15, 23-24, 262-263 (*see* also Utility of assessment)
workplace-based assessment (WPBA) (*see* Workplace-based assessment) 178-205
written 30-39
Assessment as learning 5, 20, 26, 263, 297
Assessment for learning 20, 25, 28, 233-246, 263, 266
attributes 237-240
cycle 236
effect size of feedback 235
faculty development for 242-245
methods 240-241
strengths 235
SWOT analysis 242
Assessment of learning 20-25, 234, 263

B

Bloom's levels 33
taxonomy 33
MCQ writing 56-58
Blueprinting 24
OSCE 101-102, 117
question paper setting 71-72

C

Checklists versus global ratings 358-359
Clinical competence 18
newble's model 31
COLE framework 16
Community-based assessment 221-232
4R model 223-226
clinical axis 223-224
evidence axis 223-224
personal axis 223-224
social axis 223-224
methods 224-226
direct observation of field skills 225
direct observation of professional skills 225, 230-231
directly observed procedural skills 225
family study assessment 225
logbook 225
mini-CEX 225
multisource feedback 225, 231
objective structured clinical examination 225
observation by community stakeholders 225
portfolios 225, 226
project assessment 225, 229-230
reflective writing 225, 228-229
assessment 228-229
rubrics 228-229
self-assessment of professional skills 225, 227

Paul Worley's framework 223-226
principles 222-223
Community-oriented medical education 221-223
Competency frameworks 19
Competency-based assessment 206-220
design 212-216
prerequisites 210
principles 210-212
Competency-based medical education (CBME) 206, 264
assessment, competency-based 206-220
Competency
core competencies 19
definition 206
dreyfus and dreyfus model 207
frameworks
ACGME competencies 19, 207
CanMEDs competencies 19, 207
five-star doctor 19
General Medical Council competencies 19, 207
indian Medical Graduate (IMG) 19
medical Council of India 19, 207
tomorrow's doctors 19, 207
ideal doctor 19
milestones 208
roles of Indian Medical Graduate 19
sub-competencies 207
Construct 9, 353
construct formulation 353
construct irrelevance variance 10, 353
construct underrepresentation 9, 353
Constructivism 267
Contrasting groups method (*see* Standard setting) 326-327
Cronbach's alpha (*See* Reliability)

D

Direct observation-based assessment of clinical skills 114-137
360° team assessment of behavior (TAB) 129
acute care assessment tool (ACAT) 126
directly observed procedural skills (DOPS) 125-126, 185-186, 189, 194
mini clinical evaluation exercise (mini-CEX) 117-125, 188-189, 225, 356
mini peer assessment tool (mini-PAT) 128-129
multisource feedback (360° assessment) 127-129
OSCE 90-113, 116, 131, 299, 356, 359
OSLER 129-130
professionalism mini evaluation exercise (PMEX) 127
tools (*see* Assessment tools) 115
Directly observed procedural skills (DOPS) 125-126, 185-186, 189, 225
Dreyfus and Dreyfus model 207-210, 213-216

E

Educational environment 239-240
Educational feedback (*see* Feedback to students)
Educational impact 14, 262
Educational system 236
Entrustable professional activities (EPA) 207, 213-219
    designing EPAs 208, 213-217
    EPA versus specific learning objectives (SLO) 210
    stages of entrustment 213
Ethics
    AETCOM 174-175
    attributes 166
        autonomy 166
        beneficence 166
        dignity 166
        justice 166
        non-maleficence 166
    difference between professionalism and ethics 166
    narratives 173-174
Evaluation 2
Evaluation of teaching (*see* Student ratings of teaching effectiveness) 342-351
Expert judgment (*see* Subjective expert judgment) 357, 359-361

F

Faculty development for better assessment 364-370
    assessment for learning 242-245
    for better assessment 364-370
    formal approaches 367
    informal approaches 367
    model program for training 368-370
    objective-structured clinical examination 100-101
    transfer-oriented training 368
    workplace-based assessment (WPBA) 199
Feasibility of assessment 14
Feedback (*see* also Feedback, educational; Feedback, from students; Feedback, to students) 25-26, 238-239
Feedback, educational 329-341
    attributes 332-334
    definition 329-330
    descriptive 334-335
    feedback loop 330-331
    immediate feedback assessment technique 337
    issues 338-339
    models 335-336
        feedback sandwich 335
        PCP model 335
        Pendleton model 335
        reflective model 336
        SET-GO model 336
        STAR model 336
        stop-start-continue model 336
    opportunities 336-338
    self-monitoring 337-338
    strategies for improvement 339-340
    types 332-333
        benchmarking 332-333
        correction 332-333
        diagnosis 332-333
        longitudinal development 332-333
        reinforcement 332-333
Feedback, from students (*see* Student ratings of teaching effectiveness) 342-351
Feedback, to students (*see* Feedback, educational) 6, 15, 25, 26, 63, 86, 92, 103, 115, 117, 123, 130, 170, 180, 188, 211, 234, 237, 263, 266, 268, 282, 329-341
Feed forward 25-26

H

Hofstee method (*see* Standard setting) 327

I

Internal assessment 278-284
    1997 MCI regulations 278-279
    2019 MCI regulations 279
    formative or summative 280-281
    issues 286-288
    principles 283
    quarter model (*see* Quarter model) 281, 285-295
    reliability 281-282
    strengths 255-256, 278-284, 286
    validity 282
Item analysis 308-318
    item statistics 308-313
        difficulty index 309-310
        discrimination index 309-311
        distractor efficiency 309, 311
        facility value 309-310
        point biserial correlation 311-313
    test analysis 313-318
        methods of estimating reliability 314-318
            equivalent-forms reliability 314
            internal consistency reliability 314-315
                Cronbach's alpha 315-316
                KR 20 formula 315
                Kuder Richardson formula 315
                split half method 315
                standard error of measurement 317-318
        parallel-forms reliability 314
        test-retest reliability 314
    reliability coefficient 284, 313-314

K

Knowledge
 assessment of knowledge (*see* Written assessment) 30-46
  free response type questions 30-39
  multiple choice questions (*see* Multiple choice questions) 47-64
  selection type questions (*see* Selection type questions) 39-46
 type A (declarative) 31
 type B (procedural) 31
Kolb's learning cycle 155, 330-331
Kuder Richardson formula (*see* Item analysis) 315

L

Logbook 185-187, 225
Long case 83-90
 comparison with mini-CEX 131-133
 comparison with OSCE 131-133
 issues 84-85
 OSLER 83, 260
 process 83-84
 strategies for improvement 85-89

M

Mentoring 26, 153, 244-245, 266, 271
Miller pyramid 20-23, 30-31, 92, 114-115
Mini-clinical evaluation exercise (mini-CEX) 117-125, 185-186, 188-189, 225
 comparison with long case, 131-133
 comparison with OSCE, 131-133
 form 119-120
 process 118-121
 strengths 122
Mini-peer assessment tool (mini-PAT) 128-129, 185-186, 193
Modified essay questions (MEQ) 31, 35-36
Multiple choice questions (MCQs) 47-64
 challenges of using MCQs 48-49
 conducting MCQ tests 48
 guidelines for writing MCQs 50-55
 negative marking 60-61
 optical mark reading scanners 59
 scoring MCQs 58-60
 standard setting 62
 strengths of MCQs 48
 structure of an MCQ 49
Multiple mini-interview (MMI) 111, 143-147, 249-251
Multisource feedback (360° assessment) 127-129, 170-171, 185-186, 192-193

N

Narratives 173-174
 critical incident technique 173
 portfolios 173-174

O

Objectification 357
Objective structured clinical examination (OSCE) 91-113
 admission OSCE 111
 blueprinting 101-102, 117
 checklists versus global ratings 105, 116, 358-359
 comparison with long case 131-133
 comparison with mini-CEX 131-133
 computer assisted OSCE (CA-OSCE) 110
 examiner training 100-101
 factors affecting utility 106-108
 feasibility 106-107
 group OSCE (GOSCE) 109
 key features 93
 modifications and innovations 109-111
 multiple mini-interview (*see* Multiple mini-interview) 111
 objectivity 107
 reliability 108
 remote OSCE (ReOSCE) 110
 resources to conduct OSCE online 380-381
 setup 97-103
 simulated patients 100-101
 standard setting (*See* Standard setting) 103-104
 team OSCE (TOSCE) 109-110
 telemedicine OSCE (TeleOSCE) 110
 types of stations 93-97, 116
  procedure stations 94, 95-97
  question stations 94-95
  rest station 97
 validity 107-108
Objectivity 2, 108, 212, 282
 reliability versus objectivity 352-363
Observable practice activities (OPA) 210
Online assessment 296-307
 automation 298
 cheating 305-306
 consortia 306
 designing 297-304
 electronic patient management problem 301-303
 implementation 304-307
 methods 300-301
 open-book exams 305
 plagiarism 305
 question formats 299-300

sharing resources 306
skill labs 306
take-home exams 305-306
triage 306-307
types of questions 300-301

Online resources for assessment 371-383
e-portfolios 379-380
for creating distributing and grading assessment 373
for high stakes examinations 381-382
for online collaboration 379
gamification apps 376-377
interactive tools for formative assessment 373-375
learning management systems 372-373
online security 381-382
proctor devices 381-382
quiz apps 376-377
to conduct online OSCE 380-381
to conduct online simulations 380-381
to create interactive videos 377-378
to create online polls 378-379
to create online surveys 378-379
to create rubrics 381
to enhance student engagement 373-375

Oral examination (viva voce) 138-148
cost-effectiveness 141-142
examiner training 147-148
flaws 139
halo effect 140
objectivity 139-140
reliability 140-141
strategies for improvement 142-148
strengths 139
structured oral examination 142-143, 144-146
validity 141

OSLER (*see* Direct observation-based assessment of clinical skills) 83, 129-130, 260

P

Patient management problem 301-303
Portfolios 151-164, 185-186
advantages 159-160
challenges 162-163
contents 152-154
definition 151-152
e-portfolios 379-380
for assessment 157-159, 173-174
for learning 152-157, 241
implementation 161-162
limitations 160-161
reflective writing 154-157
workplace-based assessment 185-186

Professionalism 165-177
AETCOM 174-175
altruism 166
assessment methods 169-171
  principles 167-169
attributes 166
challenges 167-169
conscientious index 175
definition 165-167
difference between professionalism and ethics 166
multisource feedback 170-171
narratives 173-174
  critical incident technique 173
  portfolios 173-174
patient assessment 170, 171
peer assessment 170, 241
professional competence 166
professional identity formation 174-175
professionalism mini evaluation exercise (PMEX) 127, 172-173
self-assessment 169-170
supervisor ratings 170, 172

Professionalism mini-evaluation exercise (PMEX) 127, 172-173

Programmatic assessment 11, 26, 243-244, 261-277
CBME 264, 270
challenges 273-276
components 264-270
implementation 271-276
principles 264-267
rationale 262-264
traditional assessment versus programmatic assessment 268-270
triangulation of data 267

Q

Quarter Model 281, 285-295
format 289
implementation 289-293
Question banking 318-321
steps 319
uses 320-321
Question paper setting 65-82
blueprinting 71-72
determining weightage 68-70
item cards 73-76
limitations of conventional practices 66
moderation 77-78
steps for effective question paper setting 67-78

R

Reflections (*see* Reflective practice)
Reflective practice
   for assessment for learning 26, 166, 173, 241, 266
   models 155
   reflective writing 154-157, 225, 228-229
   rubrics 228-229
Reliability 12-13, 262, 354-356
   equivalent-forms reliability 314
   methods of estimating reliability 313-318
   internal consistency reliability 314-315
      Cronbach's alpha 315-316
      KR 20 formula 315
      Kuder Richardson formula 315
      split-half method 315
      Standard error of measurement 317-318
   parallel-forms reliability 314
   test-retest reliability 314
   reliability coefficient 313-314
   versus objectivity 352

S

Selection type questions 39-46
   assertion-reason questions 41-42
   computer-based objective forms 45
   matching questions 43-44
   key feature test 44
   matching questions 42
   multiple choice questions 40
   multiple response questions 40
   ranking questions 41
   true-false questions 40
Self-monitoring 337-338
Self-directed learning 266
Short answer questions (SAQ) (*see* Written assessments) 31, 36
Simulated patients 100-101
Specific learning objectives 210
Standard error of measurement (*see* Item analysis) 317-318
Standard setting 24, 322-328
   absolute standards 323-324
   compensatory standards 324
   conjunctive standards 324
   criterion-referenced 323-324
   effect on learning 324-325
   MCQs 62
   methods 325-328
      for clinical skills 327-328
      for knowledge tests 325-327
         angoff method 326
         contrasting groups method 326-327

      hofstee method 327
      relative method 325
   need 323
   norm-referenced 323-324
   OSCE 103-104
   relative standards 323-324
   workplace-based assessment (WPBA) 184
Student ratings of teaching effectiveness 342-351
   design of instrument 343-344
   Dr Fox effect 347
   generalizability 347
   interpretation of data 345-346
   logistics 344-345
   misconceptions 342-343
   misuses 342-343, 348
   process 343-346
   professional melancholia 346
   purposes 348
   reliability 346-347
   validity 346-347
Subjective expert judgment 28, 122, 262, 267, 357, 359-361

T

Triage in medical education 306-307

U

Utility of assessment 15, 262
   Vleuten's formula 15, 23-24, 262-263

V

Validity 6-11, 353-354
   consequence-related evidence 8,10, 262
   construct-related evidence 8, 9-10, 353
   content-related evidence 8
   criterion-related evidence 8-9
   factors which lower validity 11
   Kane's arguments 354
   key concepts 10

W

Web resources for assessment (*see* Online resources for assessment)
Workplace-based assessment (WPBA) 170-171, 178-205
   difference from traditional assessment 180
   faculty development 199
   implementation steps 181-184
   need 178-179
   prerequisites to implementation 179-181
      direct observation 180-181

feedback, 181
practice, 181
tasks 180
problem areas 199-202
quality parameters 197-199
role of assessors 196-197
role of trainee, 197
standard setting 184
strengths 182
tools 184-196
   acute care assessment tool (ACAT) 194-195
   assessment of performance, 194
   case-based discussion (CbD) 185-186, 190-191
   clinical encounter cards (CEC) 185-188
   directly observed procedural skills (DOPS) 185-186, 189
   discussion of correspondence (DOC) 185-186, 192
   evaluation of clinical events (ECE) 185-186, 191-192
   assessment tool (HAT) 195-196
   LEADER case-based discussion (LEADER CbD) 195
   logbook, 185-187
   mini-clinical evaluation exercise 185-186, 188-189
   mini-peer assessment tool (mini-PAT) 185-186, 193
   multisource feedback (360° assessment) 185-186, 192-193, 225, 231
   patient satisfaction questionnaire, 185-186
   portfolio, 185-186, 225-226
   procedure based assessment (PbA) 185-186, 189-190
   safeguarding case-based discussion 196
   sheffield assessment instrument for letters (SAIL) 185-186, 192
   supervised learning events 194
   team assessment of behaviour (TAB) 185-186, 193-194
weaknesses 182
Written assessment 31-38
   closed-ended questions 32
   context-poor questions 32
   context-rich questions 32
   essay questions 31, 34-35
   modified essay questions (MEQ) 31, 35-36
   multiple choice questions 47-64
   open-ended questions 32
   short answer questions (SAQ) 31, 36
      best response type, 37
      completion type, 37
   open SAQ, 37-38
   structured essay questions (SEQ) 31

EU GSPR Authorised Reprsentative
Logos Europe, 9 rue Nicolas Poussin
1700, La Rochelle, France
Phone: +33 (0) 6 67 93 73 78
E-mail: contact@logoseurope.eu

www.ingramcontent.com/pod-product-compliance
Ingram Content Group UK Ltd.
Pitfield, Milton Keynes, MK11 3LW, UK
UKHW050429150426
5217IPUK00019B/1313